T0329767

The Antivaccine Heresy

Rochester Studies in Medical History

Senior Editor: Theodore M. Brown
Professor of History and Preventive Medicine
University of Rochester

Additional Titles of Interest

Beriberi in Modern Japan: The Making of a National Disease
Alexander R. Bay

The Lobotomy Letters
Mical Raz

Plague and Public Health in Early Modern Seville
Kristy Wilson Bowers

Medicine and the Workhouse
Edited by Jonathan Reinarz and Leonard Schwarz

Stress, Shock, and Adaptation in the Twentieth Century
Edited by David Cantor and Edmund Ramsden

Female Circumcision and Clitoridectomy in the United States:
A History of a Medical Treatment
Sarah B. Rodriguez

The Spanish Influenza Pandemic of 1918–1919:
Perspectives from the Iberian Peninsula and the Americas
Edited by María-Isabel Porras-Gallo and Ryan A. Davis

Infections, Chronic Disease, and the Epidemiological Transition:
A New Perspective
Alexander Mercer

Save the Babies: American Public Health Reform
and the Prevention of Infant Mortality, 1850–1929
Richard A. Meckel

Intrusive Interventions: Public Health, Domestic Space,
and Infectious Disease Surveillance in England, 1840–1914
Graham Mooney

A complete list of titles in the Rochester Studies in Medical History series
may be found on our website, www.urpress.com.

The Antivaccine Heresy

Jacobson v. Massachusetts *and the* Troubled History of Compulsory Vaccination in the United States

KAREN L. WALLOCH

UNIVERSITY OF ROCHESTER PRESS

First published 2015

University of Rochester Press
668 Mt. Hope Avenue, Rochester, NY 14620, USA
www.urpress.com
and Boydell & Brewer Limited
PO Box 9, Woodbridge, Suffolk IP12 3DF, UK
www.boydellandbrewer.com

ISBN-13: 978-1-58046-537-3
ISSN: 1526-2715

Library of Congress Cataloging-in-Publication Data

Names: Walloch, Karen L.
   Title: The antivaccine heresy : Jacobson v. Massachusetts and the troubled history
of compulsory vaccination in the United States / Karen L. Walloch.
   Description: Rochester, NY : University of Rochester Press, 2015. | Series:
Rochester studies in medical history | Includes bibliographical references and index.
   Identifiers: LCCN 2015029795 | ISBN 9781580465373 (hardcover : alk. paper)
   Subjects: LCSH: Vaccination—United States—History—20th century. |
Immunization of children—United States. | Vaccination of children—Complications.
   Classification: LCC RA638 .W35 2015 | DDC 614.4/70973—dc23 LC record
available at http://lccn.loc.gov/2015029795

A catalogue record for this title is available from the British Library.

This publication is printed on acid-free paper.
Printed in the United States of America.

Contents

List of Illustrations   vii

Acknowledgments   ix

Abbreviations   xi

Introduction   1

1   Vaccination in Nineteenth-Century America   11

2   Problems with Vaccination in the Nineteenth Century   27

3   The 1901–2 Smallpox Epidemic in Boston and Cambridge   59

4   The Hazards of Vaccination in 1901–2   79

5   Massachusetts Antivaccinationists   102

6   Immanuel Pfeiffer versus the Boston Board of Health   127

7   The 1902 Campaign to Amend the Compulsory
Vaccination Laws   146

8   Criminal Prosecution of Antivaccinationists   163

9   *Jacobson v. Massachusetts*   187

Conclusion   215

Appendix A: Boston Health Department Vaccinations,
1872–1900   221

Appendix B: Voting Records for Samuel Durgin's Vaccination
Bill before the Massachusetts State Senate   223

Notes   229

Bibliography   309

Index   329

Illustrations

Figures

2.1 Nineteenth-century photograph of vaccine erythema   29

2.2 1896 Codman & Shurtleff advertisement   45

2.3 1902 H. K. Mulford advertisement   51

2.4 1902 *Boston Evening Record* cartoon referring to tuberculosis in vaccine-farm cows   57

4.1 1901 advertisement for Howard Health Company   84

4.2 1901 Bactil advertisement   96

4.3 1901 Radam's Microbe Killer advertisement   99

4.4 1902 advertisement for Lifebuoy soap   100

5.1 Front of J. M. Greene's 1901 pamphlet   108

5.2 Back side of J. M. Greene's 1901 pamphlet   109

5.3 Sara Newcomb Merrick   119

5.4 Frontispiece from R. Swinburne Clymer's *Vaccination Brought Home to You*   125

6.1 Illustration of Pfeiffer's movements around Boston   138

6.2 Illustration depicting Boston as a prim old lady deploring the danger Pfeiffer represents   143

8.1 Illustration depicting South Boston vaccination sweep   174

9.1 George Fred Williams   198

9.2 Justice John Marshall Harlan   208

9.3 Henning Jacobson's church, Augustana Lutheran Church, Cambridge, Massachusetts   213

Acknowledgments

I could not have written this book without the advice and encouragement of so many people. First and foremost is Judith Walzer Leavitt, professor emerita at the University of Wisconsin–Madison. I benefited so much from her support, guidance, and wisdom.

Other faculty members at the University of Wisconsin's medical history and bioethics department—Ron Numbers, Rima Apple, Tom Broman, and Judy Houck—also read this work. Their perceptive questions and comments gave me the confidence to make bolder statements and conclusions than I originally planned. Ron especially gave me valuable editing advice and corrected my understanding of the history of eclectic medicine.

Two medical history librarians especially deserve my eternal gratitude. At the University of Wisconsin Middleton Library (now the Ebling Library), Phyllis Kaufman, now retired, originally handed me the vaccination files that got me started. Both she and her fabulous successor, Micaela Sullivan-Fowler, trusted me with very old, delicate books and provided space for me to work.

The archivists John E. Peterson and Robyn A. Kulp at the Lutheran Archives Center in the Krauth Memorial Library of the Lutheran Theological Seminary at Philadelphia enthusiastically dragged out box after box of material relating to Jacobson and provided the services of Dr. Kim Eric Williams, who patiently translated Jacobson's handwritten letters from Swedish to English for me. Joel Thoreson at the Evangelical Lutheran Church in American Archives in Chicago provided photocopies of many important sources relating to Jacobson's life and church.

During the course of my research, I received funding from the Maurice L. Richardson fellowship and the Cremer fellowship. I appreciated not only the money but also the honor bestowed on me by these fellowships.

Graduate students, friends, and family helped immensely. The attorney Susan M. Adams brought *Mugford* to my attention and generously shared her knowledge of constitutional law and legal research with me. Eve Fine provided some valuable information about homeopathic sources that have enriched my narrative. John Buder also shared an important vaccination source and his considerable knowledge about Henry Austin Martin. Heather Willever and Steve Farr gave me a place to stay in Philadelphia while I did some of my research. Sean Sullivan's parents also provided a wonderful apartment for me to use while I conducted research in Cambridge. Judy Bates, a great genealogical researcher, dug up fascinating biographical details about some of the persons in my history.

I would like to thank especially the reviewers of my original manuscript. One remained anonymous, but another made himself known to me: Robert D. Johnston. I took his painstaking comments to heart and I treasured his encouraging words.

Finally, to my husband, Tim, our daughter, Persephone, and my father, Bob—thank you for putting up with me in this endeavor.

Abbreviations

BDA   *Boston Daily Advertiser*

BET   *Boston Evening Transcript*

BG   *Boston Globe*

BMSJ   *Boston Medical and Surgical Journal*

BP   *Boston Post*

CC   *Cambridge Chronicle*

JAMA   *Journal of the American Medical Association*

JMABH   *Journal of the Massachusetts Association of Boards of Health*

Introduction

Soon after the British physician Edward Jenner demonstrated vaccination's immunizing power against smallpox in 1798, the practice spread rapidly through Europe and overseas to the Americas. Yet from its inception vaccination was neither simple, foolproof, nor benign. Although most physicians believed that its benefits far outweighed its risks, vaccination could, and did, go awry. Over the course of the nineteenth century, issues of efficacy and stories of infection, disease, and even death after vaccination undermined public confidence to the point that people did not vaccinate sufficiently to prevent the periodic resurgence of smallpox epidemics.

By the middle of the century, widespread avoidance of vaccination drove some states to exact compliance through legal compulsion. The authoritarian nature of compulsory vaccination troubled people who believed it subverted democratic ideals of personal liberty. In their view, vaccination represented a departure from time-honored police power methods to protect public health. Nuisance abatement, quarantine, and isolation of the sick infringed private rights to body and property, but they dealt with obvious threats to public health. Even during the eighteenth century, when inoculation with mild smallpox (variolation) became a standard method of immunizing against further attacks, colonies did not make it compulsory. In fact, they had to make rules to restrict the procedure for fear that inoculation could spark epidemics. Vaccination infected healthy individuals with vaccinia, a disease that did not spread smallpox, and that feature convinced legislators that compulsion was warranted despite the personal risk and discomfort it posed to the populace. Official proclamations to the contrary, health departments around the country at times pushed compulsion too far, routinely resorting to coercion or even force to vaccinate working poor, destitute, or nonwhite populations. By the 1890s, antivaccination societies had organized to fight compulsory laws in legislatures and courts all over the United States. General anxiety about vaccination also rendered many people sympathetic to antivaccinationists' claims and their campaign against legal compulsion.

The antivaccination legal challenge culminated in a 1905 United States Supreme Court decision, *Jacobson v. Massachusetts*. In 1902, the ordinarily law-abiding Swedish Lutheran pastor Henning Jacobson refused to get vaccinated, despite a local health department order supported by state statute. Jacobson was no libertarian intent on sticking up for his perceived rights—his life revolved around Christian principles of service. He sincerely feared vaccination, and no amount of persuasion could convince him to change his mind. With the help of a local antivaccination society, he appealed his conviction all the way to the United States Supreme Court. In a landmark decision, Justice John Marshall Harlan affirmed the Massachusetts vaccination law. It is a cornerstone of case law that to this day supports broad and sweeping state authority to compel citizens to undergo medical treatment in the interest of public health. Although Jacobson never faced forcible vaccination, only a five-dollar fine, courts have relied on the case to support all sorts of health laws, including involuntary sterilization. Such is its importance that the leading twentieth-century authority on public health law, James Tobey, appended *Jacobson* to his 1939 edition of *Public Health Law*—the only opinion he so honored.[1] Recent legal scholarship continues to affirm the importance of *Jacobson* as "an archetypal case that illustrates the scope of the state's powers in matters affecting public health."[2]

The *Jacobson* case arose from a century-long tangled history in which physicians experimented with vaccine materials and techniques, arguing about whether or not vaccination permitted the transmission of serious diseases like syphilis or tuberculosis. As vaccination technology shifted from human to bovine sources, physicians established vaccine farms to take advantage of a growing market. Unfortunately, the vaccine they sold was sometimes too weak to take or contaminated with infectious organisms. Additionally, physicians used an assortment of vaccination techniques that could result in a wide range of reactions. Swollen arms were common, and could mean days of no pay for workers who could not do their jobs. Some techniques left more scarring than others, and contamination of the lymph or the vaccination site could lead to gangrenous sores or even tetanus. By the turn of the last century many people had come to regard vaccination with wariness even when it proceeded normally.

Health authorities tried to enforce compulsory laws on a populace confused by medical disputes about vaccination as well as increasingly skeptical about the quality of the vaccinations offered. In the view of many people dismayed by political corruption rampant in their cities, compulsory laws just seemed a bit too convenient for the growing commercial interest in vaccination. Although most of the medical press portrayed antivaccinationists as irrational cranks, their contentions about vaccination had a solid factual base. By the early twentieth century, one scandal after another shook public trust in vaccination, convincing some to join antivaccination societies and many more to avoid the procedure. Jacobson's refusal was rooted in anxiety about vaccination, and the exploration of that generalized worry as well as medical uncertainty about vaccination forms one of the main topics of this book. The *Jacobson* decision was no simple, obvious police-power ruling. It has a complicated history that raises difficult medical and human rights issues worthy of detailed examination.

Antivaccinationists and their opponents regarded the controversy over vaccination as one of the great issues of their time. Several respected late-nineteenth-century British intellectuals wrote about the futility and harmfulness of vaccination, reaching a wide audience in the United States. The English pathologist Charles Creighton authored an essay entry about vaccination for the 1888 edition of the *Encyclopedia Britannica* that attracted a great deal of attention for his criticism of Edward Jenner and vaccination.[3] In 1890, Creighton also published an article summarizing his criticisms of vaccination in a widely read Boston magazine, *The Arena*.[4] Alfred Russel Wallace, who formulated a theory of evolution simultaneously with Charles Darwin, wrote a popular history, *The Wonderful Century*, in which he excoriated vaccination as one of the failures of the nineteenth century in a chapter entitled "Vaccination a Delusion—Its Penal Enforcement a Crime."[5] Herbert Spencer, one of the most highly regarded English social theorists of the time, commented unfavorably on vaccination in *Facts and Comments*.[6] Thus at the beginning of the twentieth century, literate Americans associated antivaccination with two of the most widely read British intellectuals of the age.

Historians of medicine have long noticed in passing the influence antivaccinationists exerted over public opinion by the late nineteenth century.[7] Histories that look more closely at antivaccination demonstrate a wide range of assessments. An early study of American antivaccination pamphlet literature concluded that antivaccinationists were mainly irregular physicians trying to subvert medical licensing, pawns of patent medicine manufacturers, or cranks who had experienced ill effects from vaccination.[8] Yet detailed explorations of homeopaths' attitudes about vaccination reveal that most supported it.[9] Histories paying close attention to local health politics show that antivaccinationists had varying motivations. A study of health reform in Milwaukee, analyzing the events surrounding Milwaukee's 1894 smallpox riots, found that antivaccinationist opposition coalesced around issues of class conflict and ethnic tension rather than differences between orthodox and irregular physicians.[10] Another study of middle-class radicalism in Portland, Oregon, finds local activists regarded antivaccinationism as part of a larger struggle to bring about a more democratic society, a "populism of the body" that went "far beyond a simple defensive libertarianism to develop a comprehensive, and indeed radical, democratic ideology of health and the body."[11] A history of public health immunization strategies in New York and Pennsylvania in the 1910s and 1920s depicted the controversy over vaccination as a dispute over "the role elite knowledge and scientific expertise should play in a rapidly changing democratic society."[12] One wide-ranging history of immunization declares American antivaccinationists "were fueled by a spirit of rebelliousness, a sense of being right and outside the law."[13] Another recent history of the 1898–1903 smallpox pandemic concludes that "American antivaccinationists were personal liberty fundamentalists."[14]

I believe that antivaccinationism eludes easy generalization. Some antivaccinationists were libertarians, but others espoused populism or socialistic ideals. Many antivaccinationists supported the use of quarantine and isolation—tactics far more disruptive to personal liberty than vaccination. The Massachusetts antivaccinationists especially deserve thorough study within their local context before we can determine with any accuracy who they were, what they were up to, and what effect they had on the implementation of public health policy. In order to understand their perspective, I take a different stance by focusing first on medical sources to understand what physicians thought they knew about how vaccination worked in the nineteenth century. Then I shift my gaze to the history of vaccination in Boston and Cambridge to look at the Massachusetts antivaccination network that generated *Jacobson*. Massachusetts was an early leader in compulsory vaccination legislation and public health organization, and it provides a valuable example for gauging the enforcement and extent of vaccination in the decades leading up to *Jacobson*. Antivaccination activism had a long history in that state—the Boston and Cambridge health departments' efforts to control smallpox in 1901–2 took place in a landscape complicated by public distaste for vaccination, coercive health department tactics, forcible vaccination, and vaccination tragedies. By the time Jacobson refused his vaccination, a well-organized resistance network had been operating in Massachusetts for well over a decade. He was but one of a number of men and women who openly battled compulsory vaccination in the courts and state legislature of Massachusetts.

I seek to understand vaccination primarily from the perspective of the Boston and Cambridge citizens who were on the receiving end of public health policy. My aim is to develop a more precise and nuanced characterization of antivaccination in Massachusetts by interrogating antivaccination literature, the medical and popular press, and government documents. Antivaccination publications deserve careful scrutiny. These magazines, books, pamphlets, editorials, and even advertising can yield a great deal of information when subjected to close reading. Investigating the personal histories of individual antivaccination activists reveals intriguing connections with the highest levels of American science and society, connections that indicate they melded more into the mainstream of American life than historians previously have appreciated.

Unlike their British counterparts, who had built up an enduring antivaccination organization centered in London with national scope by the early 1880s, American antivaccinationists lacked any truly national organization at the turn of the twentieth century.[15] In 1879, the founders of the first antivaccination society in the United States, Drs. Robert A. Gunn and Alexander Wilder, seemingly aspired to national scope in naming their organization the Anti-vaccination League of America and sent representatives to the 1880 Paris Congress of the International Anti-vaccination League.[16] Despite its aspirations the American League floundered, and Gunn founded a new Anti-vaccination League of New York in 1885. The Iowa banker L. H. Piehn established yet another purported national organization, the Anti-vaccination Society of America, after his daughter died from blood poisoning after her vaccination in 1894.[17] In 1902, Frank D. Blue of Terre Haute, Indiana, took over as its president. Frank Blue was the appellant in *Blue v. Beach* (1900), a Supreme Court of Indiana decision that upheld the legality of the Terre Haute Board of Health's exclusion of Blue's unvaccinated son from school during a smallpox epidemic.[18] Later, in 1908, the wealthy industrialist John Pitcairn of Bryn Athyn, Pennsylvania, and Charles M. Higgins of Brooklyn, New York, established the Anti-vaccination League of America. Although ostensibly organized as a national confederation of state and local antivaccination societies, its campaigns focused on Pennsylvania (especially its 1910–13 Vaccination Commission) and New York, and the confederation remained more an ideal to work toward than a political entity with truly national reach.[19] The antivaccinationist editor and writer Lora C. W. Little worked in various American cities, first publishing an antivaccination journal, *The Liberator*, in Minneapolis, Minnesota, from 1900 to 1905. She moved to Portland, Oregon, where she led a campaign against compulsory vaccination from 1909 to 1918, and then wound up in Chicago, Illinois, during the 1920s as the secretary of the American Medical Liberty League.[20] This organization claimed "affiliates in thirty-six states" in 1922, but as the historian James Colgrove notes, "the extent of the membership in these local societies is difficult to determine."[21] None of these societies achieved the same level of national prominence and organization as the British National Anti-vaccination League, with its long-running journal, *The Vaccination Inquirer*.

Instead, small antivaccination societies popped up from time to time in towns and cities all over the United States in response to local issues, with no overarching national antivaccination organization to direct their protest. For instance, the Massachusetts Anti-compulsory Vaccination Society operated quite independently of any larger national organization. An earlier attempt at a regional antivaccination society, the New England Anti-compulsory Vaccination League, which held its inaugural meeting at Hartford, Connecticut, in 1882, seems to have had no relation to the Massachusetts society.[22] The New England organization was probably defunct by the end of the century, since Connecticut antivaccinationists established a new organization in 1902, the Connecticut Anti-compulsory Vaccination League, to work against that state's vaccination laws.[23] In Minnesota, St. Paul and Minneapolis each had antivaccination societies that worked independently of any national society. Little societies like them were scattered throughout the United States, and they certainly communicated with one another, but they operated on their own. The one under consideration here, the Massachusetts Anti-compulsory Vaccination Society, was thus an entirely independent entity.

In the American context such ephemeral, sporadic, and disperse development made a lot of sense. Whereas European nations tended to lodge the responsibility for public health legislation with the central government, the United States Constitution left that authority to each state as a "police power," that is, "a power which the state did not surrender when becoming a member of the Union under the Constitution."[24] Thus by 1902, each state had developed its own unique legislation concerning vaccination and dealt with controversy over vaccination according to its internal political dynamics. In 1901, for instance, Utah completely rejected compulsory vaccination by passing legislation (over its governor's veto) that prohibited any law that *compelled* vaccination. A Salt Lake City resident concluded that Mormon beliefs, which prevailed in that state, had tipped the balance against vaccination: "The great majority of Mormons do not use tobacco nor intoxicants, nor tea and coffee, nor are they great meat-eaters. They therefore decidedly object to having themselves or children poisoned with anti-toxin or other disease matter."[25]

In 1902 (as is the case today) vaccination laws varied a great deal from state to state. Although Massachusetts had had a general compulsory vaccination law since 1855, other states had no vaccination law at all, or linked compulsion only to public school attendance.[26] Most states had nonspecific statutes that simply granted boards of health the power to make whatever regulations they deemed necessary.[27] Only a few other states mandated compulsory vaccination of adults.[28] As in the case of Utah, some states even explicitly banned compulsory vaccination.[29]

Legislation alone, however, gives only a partial impression of the extent of popular concern over vaccination. Historians also need to look at *failed* bills—attempts to create, abolish, or amend vaccination laws—in order understand the level of concern over vaccination in each state. Rhode Island, for instance, nearly abolished its compulsory vaccination law in 1894. The abolition bill passed its Senate and failed in its House only because the Speaker cast the deciding vote against it.[30] Massachusetts likewise nearly abolished its compulsory law in 1902.[31] Such close votes indicate that compulsory vaccination polarized Americans in the late nineteenth and early twentieth centuries. Only a small number of activists organized to publicize the dangers of vaccination and oppose compulsory laws, but they had a wide and lasting influence in the creation of a great public distaste for compulsory vaccination. In state legislatures and town councils throughout the country, people fought fiercely over vaccination statutes and regulations.

The movement thus remained firmly situated in localities and states where antivaccinationists worked at the roots of the American political system to gain their ends. In state after state, local antivaccination societies lobbied their legislatures or town councils for changes in vaccination laws and supported antivaccination candidates for local boards of health, schools boards, and town councils. Working through each state judicial system, they financed individual appeals from convictions stemming from refusals to obey these laws. These local organizations and campaigns formed the heart of the antivaccination movement in the United States. In Massachusetts, the Boston general vaccination order so infuriated laypersons and physicians opposed to compulsory vaccination that they organized as the Massachusetts Anti-compulsory Vaccination Society to lobby for repeal of the law in early 1902. Their activism forms the backdrop for Reverend Henning Jacobson's refusal, trial, and appeal, providing the financial support and legal talent for his defense.

Boston and Cambridge, home to the most prestigious universities, hospitals, and medical schools in America, provided an intellectual climate that stimulated spirited public discussion on many issues, including vaccination. Although the Massachusetts Anti-compulsory Vaccination Society never established its own journal to document its activities, two Boston publications, *The Animals' Defender* and *Our Home Rights*, covered antivaccination news and perspectives extensively in the late nineteenth and early twentieth centuries, documenting the antivaccination movement in Massachusetts and its role in *Jacobson*.[32] The flamboyant physician Immanuel Pfeiffer, who owned and edited *Our Home Rights*, founded his magazine in part as a platform for opposition to vaccination in Boston. But more important, Joseph M. Greene used his editorship of the antivisection journal *The Animals' Defender* to create a network of antivaccination physicians and information in Massachusetts. Although he worked in less openly confrontational ways, Greene was crucial in organizing the antivaccination movement in Massachusetts. Another prominent Boston physician and popular author, the homeopath Charles Fessenden Nichols, argued against vaccination in *A Blunder in Poison*, a book inspired by the 1901–2 resistance in Boston and Cambridge. Boston also had one of the highest percentages of women physicians in the nation, 18.2 percent, in 1900.[33] Two of them, Caroline E. Hastings and Sara Newcomb Merrick, took on prominent roles in organizing antivaccination work there. Of these individuals, only Pfeiffer had a questionable background. The rest all possessed credible (some even sterling) medical, academic, and social credentials.

Massachusetts health officials were some of the most influential leaders in public health at the turn of the century. Through their organization, the Massachusetts Association of Boards of Health, they sponsored annual conferences and published a journal that became for a time the voice of American public health.[34] The longtime head of Boston's health department Samuel Holmes Durgin served for many years as vice president of the Association. As an acknowledged leader in the field, he had a national reputation to uphold. He and other public health officials perceived antivaccinationists as a serious threat both to their authority and to community health, a threat precisely because they disputed compulsory vaccination on medical terms as well as those of civil liberties. Many people—not just antivaccinationists—felt that health departments exceeded both the mandates of common sense and constitutional law by attempting to compel a risky procedure on those who did not choose to take such a chance. Historically, health departments had great latitude to quarantine and to isolate sick persons. But compelling vaccination—giving a disease, vaccinia, to a healthy person—was a different matter altogether. To a large degree, health officials demonstrated sensitivity to these concerns by openly acknowledging the relative uselessness of compulsion compared with voluntary compliance achieved through education, and they structured their policies accordingly. Nevertheless, antivaccinationists' determined opposition hindered vaccination campaigns, undermined public acceptance of health departments' authority, and challenged the legitimacy of their professional control over the direction of public health. Durgin and his Cambridge counterpart, E. Edwin Spencer, thus battled both the disease and local politics to control smallpox in their communities. Whereas Durgin relied routinely on coercion and even force to gain compliance with his vaccination order, Spencer took a softer approach, stalling on legal action until criticism from politicians pushed him to reluctantly bring Jacobson and other Cambridge resistors to court.

The Massachusetts antivaccinationists believed that they were fighting for a fundamental right to preserve individual health choices against a corrupt group of medical elitists who sought to establish a state-supported monopoly over medicine. Robert Johnston aptly called antivaccinationism "populism of the body" and that characterization applies well to the people I study here.[35] Antivaccinationists disputed the conclusions of health department statistics and academic studies that supported vaccination. They confronted provaccinationists with their own experts and scientific studies to refute the validity of vaccination. Thus they quarreled with medical and scientific authority not only about civil rights but also over who could legitimately wield scientific knowledge as a weapon in their debates. I give their evidence the same credence I give to that proffered by those who supported vaccination. Some readers may find this decision disturbing, but I think that both sides sincerely believed in the correctness of their position and they equally had a tendency to exaggerate or minimize certain facts and statistics to enhance their arguments. Even at the highest levels of medical inquiry, there were unresolved and unsettling questions about the nature of vaccinia and vaccination throughout the nineteenth century. Most antivaccinationists were not ignorant medical reactionaries. Some of them were physicians with degrees from reputable, even prestigious medical schools at a time when most physicians received abysmal medical training in the American system of proprietary medical schools. Others held professional positions that required higher education. They also provided scrupulous details when reporting adverse outcomes in the vaccinated, giving names, addresses, specific dates, and names of attending physicians. They certainly had a tendency to blame vaccination for nearly every subsequent illness, but at the same time the medical establishment resisted considering that vaccination might convey other diseases. The medical community, for instance, was very slow to arrive at a consensus about the possibility of syphilis or tetanus transmission through vaccination.

The *Jacobson* case arose in the context of Progressive-era political, social, and intellectual ferment. Public health at the turn of the century underwent a transition in its theoretical understanding of disease causation. For most of the nineteenth century, public health officials believed that disease originated from filth and stench. Foul-smelling air, dirty water, garbage, and other waste were thought to carry toxins that produced disease. Throughout the century, concerned citizens, charities, physicians, and politicians organized in a great sanitary reform movement to combat disease by regulating the disposal of waste, instituting building codes, and providing pure water. In the late nineteenth century, however, germ theory began to link the presence of specific microbes to certain diseases. Bacteriologists and other health professionals promulgated a "new public health" dedicated to controlling the spread of germs. They advocated turning health departments' concerns away from general sanitation efforts and re-aiming them at individuals who could harbor and transmit disease-causing microorganisms. They now saw vaccination as a far more potent and effective weapon than quarantine or disinfection in their battle against smallpox.

By the late nineteenth century, American cities faced severe problems. Unprecedented numbers of new immigrants, political corruption, and economic depression hindered their ability to function. Political machines had subverted middle-class control of political life. Political bosses doled out city jobs and contracts to the party faithful regardless of their lack of qualifications or intention to perform the work. Boston, which had hosted a large German and Irish immigrant population since the middle of the century, now also attracted many Russian and Polish Jews and Italians. To "native-born" Americans, the new immigrants from central and southeastern Europe seemed almost incomprehensible in their ethnic and cultural differences. Their need for housing and jobs drove up rents, depressed wages, and overwhelmed city health services. Crowding the North End, South Boston, and Roxbury districts, they crammed into tenements and lodging houses. Pneumonia, tuberculosis, and infant mortality scourged these slums, driving up death rates in these districts to the highest levels in the city.[36]

All of these problems seemed to erode the ideals of health, democracy, and morality that Americans valued as integral components of their culture in the late nineteenth century. Long regarding health as a symbol of individual, civic, and national virtue, many Americans associated it also with the cleanliness and discipline epitomized by middle-class life, and by the late nineteenth century they campaigned for state regulation to enforce those standards in American society generally.[37] Bacteriology taught that germs did not balk at boundaries of class, race, or national origin. Microbes threatened everyone, no matter who they were or where they lived. Reformers argued that trained professional health experts who possessed objective bacteriological knowledge about disease ought to run health departments instead of political cronies.[38] Smallpox posed a threat to community health that many Americans could no longer abide. Traditional measures of quarantine and disinfection to control outbreaks were expensive, inefficient, and an unnecessary disruption of commerce. To many proponents of public health reform, it seemed ridiculous to allow an old, preventable disease like smallpox to run rampant in the modern world and compulsory vaccination seemed to provide the perfect solution—an efficient means of disease control that fit very nicely with the developing paradigm of "new public health" based on bacteriology.

Nevertheless, this vision had its critics. Antivaccinationists questioned the safety of vaccination and the propriety of compulsion in a democratic society. Their allegations of scientific subterfuge and political shenanigans embarrassed officials who presented themselves as disinterested parties in city political life. Even supporters of vaccination questioned whether compulsory vaccination truly fit in with American democratic ideals of individual liberty, especially when no one could guarantee its safety. Antivaccinationists reported on vaccination injuries and deaths in their literature, refusing to accept official denials that contaminated lymph had anything to do with these incidents. They kept the issue before the public, thus playing a crucial role in convincing legislators at both the state and federal level of the need to regulate biologic products. Consequently public health leaders lobbied for state and federal regulation of vaccine production partly in an attempt to quell fear antivaccinationists raised about the purity of vaccine lymph. The federal government asserted control over vaccine sold in interstate commerce after a number of tetanus deaths from contaminated vaccine and antitoxin impelled Congress to pass the Biologics Control Act in 1902, and in that year the state of Massachusetts likewise took steps to regulate vaccine production within its boundaries.

Challenges to public health and social authority at the beginning of the Progressive era fill the landscape surrounding *Jacobson*. Filthy cities crowded with immigrants, political radicals, and working people demanding economic and political change seemed to threaten the basic order of society. Additionally since 1877, the United States Supreme Court produced a series of rulings based on the theory of substantive due process that valued free enterprise over police power.[39] Jacobson's attorneys argued that it was time to extend that powerful constitutional concept to individuals as well as corporations to protect them from the predations of state laws. Jacobson's attorneys asked the Court to place the same value on individual rights, at least over matters of health. By asserting that individual citizens also had federal civil rights that states may not invade, they declared an antagonistic relationship between states and their residents, one in which individuals could overturn police power in the name of individual liberty. They sought to upset the former balance of rights in which states traditionally used police power to create a "well-regulated society" that controlled markets, production, morals, and health for much of the nineteenth century.[40] The Court rejected their argument, and the *Jacobson* opinion set the precedent for notorious eugenics laws that allowed involuntary sterilization of those deemed to threaten society by virtue of their ability to procreate.

We could choose to consider *Jacobson* as a timeless expression of the contradictions inherent in civil liberty. But that choice ignores a complex history and invites careless use of *Jacobson* to justify extreme measures on the part of states to control their citizens' health decisions. When Reverend Jacobson refused to get vaccinated, he was reacting both to local events and to a controversy that had been a century in the making. Only by exploring overlapping contexts of his case can we begin to understand how and why a case about a five-dollar fine was important enough to reach the highest court of our nation.

Chapter One

Vaccination in Nineteenth-Century America

Smallpox in America before Vaccination

Smallpox infects only humans, and only humans transmit smallpox. It comes in many forms, from a hemorrhagic variety that kills all of its victims to milder types with very low death rates. Physicians now categorize smallpox into two main groups, variola major and variola minor. Variola major has afflicted humans for thousands of years. Variola minor first appeared in the late nineteenth century. Individuals suffering from variola major tend to have harsher symptoms, a higher mortality rate, and more severe scarring than variola minor victims. Nineteenth-century physicians also recognized another form of smallpox, varioloid smallpox, which appeared in vaccinated individuals. Like variola minor, varioloid smallpox usually ran a mild course with a very low mortality rate.[1]

Most victims acquire smallpox by inhaling the virus through the respiratory tract, but it also spreads by contact with infected clothing. Smallpox usually incubates eleven to twelve days before the victim shows any signs of the disease. Then, as one late nineteenth-century smallpox expert noted, "smallpox sets in suddenly and with violence."[2] Victims endure "chills or rigors, and in young children convulsions." Signs and symptoms include a bad headache, severe backache, and a fever that breaks temporarily when lesions erupt on the victim's skin, mouth, throat, and eyelids, but rises again as the lesions mature into pustules—small pus-containing protrusions—over the next few days. "Constant profuse sweating" rapidly dehydrates smallpox patients, and they suffer greatly from thirst. Depending on the type—variola major, variola minor, or varioloid—lesions can vary from just a few scattered pustules to hundreds of malignant pustules that coalesce over large areas of skin. Breaking out first on the face, palms, and soles, spreading up the legs and arms, they eventually develop into hard, pearly pustules. In cases of confluent smallpox, pustules blend together in pools on the victim's skin, and "the face swells to a shapeless mass, rendering the patient absolutely unrecognizable."[3] An 1892 medical textbook commented that "at this stage the patient presents a terrible picture, unequalled in any other disease; one which fully justifies the horror and fright with which small-pox is associated in the public mind."[4]

Even "discrete" pustules caused great irritation, becoming "extremely painful . . . accompanied by great swelling of the affected parts—greatest where the tissues are loosest or most relaxed, as in the eyelids and lips, and about the prepuce." They also formed internally, and "the conjunctivae, the mucous membranes of the nose, mouth, pharynx, and adjacent parts, are nearly always affected." They could itch, prickle, rot, and stink, leaving the poor victim desperate to scratch, but only at the cost of worsening his or her condition. About three weeks from the onset of symptoms, if the victim survived, the pustules would dry up, scab, and fall off to leave characteristic pockmark scars. Smallpox was often called a loathsome disease for good reason: as pustules ruptured, they exuded "a pungent and abominably fetid odor." Confluent smallpox victims especially reeked as the "purulent contents" of their pustules soaked "into the bedclothes and body linen . . . causing an overwhelming stench."[5] Adding to their misery, their coalesced crusts formed such large scabs that "the tough epidermis of the hands and feet may be shed entire." Pustules also could turn septic, "a most constant and troublesome complication," afflicting the patient with gangrenous painful boils. Sometimes smallpox victims lost their sight or hair, although less frequently by the 1890s with good nursing.[6]

Fortunately, survivors emerged from their bout with the disease practically immune to further attacks. This immunity was not absolute—people who had smallpox once could get it again, according to a twentieth-century source, with second attacks tending to land at one of two extremes, either "malignant and frequently fatal, or exceedingly mild and abortive."[7] Nineteenth-century physicians also understood that "exemptions from second seizures . . . are by no means invariable."[8] One expert, for instance, remarked in 1898 that "vaccination, like a previous attack of smallpox itself, is only a *temporary and therefore imperfect preventive* against smallpox."[9]

Smallpox has played an important role in American history, coming to North America shortly after the arrival of the first Europeans in 1492. One of the most deadly diseases unwittingly imported to the Americas, smallpox routinely killed at least 30 percent of Native Americans exposed to its ravages. They lacked both biological immunity and cultural experience with the disease, and epidemics wiped out villages, uprooted tribes, and undermined resistance to European incursions. From New England to the Pacific Northwest, through the Great Plains to California, historians have found that this pattern continued whenever and wherever Native Americans encountered settlers and traders of European and African descent for the next four centuries.[10]

Smallpox also afflicted English colonists in the eighteenth century, forcing them to develop rules of notification, isolation, and quarantine—the first systems of organized public health law in America. In 1721, Lady Mary Wortley Montagu promoted a new method of smallpox control, inoculation, in England, while the Boston minister Cotton Mather and the physician Zabdiel Boylston introduced it to the Massachusetts Bay Colony.[11] Practiced in Africa and the Middle East for generations, deliberate inoculation of smallpox induced a controlled attack of the disease. Inoculation consisted of extracting the viscous liquid from smallpox pustules of a mild case and inserting that liquid (often soaked up in a thread) just under the skin to induce a milder version of the illness that conferred the same immunity as natural smallpox. Although most inoculees experienced a mild case, some developed a severe one that killed a small percentage.

Inoculation had several disadvantages. Even inoculees with the mildest symptoms could spread virulent smallpox to others if they were not isolated. Inoculation also required weeks of special diet and purges to prepare for the ordeal, then weeks of nursing care and time away from work that the poor could not afford. Relatively few people could afford to undergo such an expensive procedure. As towns and colonies decided whether or not to permit inoculation, debate revolved not just around its medical merits but also around issues of class and authority in colonial society. The acceptance of inoculation involved an intense process of political and cultural negotiation. Despite its promise as a medical innovation, many colonial towns initially greeted the prospect of inoculation not with enthusiasm but rather with apprehension, and some, but not all, formulated strict controls over the practice.[12]

Widespread adoption of inoculation greatly reduced smallpox mortality by the late eighteenth century. Nevertheless, inoculation perpetuated smallpox as an endemic disease that occasionally broke out in epidemic form when inoculated patients mingled too soon with their neighbors, especially in towns that had lax controls. One physician writing in the late nineteenth century remarked that inoculation "spread smallpox just as the natural disease did" and "often with great virulence."[13] An 1866 American Medical Association report explicitly linked the decrease of smallpox epidemics in the nineteenth century to the abandonment of inoculation: "the epidemic influence of smallpox greatly increased during the practice of inoculation, and greatly decreased since vaccination has been adopted."[14] In 1871, the British smallpox expert J. F. Marson testified before Parliament that "the discontinuance of inoculation, rather than the practice of vaccination, was the cause of the lesser prevalence of smallpox" from 1800 to 1830.[15] In 1894, the Boston city physician John H. McCollom also recalled that "inoculation diminished the number of deaths from smallpox, but it also served to keep alive the disease."[16] Smallpox, both natural and inoculated, spread so far and wide throughout Massachusetts during the eighteenth century that one early twentieth-century physician reckoned that "almost all of the inhabitants of the state had passed through an attack of smallpox" in their lifetimes.[17] Although inoculation reduced smallpox mortality, it did not lesson the incidence of the disease. It conferred immunity but encouraged the continued spread of smallpox.

The Advent of Vaccination in America

When the English physician Edward Jenner announced in 1798 that inoculation with cowpox virus could provide immunity to smallpox, the public and medical men alike quickly realized its potential.[18] The new method seemed promising because it induced vaccinia, a much milder disease than inoculated smallpox. Jenner called his innovation "vaccination" and the old way of inoculating smallpox "variolation." Vaccination possessed considerable advantages over variolation in that vaccinated individuals could not transmit smallpox, nor could they easily spread vaccinia without direct physical contact. Even more important, vaccination ideally left just one minor scar at the point of inoculation and suffering seemed limited to mild fever and discomfort at the site of insertion.

Jenner's innovation promised to suppress smallpox altogether, supplanting expensive inoculation practices that perpetuated smallpox. Medical authorities, royalty, and political leaders sent vaccine lymph all over Europe and the Americas within the course of a few years.[19] Many years later, one physician linked this initial enthusiasm for vaccination to the "great fear . . . especially of the educated and wealthy class" of smallpox epidemics sparked by careless inoculators. Noting that "it was utterly impossible for Jenner or anybody to know whether it would protect for a lifetime," he argued that convenience rather than proof of its effectiveness over the long term helped establish it as "accepted medical dogma."[20] Another physician, C. H. Stedman, preferred a less cynical explanation for the rapid acceptance of vaccination: "perfect isolation . . . necessary after inoculation placed the benefit of this discovery entirely out of the reach of the masses of the people," but vaccination "furnished perfect protection to every one."[21]

Vaccination reached the United States almost immediately, with leading medical men in the eastern seaboard cities of Boston, Philadelphia, Baltimore, and New York adopting it quickly. The Harvard Medical School professor Benjamin Waterhouse introduced vaccination to America in 1800 by inoculating his own son with virus he had obtained from a colleague in England. By the summer of 1802, he convinced the Boston Board of Health to try out the procedure in a public demonstration. Nineteen boys were vaccinated and then tested by smallpox inoculation. None of them came down with smallpox. Waterhouse declared that "this decisive experiment has fixed forever the practice of the new inoculation in Massachusetts."[22]

Personal and proprietary disputes over vaccination impeded the distribution of vaccine at a cost low enough to reach the poorer classes. In Boston, for instance, Waterhouse's attempt to monopolize the supply of vaccine material tarnished his reputation so irreparably that he could not convince Boston to establish a vaccine institute to furnish low-cost vaccine to local physicians.[23] In Baltimore, Dr. James Smith fought for years with municipal authorities over the proper management of smallpox epidemics. His contentious personality alienated many who would have supported his efforts to obtain permanent federal and state support for vaccine production and distribution.[24] From its inception, greed and professional rivalries undermined early efforts to promote vaccination to the wider public.

Vaccination spread rapidly among the medical elite, however, as physicians sent vaccine matter to their colleagues in other towns and cities in the early nineteenth century. Benjamin Waterhouse sent vaccine to Thomas Jefferson, who used it to vaccinate "seventy to eighty of my own family," as well as his neighbors.[25] Jefferson sent some of his supply to the Philadelphia physician John Redman Coxe, who used it to vaccinate himself, his own infant son, and Dr.

Benjamin Rush's children. Rush declared that "the vaccine inoculation is generally adopted in our city and its success has hitherto equaled the best wishes of
its most sanguine and zealous friends."[26] Almost all of Philadelphia's eminent
physicians embraced vaccination wholeheartedly: by April 1803, forty-nine out
of fifty members of Philadelphia's College of Physicians endorsed vaccination
publicly (Adam Kuhn refused); in 1809, the Pennsylvania Hospital began offering free vaccinations to the poor; and by 1816, Philadelphia created the post of
city vaccine agent.[27]

Initial medical enthusiasm for vaccination did not automatically guarantee
that it reached everyone over the course of the nineteenth century. Vaccination
was not necessarily cheap or easily available: most people had to go to some
lengths to obtain vaccinations, either by seeking out a private physician or by
going through a certification process to prove their moral worth and lack of
means to receive a free vaccination. Spotty and sporadic, public provision for
vaccination depended on the efforts of private charities, city physicians, state
legislatures, and town councils. Town councils dealt with public health threats
on an ad hoc basis, forming a temporary board of health to provide vaccination
in times of epidemics. Free vaccination apparently did not become that common
until after the Civil War, when a committee of the American Medical Association
observed that "gratuitous vaccination in our large cities is . . . fast becoming
the rule instead of the exception as heretofore."[28] Some cities employed a city
physician to give free vaccinations to the poor, but dispensaries—charitable outpatient clinics funded usually with private donations—also offered free vaccinations, performing "an important public health role in providing vaccination for
the poor and vaccine matter for the use of private practitioners."[29] One New
York City dispensary became a mainstay for vaccine supply both during and after
the Civil War, distributing "great quantities of lymph . . . to the surgeons of the
United States service" and private physicians alike.[30]

Despite these efforts to offer free vaccination to the urban poor, we know
very little about the extent to which vaccination actually spread throughout the
United States in the nineteenth century. Sources for vaccination statistics are
scant, scattered, and cover only a part of the total population of some cities.
Data for smallpox and vaccination is simply lacking until much later in the nineteenth century. Cities and states did not establish health departments capable of
collecting consistent records until the 1860s, and even then they did not collect
statistics on vaccination for the whole population. Nearly all nineteenth-century
vaccination records pertain to those given to the poor at public expense in major
cities like Boston, Philadelphia, New York, Baltimore, and New Orleans. What
went on in rural areas is even more problematic. A 1902 medical journal editorial commenting on the progress of vaccination in America noted that "in the
rural districts vaccine material was not easily obtained, and does not appear to
have been made a commercial article of sale for many years, to a great extent."[31]

When the homeopath George Winterburn attempted to track the progress
of vaccination in America up until 1885, he found "few vital statistics in the
United States worthy of credence, and none that are any help in this inquiry."[32]

The Massachusetts State Board of Health, established in 1869, did not compile data on smallpox until 1883 and did not record the vaccination status of smallpox victims until 1885.[33] The Boston health department physician Frank Morse pointed out in 1903 that "accurate records have been kept" only since 1888.[34] Even so, such numbers still gave no information about how many people were vaccinated and revaccinated out of the total population. In 1894, Samuel W. Abbott, secretary to the Massachusetts State Board of Health, complained, "in America, almost throughout the whole country, statistics are entirely wanting on this subject."[35] Although some cities kept records of the free vaccinations they performed as a public service, they could not ascertain total vaccinations for the population because no law required private physicians who performed most of the vaccinations to report them.[36] In a 1902 paper delivered to the Massachusetts Medical Society, Abbott still found American laws "defective" in respect to requiring records of vaccination. He argued that even public authorities did not keep adequate accounts of vaccinations they performed: "Boards of health often make wholesale vaccinations upon the population of large districts, institutions, schools, the employees of corporations, etc., without even a slight record of the names only of those who have been vaccinated."[37] Without accurate records, it was impossible to know who got vaccinated and whether or not he or she encountered any difficulties after the procedure.

We may not have comprehensive statistics on vaccination, but we do know that smallpox continued to plague American cities and towns throughout the nineteenth century. Time and again, histories of public health note that general apathy and even downright hostility to vaccination limited its spread among Americans from the beginning.[38] In 1886, George Winterburn remarked that "the most silly and extravagant charges are brought against vaccination. Mothers, in our tenement-house class, are prone to refer back to the 'time when baby was vaccinated,' as from whence came every subsequent ill."[39] Only epidemics seemed to excite much interest in vaccination, as for instance when the New York Dispensary provided a total of almost fifty-eight thousand free vaccinations in epidemic years 1854 to 1858.[40]

If a significant number of people rejected a primary vaccination, even more neglected to get a second one. Although Jenner initially asserted that one vaccination would suffice for a lifetime's protection against smallpox, cases of smallpox among the vaccinated soon appeared. By the 1820s, smallpox epidemics in Europe overwhelmingly confirmed the need to periodically renew immunity.[41] Yet the American medical profession did not strongly advocate revaccination until the second half of the century. In an important 1865 paper, a leading member of the American Medical Association, Joseph M. Toner, remarked that although the public "almost universally conceded" the need for one childhood vaccination, "conviction is by no means so general in favor of secondary vaccination," and the medical profession only recently had "reluctantly conceded" the need for revaccination. Toner observed that "revaccination is often refused by the people, and . . . is thought to be unnecessary by some of the medical faculty."[42] In 1866 an American Medical Association committee reported that "in the United States revaccination has received but little attention," recommending "it is incumbent to revaccinate at intervals not exceeding five years."[43] Although widely distributed to medical journals and newspapers, this advice apparently did not substantially affect rank-and-file practitioners. Throughout the rest of the century, leading physicians and public health officials repeatedly brought up the need for revaccination. At an 1882 American Public Health Association conference, for instance, an Indiana practitioner proposed that "revaccination should be repeated, say every five years," as if the message had not yet gotten out sufficiently.[44] By 1900, Massachusetts State Board of Health Secretary Samuel Abbott estimated that about 90 percent of the American public may have received one vaccination, but only about half ever got another one.[45]

By the late nineteenth century, most physicians understood that even recent vaccination did not always prevent smallpox, just as one attack of smallpox did not confer absolute immunity. Vaccination lowered the risk of contracting smallpox, however, and it substantially lowered the risk of dying from it. An 1898 textbook author figured the probability of a vaccinated person contracting smallpox at one in four compared with one in two for the nonvaccinated. He posited the chances of dying from smallpox at ten times less for the vaccinated than the unvaccinated.[46] Another contributor to this textbook noted that smallpox in the vaccinated usually took a mild course of the discrete variety, thus "vaccination *prevented* a large number of these cases from being confluent."[47] In 1902, an El Paso, Texas, surgeon admitted "that it is possible to contract severe smallpox after comparatively recent successful vaccination." Along with most public health experts at that time, he believed that a primary vaccination in infancy, followed by one at puberty conferred immunity that "will last during the remainder of life," but that "it is best to revaccinate whenever one is exposed to the disease or whenever there is an epidemic in one's locality."[48]

As various European nations instituted compulsory vaccination laws in the nineteenth century, American physicians and public health officials began to argue for similar legislation in the United States. Joseph M. Toner acknowledged that many of his colleagues thought "that the temper of the American people would not tolerate any interference on the part of government in matters of a purely personal and domestic character," but he declared that the Civil War had demonstrated "us to be as submissive to the will of rulers and governments as any people on earth." He argued that "a compulsory mode is the only one that will ever secure protection to those whose indifference or prejudice causes them to neglect themselves, and thereby endanger the safety of the communities in which they live."[49] Yet some of Toner's colleagues approached the idea of compulsory vaccination warily. Just one year later, an American Medical Association committee warned that the American public had "much prejudice still to be overcome," and "people must be first educated into the belief that the right of doing as they please does not include among its privileges the right to have smallpox, and thereby trespass upon their neighbors."[50]

Medical wavering on compulsion persisted throughout the nineteenth century. In 1879 two city health department physicians blamed "the concealment of cases, and prejudice against vaccination" for the continued propagation of smallpox. Their experiences convinced them that "force is worse than useless" when it came to vaccination, and "it is certainly not suited to our own country, where cosmopolitan prejudices and a republican form of government exist."[51] The physician James F. Hibberd admonished his colleagues at an 1882 American Public Health Association meeting to tread cautiously: "An attempt at compulsory vaccination will not only fail of success in the existing state of public opinion, but will seriously retard the growth of faith among the populace that universal vaccination is a reasonable service."[52] One year later, the physician Eugene Foster reported to the Association that although "compulsory vaccination is just and necessary, . . . the masses of the people are not yet sufficiently well informed to understand the necessity of vaccination." Even worse, "some physicians are not sufficiently versed either in the history or the practice of vaccination to enable them to form a deep-settled conviction of the necessity of the measure, except in communities imminently threatened with an epidemic."[53] In 1890, the Michigan physician Henry B. Baker complained that although he supposed "it is true that many physicians favor compulsory vaccination," he believed "this is one of the many instances in which a pet theory does not 'work' as it should." He proposed "educational methods" rather than laws to promote vaccination, arguing that "compulsory vaccination of an intelligent adult person is such an interference with the liberty of the individual relative to his own person" that people then "decline to listen to facts and reasons supporting the belief in the beneficence of vaccination."[54] In 1897, C. S. Lindsley, secretary of the State Board of Health of Connecticut, declared he was "positively opposed" to compulsory vaccination "wholly on the ground of expediency" because "the people in this country are too thoroughly imbued with a sense of personal independence to submit patiently to personal compulsion."[55] By 1900 another American Public Health Association committee despaired that "the experience and practical demonstrations of a century have failed to establish, in the public mind and among governmental authorities, the beneficent necessity of self-protection from this loathsome disease by uniform and more energetic compulsory vaccination laws."[56]

Vaccination in Massachusetts

Boston provides a case in point to outline some of the problems a nineteenth-century municipality faced in assuring the vaccination of its inhabitants. Its 1822 city charter gave the City Council authority to appoint health commissioners to enforce health ordinances. But then, in 1824, the Council turned that duty over to the police. By 1833, it had added five elected consulting physicians to the roster, but the City Council usually ignored their recommendations, since they possessed only advisory power. In 1853 the city created the office of Superintendent of Health, but mostly to direct street cleaning operations. Boston did not establish an independent Board of Health until 1873, when the fallout from a scandal involving tainted meat, followed by a devastating fire and the 1872 smallpox epidemic, forced the City Council to take real action.[57] Boston's situation was not at all unusual: other cities likewise lacked a public health office with sufficient authority to consistently enforce existing vaccination laws or to effectively encourage its practice until the last third of the nineteenth century. New York City, for instance, established the first permanent municipal health department in 1866 only after an arduous process of political negotiation.[58]

John Blake provides the most detailed account of the early progress of vaccination in Boston up to 1822, and many of his findings indicate that it may not have spread that thoroughly throughout the population. A free vaccination program initiated in 1802 failed within the year "apparently because people stopped coming."[59] The Boston Dispensary attempted to stir up interest by recommending vaccination in local newspapers in 1803 and providing vaccinations on demand to the worthy poor.[60] Blake depicts Bostonians' interest in vaccination quickening mostly when epidemics threatened and flagging otherwise. He thought that vaccination spread slowly, and he explained low smallpox mortality from 1800 to 1820 as a consequence of overall immunity derived from the 1792 smallpox epidemic rather than widespread vaccination.[61] Vaccine quality also proved problematic in the years immediately after its introduction—some early vaccinations failed to protect against smallpox and an epidemic of smallpox broke out in Marblehead among the vaccinated. In 1808, the Massachusetts Medical Society endorsed vaccination wholeheartedly, but it urged revaccination to protect those who might have received ineffective vaccines earlier, "particularly in cases where the inoculators have not been well instructed in this practice."[62]

Blake produces much evidence that indicates a favorable attitude toward vaccination, but he also finds only sporadic government initiatives to provide it for the general population. For the most part, vaccination remained an expensive proposition in Massachusetts. Some towns, like Milton, experimented successfully with reduced-price vaccination campaigns. In 1809, it offered 25-cent vaccinations to its residents for three days. Almost everyone (337 out of 357) took advantage of this opportunity. Milton's enthusiastic response indicates that people would seek vaccination for the right price, but other towns like Boston had difficulty persuading physicians to reduce their fees. Boston physicians set prices as high as five dollars apiece for vaccinations, and only intense negotiation convinced them to drop the price to two dollars temporarily in 1811. In 1810 the General Court of Massachusetts passed a law requiring every town to appoint a vaccination committee to provide low-cost vaccinations, but since it lacked penalties for failure to comply, "the act was in effect no more than an expression of benevolence toward vaccination," and "as a whole it failed." By 1816, a canvass revealed that about 14 percent of Boston's population lacked protection from smallpox. The city formed ward vaccination committees that sent physicians to every susceptible household, offering either cheap or free vaccinations, depending on certification of poverty.[63]

Despite Blake's gloomy assessment of the effect of the 1810 law, Massachusetts towns apparently offered public vaccination to their residents on a regular basis at least until the late 1830s. The statistician Lemuel Shattuck later claimed in his 1850 *Sanitary Survey of Massachusetts* that "under the old law many towns were accustomed, once in five or more years, to have a general vaccination." In 1836, however, the legislature amended the 1810 law to read that each town *may* rather than *shall* provide vaccination for its inhabitants. Shattuck believed this amendment, which "left it optional with towns to do or not to do it," rapidly sent vaccination into decline and "probably caused the loss of many lives." By the 1840s, few towns undertook regular vaccination operations anymore, and "this custom, as far as our knowledge extends, has been generally discontinued."[64]

Even worse, in 1838 the General Court "at the earnest request of the Massachusetts Medical Society" also repealed sections of the *Revised Statutes* that required quarantine and isolation of smallpox victims.[65] Smallpox, which had killed only 37 persons in Boston from 1807 to 1837, resurged with a vengeance, taking 533 individuals from 1837 to 1849 and slaying 146 in the first half of 1850 alone. Although the Massachusetts Medical Society officially supported vaccination, Boston residents apparently did not get the message even though the city required vaccination for school attendance and offered free vaccinations to the poor at the office of the city physician.[66]

Lemuel Shattuck asserted that Massachusetts needed a new vaccination law. He blamed rising smallpox rates partly on citizens who left their bodies "open to be entered and pillaged" by smallpox. Although "chargeable with ignorance, negligence or guilt," these individuals should not have to shoulder the entire burden of blame. Government also ought to encourage and even compel vaccination: "And upon that state, city, or town, which does not interpose its legal authority to exterminate the disease, should rest the responsibility, as must rest the consequences, of permitting the destruction of the lives and the health of its citizens." Still the legislature did not act immediately. Smallpox deaths in Boston declined abruptly to a low of six by 1853, and the need for any special legislation probably seemed remote.[67]

In 1854, however, smallpox deaths rose precipitously to 118 and then to 132 in 1855.[68] This change prompted comment among local physicians. In October 1854, the editors of the *Boston Medical and Surgical Journal* warned that "smallpox is gradually showing itself, on the approach of cold weather, as it did last year."[69] Anxiety about immigrants arriving sick with smallpox and cholera also filled its pages that year. A United States Senate Report about conditions on immigrant ships revealed that passengers endured abhorrent conditions, "festering in filth," and provoked a *Journal* editor to call for "rigid enforcement of stringent enactments" to "remedy the evil."[70] Other editorials complained about the preponderance of smallpox "when the remedy is at hand, and to the poor always free. . . . Massachusetts, New Hampshire, Maine and Vermont, lose many citizens annually, who either obstinately refuse the blessing of vaccination, or haggled at the pittance of it."[71]

By early 1855, momentum built for legislation to address the growing danger from smallpox as citizen groups filed five separate petitions for vaccination bills. As a result, the General Court commissioned the Boston physician Charles H.

Stedman to write a report on vaccination in order to frame a new compulsory law. He acknowledged that some people possibly received ineffective vaccinations in the first place, but he thought it more likely that many neglected revaccination because they erroneously believed that one vaccination would provide lifelong protection. He also noted that people worried that vaccination would render them "liable to all the constitutional diseases of the one from which the virus was taken." By "constitutional diseases," he referred mainly to syphilis and tuberculosis, two diseases that induced much anxiety in nineteenth-century society. After reviewing the experiences of European countries with compulsory vaccination laws, Stedman concluded that Massachusetts needed a law that not only mandated a primary childhood vaccination but also called for revaccination.[72]

Stedman articulated two important reasons—ignorance of the lapse in immunity and fear of tuberculosis or syphilis—that might cause people to avoid vaccination. Whether people simply avoided vaccination because they feared ill effects or because they mistakenly trusted in the sufficiency of one vaccination, we cannot know. Additionally, since the Boston city physician supplied only primary vaccinations for free, getting revaccinated involved a personal financial commitment that many people balked at in the absence of smallpox.

Stedman's report convinced the Massachusetts legislature to enact one of the strictest and most comprehensive vaccination laws in the United States. One historian later called it "the most advanced stand ever taken by any of the States" to promote vaccination, and in 1901 it still stood out as one of the strictest vaccination laws in America.[73] The new statute required parents or guardians to vaccinate all children before the age of two and forbade the admission of unvaccinated children to public schools. It charged factory and mill owners with the duty of vaccinating their employees. It mandated vaccination for the inmates of public institutions like jails, orphanages, and insane asylums, too. The statute also authorized the selectmen, mayors, or aldermen of towns and cities to enforce revaccination whenever they judged "the public health requires the same," by penalizing with a fine of five dollars any who would not comply.[74]

Despite the sweeping authority granted by this law, Boston seemed reluctant to implement it. In 1856, Lemuel Shattuck appealed to the Boston City Council to use this new law to enforce a "general, compulsory vaccination of the whole of the inhabitants." Nothing, however, happened despite the approbation Shattuck's view received from the *Boston Medical and Surgical Journal*, whose editors proclaimed that "foreign immigration has undoubtedly had an influence in increasing smallpox amongst us . . . yet doubtless this great mortality might be very essentially diminished—perhaps, finally, annulled, by thorough vaccination on the plan proposed."[75] Perhaps the Boston City Council shied away from enforced vaccination at that time because (as one correspondent put it) "the expediency of compulsory vaccination has been much doubted."[76]

The Council may have believed compulsion unnecessary. An 1869 canvas of Boston police districts claimed it found only 8,411 unvaccinated persons out of a total population of 250,000, representing around 3 percent of the population.[77] In 1871 the City Council smugly proclaimed that free vaccinations, "combined with the rule that all children entering public schools shall produce evidence of vaccination, has kept small-pox under control."[78]

Such complacency belied reality. Since the state did not keep records of vaccinations for each smallpox case until 1885, health officials had no hard data "to gain fairly accurate information as to the protection afforded by vaccination."[79] Thus they resorted mostly to guessing when gauging the extent of vaccination in the state. By 1872, any optimism about vaccination was wiped out as smallpox reached epidemic levels not seen in a generation. Towns and cities throughout Massachusetts relayed disquieting evidence of inadequate vaccination. Worcester authorities found "large numbers of persons of all ages . . . unprotected by vaccination, and Holyoke reported "indifference and neglect of the people in regard to vaccination."[80] Town officials all over the state complained that large percentages of their residents "have not been vaccinated since childhood," that "there have been many unvaccinated children attending school," and that "there is criminal indifference to the subject."[81] One correspondent blamed French Canadian immigrants, claiming "these people are notoriously perverse in refusing vaccination, and when sick with small-pox conceal if possible the nature of their disease."[82] Other towns reported resistance to vaccination among Irish immigrants as well as the French Canadians.[83] Even supposedly well-vaccinated Boston suffered greatly from smallpox, reporting 3,367 cases with 996 deaths from 1 May 1872 to 30 April 1873.[84]

Yet when the newly formed Boston Board of Health faced this terrible epidemic, it did not rely on the 1855 law to issue any vaccination order. Instead it merely stated that "vaccination and re-vaccination . . . are the principal and most important means . . . to diminish the spread of this loathsome disease" in its official statement of regulations.[85] Even so, in 1874, the Massachusetts State Board of Health deplored the insufficiency of the 1855 law: "the protection of the community from so dreadful a disease as small-pox requires something more than the imposition of the trifling fine of *five dollars*," and the law ought to "as well as provide for vaccination at an earlier age than *two* years."[86] The State Board never got its desired amendments, possibly because of public distaste for compulsory vaccination. At the end of the century, it even found some mills and factories that failed to enforce vaccination among their employees, despite clear state requirements for it. In 1899, for instance, the State Board of Health complained that smallpox outbreaks among mill operatives at Fall River "revealed a gross violation of certain specific laws relating to vaccination," and it grumbled that in general, "a considerable portion of the population is still without protection."[87] Although the law, leading medical authority, and editorial opinion show overwhelming official support for vaccination, these reports of neglect and resistance indicate that it had not truly saturated the state's population.

Another factor—accessibility—played a part too. People had to go to some trouble to obtain a free vaccination. Although the Boston city physician Henry G. Clark advertised free vaccinations daily in 1854 at his office in Court Square, they were offered only from "Twelve to One o'clock," a time hardly conducive for working people who might have to walk a long way (often with children in tow) to the office.[88] Although the *Boston Medical and Surgical Journal* defended the arrangement, claiming that "this office is central, and well known to that class of the community who generally avail themselves of this public charity," the Boston City Council decided in 1855 to add seven physicians, one for each police district, "to vaccinate gratuitously any inhabitant who may apply" in order to reach more people.[89] This restructuring indicates that Boston politicians recognized that vaccination had not spread sufficiently and they needed to do more to make it available to "any inhabitant," not just those who had to demonstrate moral worth to secure charity from private dispensaries. Still, the city physician did not offer free revaccinations until 1873.[90] And by 1877, the city physician's office had added only one hour for vaccinations: "from 10 to 12 a.m., six days in the week."[91] Around twenty-five years later, this situation had not changed, with very similar hours of operation in effect.[92] Dispensaries also provided free or cheap vaccinations, but they similarly restricted their hours of operation and often required a certificate of recommendation from a subscriber who had donated money. Thus obtaining a free vaccination involved considerable effort, along with the burden of proving moral worthiness for such charity. During epidemics the city went to greater lengths to make vaccination available, but only for a short time. As smallpox cases mounted into the thousands in late 1872, for instance, it authorized physicians to vaccinate throughout the city. No agency kept track of the vaccinations they performed until the Board of Health assumed its duties in early 1873, when it appointed a medical inspector and assistants to undertake vaccination for each ward starting in late January. These inspectors and their assistants ultimately vaccinated 14,977 persons over the course of the next six weeks, but then the health department laid them off.[93] The city physician also provided over two thousand gratuitous vaccinations from May 1872 through April 1873.[94]

Yet for the rest of 1873, interest in vaccination lagged: the Boston city physician provided only 484 primary vaccinations and 29 revaccinations.[95] The city physician also provided only 143 certificates of vaccination to schoolchildren and furnished only 15 physicians with vaccine virus.[96] Perhaps many Bostonians had recently obtained vaccinations—Boston had just endured the worst smallpox epidemic of the century in 1872–73. Perhaps many people lacked confidence in city lymph: the reported success rate of the 1872–73 vaccinations was disappointing—just 55 percent.[97] Undoubtedly also many more Bostonians got their vaccinations from private physicians. Yet how many sought out that first vaccination *before* their children reached school age or obtained *second* vaccinations routinely? Disquieting statistics from the Boston City Jail for 1873–74 showed that only slightly more than half of the inmates "were already protected by a previous attack of smallpox, or a recent vaccination," a strange situation given the recent smallpox epidemic.[98]

The numbers of free vaccinations given by the city over the next decade indicate that interest in vaccination depended on the presence of smallpox. When smallpox cases were low or nonexistent, relatively few sought free vaccination, such as the 673 persons (of which "10 were persons revaccinated") in

1874–75, when seven cases appeared.[99] During 1881–82, however, mounting cases of smallpox "served to arouse the inhabitants to the necessity of vaccination," creating such demand that the health department opened ten additional offices temporarily to deal with the rush. Some 25,340 applied for free vaccinations at these special offices, while another 12,001 got them from the city physician.[100] This time the health department kept records of the vaccinated. By counting and assessing vaccination scars as a way to calculate revaccination rates, it reckoned that 454 out of every 1,000 persons in Boston—almost half the population—had not been vaccinated in the last fifteen years. Then it realized that this ratio came from a population that *deliberately* sought out vaccination, that is, the 37,341 persons noted above who had shown up for free vaccinations. Using past smallpox cases as a guide instead, it recalculated that the true number of those needing revaccination was much higher, 968 out of every 1,000 persons. The health department also noted that "nearly all applying for public vaccination belong to the laboring class, and, naturally, those of adult age are unwilling to run the risk of losing several days work, to which they are liable, if the vaccination is successful." It found it "difficult . . . to induce laboring people, of both sexes, to submit to vaccination, even after being exposed to smallpox," complaining that working people resisted, resorting to "every kind of deception" to evade the vaccinators. It suggested "for the public good to have every child of fifteen years of age revaccinated on graduation from school," but the state legislature never acted on that proposal.[101]

Although we cannot know with any certainty, revaccination rates probably remained low for the rest of the century. As late as 1901, an Ohio physician observed, "it is only of late years that the importance of revaccination is beginning to be fully understood."[102] When the Boston city physician's office began to offer revaccinations in 1873, few people took advantage of the service, declining from a high of 203 in the first year to just 6 by 1877.[103] In 1894, the State Board of Health observed that among smallpox case data they had accumulated for the last ten years, in "very many of the cases recorded as vaccinated, and especially among adults, there had been but one vaccination, and often of a single scar only, and that of an imperfect character."[104] It appeared that people would get a primary vaccination in childhood for school, but after that few sought out more vaccinations to ensure immunity.

The 1893–94 epidemic also revealed a disturbing trend when health authorities in South Boston found "that many children were attending the public schools without ever having been vaccinated."[105] As a result the superintendent of schools sent medical inspectors to examine and vaccinate every single student "who permitted it" in early 1894. Out of nearly 60,000 children, they gave 4,120 primary vaccinations and 10,152 revaccinations. Absent at the time of inspection were 3,400 children, while 1,678 pupils refused vaccination. Assuming that most of the parents who kept their children away from school did so to avoid the examination, over 15 percent of Boston parents thus neglected, avoided, or outright rejected vaccination. Even worse, many high school students must have lacked a second vaccination since the 10,152 revaccinations amount to nearly

17 percent of the total school population—just that proportion accounted for by high school students, since only older children would need revaccination.[106] A significant proportion of Boston's population not only quietly evaded vaccination but also neglected revaccination at adolescence. This vaccination campaign probably stirred up resentment about compulsory vaccination to the point that the state legislature amended the law later in the spring of 1894 to allow children medical exemptions from vaccination.[107]

Another factor added to the complexity of getting vaccination to the masses. Although the Boston Board of Health repeatedly proclaimed the need for a well-vaccinated population, it also clearly organized its free vaccination service so as not to tread on private medical practices. Private practitioners and druggists resented both public and private provision of free vaccination because they believed it cut into their businesses, attacking dispensaries "as purveyors of ill-considered charity to the unworthy."[108] Public health officials sensitive to this issue did not question the precept that people able to pay ought to pay, and they limited free vaccination by restricting it to one central office, for just an hour or two a day in years of low smallpox incidence.

In 1880–81, for instance, despite "alarm . . . as to the immediate danger of another epidemic of smallpox," the health department decided against a general vaccination order "as allowed by the statute law, at the city's expense, while we know that the work is being rapidly done, as it should be, by physicians at the request and expense of individuals who are able and willing to pay for it."[109] Even though the Boston Health Department clearly had the power to order vaccination during times of crisis, doing so meant that it had to mount a citywide free vaccination campaign. The Board of Health's reluctance to utilize its power came not from any apprehension that a general vaccination order might lead to public unrest, but rather because it feared to upset the balance sheets of local physicians.

As smallpox cases rose in the 1881–82 outbreak, the health department opened temporary vaccination stations that kept evening hours in each major district to accommodate workers. That year the city gave out 37,341 vaccinations without charge. Nearly overwhelmed by "the large number of persons who crowded the offices in the evening," only a few offices could keep complete, accurate vaccination records that year.[110] These stations and their convenient evening hours disappeared, however, after the threat abated. Not until smallpox resurged in 1893–94 did the health department again provide free vaccinations at places and times conducive to workday schedules. At first, it sent physicians to locate and vaccinate just those exposed to a smallpox case. As smallpox cases rose in November 1893, however, the Board of Health decided "to offer free vaccination in those sections of the city where cases of this disease were most frequently found."[111] By opening the schoolhouses during evening hours, the health department managed to vaccinate 127,303 persons over the course of the next few months.[112]

Despite some impressive numbers for free vaccination in 1893–94, 1881–82, and 1872–73, in nonepidemic years often less than 1 percent of Boston's residents got vaccinations from the city physician.[113] Only when smallpox reached epidemic levels did the health department open free vaccination stations with hours conducive to working people. At other times, despite rhetoric about the need to secure universal vaccination, the Boston Health Department's policy was to provide limited access to free vaccination for fear of undermining the profits of private practitioners.

Chapter Two

Problems with Vaccination in the Nineteenth Century

Although physicians touted vaccination's relative harmlessness compared with the rigors of variolation, it did induce a disease, vaccinia, which could provoke great discomfort and temporary disability. Vaccinations sometimes went terribly wrong, leading to disastrous infections that maimed or even killed. Throughout the nineteenth century, physicians argued about the merits of various vaccination techniques, equipment, vaccine strains, and appropriate aftercare. Vaccination additionally underwent substantial technological change during the course of the century as practitioners shifted from propagating vaccine virus in humans (humanized lymph), to cultivating it solely by transfer in calves and heifers (bovine lymph), and then to treating the lymph with an antiseptic, glycerin (glycerinated lymph).

Medical Knowledge about Vaccination

In 1897, the physician-proprietors of the New England Vaccine Company described the stages of an ideal vaccination in their instructional booklet *Variola and Vaccinia*. Vaccinators usually scratched or abraded the upper layer of skin on the arm or leg, and then smeared vaccine lymph into these superficial cuts. Three days after the vaccination, a small, firm reddish skin lesion called a "papule" would appear on each scratched site. By the fourth to sixth day it became "a distinct vesicle of a pearly color, with edges a little elevated," and by the eighth day swelled to its maximum height, "filled with clear lymph, its elevated margin and depressed center being more clearly marked." As the area around the vesicle swelled and became inflamed, "constitutional symptoms, fever, headache and backache" appeared and could last for several days. Then as the vesicle slowly faded away, it dried up into "a hard, brown scab," falling off three to four weeks after the initial inoculation to leave "a depressed foveolated scar, having small pits, or apparent pin-holes, in its center."[1]

Yet the pamphlet also warned that "many deviations from the normal course of the vaccine disease may occur."[2] Vaccination vesicles did not always replicate perfect textbook descriptions to yield Jenner's classic vesicle that looked like "the section of a pearl upon a rose-leaf."[3] Edward Cator Seaton, a respected mid-nineteenth-century British vaccinator, advised that "older children and adults tend to get vesicles that are not perfectly colored or shaped."[4] Different techniques of scratching the virus into the skin also yielded different results from the perfectly round, pearl-like textbook vesicle.

Experts thus looked to the areola, the expanding ring of inflammation around the vesicle, as the hallmark of vaccination. Seaton regarded its "establishment . . . as the anatomical evidence that the Cow-pox has produced its specific effect on the constitution."[5] The American homeopath George Winterburn noted that the development of the aerola "varies greatly," sometimes confined to a "clearly circumscribed round spot less than three inches diameter," but then occasionally "it extends irregularly, involving perhaps the entire limb." Winterburn declared that "in extreme cases the arm may become enormously swollen, and so rigid as to be practically immovable." He remarked that most physicians expected rather severe systemic disturbance to ensue from vaccination: fever, headache, nausea, diarrhea, and swelling were "never altogether absent, even in the mildest cases," and they were seen as "marking the effectiveness of the protection afforded by vaccination."[6] An 1898 medical textbook described the "usual course" of temperature after a vaccination done "with the ordinary precautions" as ranging from 102.2° F. to 104° F.[7] A Texas surgeon recalled, "formerly it was thought by the majority of physicians that the greater the disturbance produced by the vaccination, short of death, the more efficient was the protection against smallpox."[8]

Vaccinations could provoke disquieting results. The New England Vaccine Company noted that "cases of intense inflammation" often resulted "in ulceration, many times indolent and slow in healing." It cautioned that vaccinations giving rise to vaccine roseola (a rose-colored rash) and lichen (thickened, hardened lesions grouped closely together) "are so often seen in the practice of all physicians that it is unnecessary to describe them."[9] Other experts described cases of generalized vaccinia in which vesicles broke out all over the body, causing disfigurement and even death.[10] One physician in 1901 described a patient's face as "badly pitted" and "marked for life" after his nasty bout with it.[11]

Over the course of the nineteenth century, physicians learned that existing illness or conditions like herpes or eczema could interfere disastrously with the course of a vaccination. Edward Seaton warned in 1866 that "special attention must be given to the health of the child to be vaccinated."[12] J. F. Marson, resident physician at the London Smallpox Hospital for thirty years, cautioned that some children "do not take vaccination well."[13] The Massachusetts State Board of Health reminded practitioners in 1894 to delay vaccination "for a month" when "there has been recent exposure to the infection of measles or scarlet fever, and where erysipelas prevails in the place of residence."[14] The smallpox expert John William Moore also advised his readers in 1898 never to vaccinate in the "presence of skin diseases and the propinquity of scarlet fever or erysipelas." He also recommended avoiding vaccination during "periods of teething and of weaning" infants.[15]

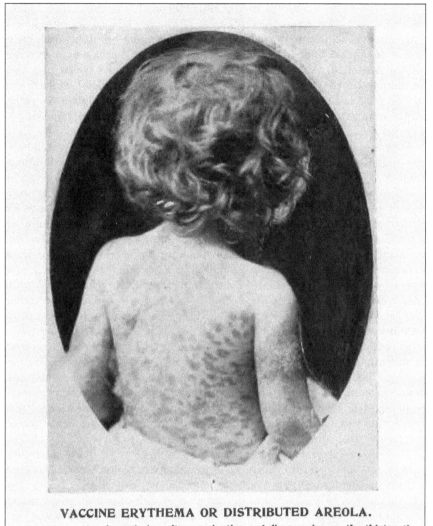

VACCINE ERYTHEMA OR DISTRIBUTED AREOLA.

Appearing on the eleventh day after vaccination and disappearing on the thirteenth.

Figure 2.1. Nineteenth-century photograph of vaccine erythema. William C. Cutler and J. F. Frisbie, *Variola and Vaccinia* (Boston: New England Vaccine Company, 1897), 38.

Many nineteenth-century physicians also observed that vaccination could provoke all sorts of diseases and complications. Although Edward Seaton asserted that most vaccinations went well, sometimes they wound up inflicting a great deal of discomfort. "The local and general symptoms of Vaccination seldom call for any treatment. Occasionally, however, they run an active course; the arm becomes inflamed; erythema, or sometimes true erysipelas, develops itself; the vaccine vesicle degenerates into a purulent ulcer or sometimes into a sloughing sore, leaving a cicatrix which has none of the characteristic pittings, but is simply a puckering, or a flat, smooth, shining scar."[16]

Even as staunch an advocate for vaccination as Henry Austin Martin admitted in 1882 that there were "a considerable number of diseased conditions liable to complicate and follow vaccination." Martin believed that "the slight constitutional disturbance incident to *vaccinia*" sometimes provoked "an eruption of disease already latent in the system." Other bad effects, however, he attributed to "filthy habits of life, gross neglect of ordinary care, very morbid condition of patient, and, above all, and in the most severe cases, malpractice, gross and often incredible, of physicians; in improper methods, and in use of virus taken from improper subjects, at too late a period of the disease, or in a state of decomposition."[17] In 1892, the eminent medical professor and clinician William Osler also described various vaccination complications, noting that "vesicles inflame and deep excavated ulcers result. Sloughing and deep cellulitis may follow. . . . Erysipelas may occur, or there may be deep gangrenous ulceration. Such instances are rare, but I have seen two which proved fatal."[18] An 1898 medical textbook also described erysipelas as a "grave complication" among "debilitated children," one that occasionally attained epidemic proportions in foundling hospitals during the nineteenth century.[19] Sometimes inexplicable, sometimes the result of improper technique, bad results after vaccination reminded nineteenth-century physicians never to take vaccination for granted as a foolproof operation.

Medical texts also taught that revaccination could prove far more uncomfortable, even more dangerous than a primary vaccination. Seaton observed that the scabs itched more, with "considerable constitutional irritation . . . and in very exceptional cases the vaccine lymph may act as an animal poison, giving rise to phlegmonous erysipelas; some still rarer cases have occurred of pyaemia, terminating fatally."[20] Winterburn also observed that some vaccinated individuals "are so susceptible to the influence of this virus that they will be severely afflicted by it whenever it may be re-introduced."[21] Osler agreed that "the constitutional symptoms in revaccination are sometimes quite severe."[22] The French vaccination expert Paul Brouardel warned in 1898 that "an inability to use the arm for several days may be the consequence of this rather intense reaction." He advised revaccinating on just one arm for "soldiers, laborers, and others who are more or less dependent on the free use of their arms."[23]

In 1897, the New England Vaccine Company noted that "secondary vaccinations seldom run a uniform course of development."[24] It contended, however, that many rather frightful vaccination reactions were actually relatively harmless.

"It is not unusual for the areola accompanying a vaccination to extend far below the elbow and even to the wrist, giving rise to the often reported instances of erysipelas. Many of the older vaccinators called this erysipelas, but according to later observations, the constitutional symptoms of that disease, such as rigors, rapid pulse and high temperature, are not found present. Therefore, the conclusion that the case is simply intensified areola and nothing more should be formed. True erysipelas will, in a certain very small proportion of cases, follow vaccination, regardless of purity of lymph used, or care the surgeon may have taken in applying it."[25]

Writing from the standpoint of the late 1890s, these authors casually corrected the "older vaccinators" for mistakenly diagnosing erysipelas in the past. Erysipelas, however, was a rather alarming and often fatal infection in the nineteenth century.[26] The Boston physician and staunch vaccination advocate John H. McCollom acknowledged that "erysipelas may follow vaccination, but there is no proof that the specific organism of this disease is in the vaccine lymph. Erysipelas also frequently follows the scratch of a pin or any slight abrasion."[27] Patients afflicted with the reddened, swelling arms and legs, fever, pain, and skin lesions characteristic of erysipelas, whether true or false, whether acquired from their vaccinations or some scratch afterward, suffered nonetheless, and they certainly learned to regard vaccination with wariness. Those few who actually got erysipelas undoubtedly felt bitter about their vaccination experience, if they survived it. Nineteenth-century physicians thus regarded vaccination not as a trivial procedure, but rather as one fraught with all sorts of complexities and risks. This attitude prevailed both before and after the advent of germ theory.

The Many Sources of Vaccine Virus in the Nineteenth Century

Smallpox vaccines came from different sources, and they could differ enormously in their effects. By the 1880s, one American practitioner complained that "millions of vaccinations are made every year, and nobody knows what they are made with. The whole process is a haphazard game of chance."[28] Jenner originally derived his vaccine material from fluid ("lymph") extracted from vesicles on the hands of dairy workers supposedly infected with cowpox, a comparatively rare disease found only in a few places in Europe.[29] Jenner transferred the lymph from one human subject to another—he did not just take it straight from the cow. Jenner conjectured that a disease of horses called "grease" had provided the true source for the vaccine because he found evidence that stable workers infected by horses had infected the cows they milked, who in turn infected others who milked them.[30] Unfortunately, Jenner's original vaccine strains "of 1796 and 1798 were soon lost," and variolators William Woodson and George Pearson developed several vaccines of their own at the London Smallpox and Inoculation Hospital from cases of cowpox in 1799, some of which they sent to Jenner.[31] Their strains of vaccine became contaminated with variola yet circulated widely throughout England even though they caused eruptions of pustules and rashes.[32] When an Italian physician, Luigi Sacco, discovered cowpox in Lombardy in 1801, he developed his own vaccine strain, sending samples to Jenner and many others. His vaccine reputedly "did not cause eruptions and produced a less severe local lesion than the English strains."[33] By 1803, practitioners were using this vaccine extensively throughout Europe, the Middle East, India, and England.

Over the course of the nineteenth century, these early strains lost much of their effectiveness after a generation of arm-to-arm transfer. After passage through many subjects, vaccine lymph became "humanized" and lost some of its previous potency. In 1845, the British chemist John Badcock declared that "the vaccine lymph, *that most precious boon of Jenner to a suffering world,* has become greatly impaired in value, and is even still advancing in the process of deterioration."[34] Badcock had personally experienced this deterioration: he came down with smallpox shortly after his own revaccination in 1836. A few Italian physicians avoided this problem by inoculating humanized lymph back into cows to refresh it in a process called retrovaccination. After 1842, they abandoned retrovaccination for simple propagation from cow to cow, creating bovine lymph.[35]

Uncertainty about the origin of vaccinia led to all sorts of experiments to create effective vaccine lymph from various sources. Some researchers believed that the lymph originated from smallpox attenuated by passage through a cow or other animals; others, like Jenner, thought that passage through humans had somehow transmuted cowpox or horse "grease" into a new form.[36] By the mid-nineteenth century, medical opinion leaned toward the smallpox theory. In 1866, for instance, an American Medical Association report on vaccination confidently proclaimed current medical understanding of vaccinia's origins as smallpox of the cow, "knowing, as we do, that smallpox and cowpox are in reality the same disease, the latter being merely deprived of its virulence by having previously passed through the system of the cow."[37] Nevertheless, some experimenters continued to seek new vaccine strains in outbreaks of cowpox. Yet finding true Jennerian cowpox, a relatively rare disease, proved difficult, leading John Badcock to complain "that the hope of thus procuring it is almost illusory."[38] Finding a new strain of Jennerian cowpox and extracting usable lymph from it depended mostly on luck.

Physicians thus rushed to develop new vaccines whenever they discovered a new outbreak of cowpox. Direct inoculations into humans of lymph extracted from a cowpox pustule initially induced severe reactions, causing "a great deal of temporary disfigurement and annoyance."[39] An 1836 French vaccine derived from cowpox produced vesicles that "hollowed out the skin so deeply that they left *regular holes.*"[40] Another 1838 British vaccine at first yielded a "'larger and longer-contained areola, more constitutional disturbances, and a much deeper indentation left on the arm.'"[41] Successive transmissions through humans could modify these effects, however. According to Edgar Crookshank, a nineteenth-century historian and critic of vaccination, the 1838 British vaccine eventually achieved such acceptance that "it was also sent to America and other parts of the world."[42]

These problems inspired many to inoculate cows with smallpox to establish new vaccine strains. In late 1840, John Badcock successfully inoculated "a fine young cow, with Small Pox matter taken from a strong healthy girl, and was singularly successful." He then vaccinated "my own little boy," reporting "from this and subsequent operations I have carefully kept up the supply of vaccine."[43] Practitioners eventually used Badcock's vaccine for over fourteen thousand vaccinations. Despite the danger of transmitting smallpox in such vaccine, a number of nineteenth-century researchers inoculated smallpox virus into calves, transferring it "two or three" times through calves and then "five or six" times through humans to produce "entirely normal vaccinations in children." The British surgeon Robert Ceely also produced a reliable strain derived from variola "used in large-scale vaccination" in the 1840s.[44] In Waltham, Massachusetts, the physician Horatio Adams successfully replicated Ceely's experiment in 1840.[45] And the Baltimore physicians C. Van Bibber and Samuel Knight established strains in 1852 that were "still handed down from arm to arm" into the 1880s.[46] Some researchers, however, failed miserably when subjects developed smallpox from their vaccinations. In 1836, for instance, the Massachusetts physician John C. Martin "became at once the most unpopular of men," destroying his practice, after a smallpox epidemic ensued from vaccinations with his experimental variola-derived strain.[47] Others, like Ephraim Cutter of Woburn, Massachusetts, determined that the method was just too difficult and "cannot be relied on in urgent circumstances."[48] He recommended the practice of retrovaccination instead.

Many practitioners felt uneasy about these vaccines. In 1886, George Winterburn recalled a growing "widespread dissatisfaction with the prevailing vaccine material" such that when natural cowpox broke out in Beaugency, France, in 1866, "there were hundreds of practitioners who were willing to give the new brand a trial."[49] One of these practitioners, Henry Austin Martin, imported this vaccine lymph in 1870 to Boston, where he established a vaccine farm to become a major supplier of bovine lymph (lymph drawn from cowpox vesicles propagated only on cows or calves rather than by arm-to-arm transfer) for New England.[50] For many years until his death in 1884, Martin touted "the typical perfection of the *vaccinia* induced by true animal vaccination, and its entire freedom from those irregular and unprotective developments."[51] Martin distinguished his lymph as "true animal vaccination" from other bovine lymph because it had originated from cowpox rather than from humanized lymph inoculated and propagated on cows and calves. Martin's Beaugency lymph apparently gained quite a following among late-nineteenth-century practitioners. Nevertheless by 1897, Samuel W. Abbott, secretary of the Massachusetts State Board of Health, criticized Martin's claims: "The original source of the disease in the cow is undoubtedly some exposure to smallpox infection. Experiment has definitely settled this point. The term 'spontaneous cowpox' has often been used in this country and abroad in connection with this subject. No progressive physician, however, at the present day, would for a moment admit the use of such a term. Infectious diseases have an origin, and that origin is an infectious disease of the same kind. As a matter of fact, the term is simply used as a catch-penny dodge for lining the pockets of some particular producer of vaccine lymph."[52]

In the early twentieth century, one medical journal editor recalled, "for many years, in America, succeeding the introduction of animal vaccination, a superstitious reverence for the so-called Beaugency stock appears to have prevailed, and an unbroken pedigree from this historic heifer was considered a *sine qua non* of vaccinal purity." He disparaged this preference for the Beaugency lymph, calling it a "curious fetish of the 19th century," especially when German authorities successfully inoculated calves with "humanized lymph from healthy infants" all the time.[53]

Vaccines thus originated from many sources and they produced markedly different reactions. During the Civil War, Ephraim Cutter, for instance, sold to the United States Army both vaccine derived from retrovaccination and some obtained from his serendipitous discovery of natural cowpox.[54] Cutter later found that 30 percent of the five hundred physicians he queried complained that the vaccine he sent them was inert. Although most had no problems with it, declaring that "the effects were as severe as ordinary virus," one vaccination ulcerated in a "deep conical cavity" that took several weeks to heal.[55] Over the course of the nineteenth century, experimenters developed vaccine strains from cowpox, equine pox, swine pox, goat pox, as well as variolated cow vaccine. By the 1880s, George Winterburn declared that so many different vaccine strains had circulated that "it is impossible for anybody to tell what he is using."[56]

In 1903, a confused Indiana physician asked the editors of the *Journal of the American Medical Association* to clear up the mystery: "From what source do vaccine laboratories or vaccine farms obtain their original vaccine virus? Do they use the smallpox lymph, or the cowpox lymph, which comes originally from the 'grease heel' of the horse?" The editors queried several vaccine manufacturers and found considerable differences among them. The H. K. Mulford Company did not worry about the original source, but instead procured vaccine from a variety of European and American sources, tested each one, and chose the one that produced "the most typical physiological effect" to propagate its virus. Parke, Davis & Company insisted that "all our seed" came from "the calf or heifer—not in any instance the virus obtained from human smallpox pustules." Yet it acknowledged that "cowpox is the result of the direct introduction of smallpox virus into the animal organism," and described experiments in which German researchers had derived lymph from smallpox inoculated into calves that "produced in human beings perfectly normal vaccinations, affording full protection." It also noted that a "great English authority, Copeman," had produced a successful vaccine by "repeatedly inoculating monkeys with the virus of human smallpox," which he then inoculated into calves to produce lymph that he had used on "hundreds of people." Frederick Stearns and Company used vaccine virus "from heifers . . . previously inoculated with smallpox lymph taken from a human being." It dismissed natural cowpox as source for vaccine: "in our opinion there is no such thing as a cowpox which will confer immunity to smallpox which had not originally a human source." H. M. Alexander also denied "most emphatically" that cowpox or horse grease were sources for vaccine: "My experiments proved to me beyond any reasonable doubt that vaccine virus was simply smallpox passed through the cow."[57] Yet in an 1898 medical textbook, the French vaccination expert Paul Brouardel confidently asserted that "we know then to-day that horsepox is a source of vaccina [sic]," and he disparaged any notion that inoculating cows with smallpox produced anything except "the ancient smallpox inoculation," referring to the older practice of variolation.[58] Thus over a century after Jenner introduced vaccination, physicians derived vaccines from a variety of sources, and they disagreed vehemently about which ones worked best or even what they actually were.

Methods of Lymph Extraction and Preservation

The source was but one factor that could affect vaccine quality, however. The timing of lymph extraction was also crucial. Classic Jennerian doctrine dictated removal at the eighth day after inoculation, when the fluid in the vesicle was clear. After that point, as the fluid became more opaque, it lost its potency. Yet rules sometimes fell by the wayside when practitioners succumbed to the temptation of convenience. Under pressure to accumulate a large volume of lymph quickly, they harvested it after the proper maturation date. Seaton agreed that lymph taken later "flows then more freely, and may be got in greater abundance." This convenience, in his opinion, came at a price: "very often it takes; but it does not do *this with anything like the same certainty*."[59] He disparaged this practice as "the source of much current inferior Vaccination," observing that some practitioners "will often be induced to take their lymph from second-rate vesicles, rather than lose the opportunity of vaccinating direct from an arm."[60] Crookshank observed that patients sometimes paid a high price for a physician's laxness: "under certain conditions, such as a peculiarity in the subject inoculated, or if lymph be taken too late, there will be, just as in variolation, a tendency to revert to the full intensity of the natural virus."[61]

Storage of lymph also presented a problem. According to the vaccination expert John Buist, best medical practice dictated that the "most perfect results" obtained when the vaccinator used "fresh lymph transferred directly from a typical vesicle on the arm of a healthy child to the arm of another."[62] Although Seaton insisted that "lymph should in every instance (where practicable) be inserted direct from arm to arm," this was not the practice everywhere.[63] In reality, physicians often could not control vaccination so precisely. Bringing subjects to a donor took time and effort. It was much more efficient to collect lymph in capillary tubes or dry it on ivory points for use later, even though experts understood that "storage of lymph, even for the shortest period, exerts an injurious influence upon its activity."[64] Thus when vaccinators used stored lymph, their vaccinations failed to take more often than those from fresh lymph.

American physicians, with no state-sponsored system of vaccine propagation, lacked easy access to human donors and fresh lymph. Where European vaccinators favored direct inoculation of fresh lymph, by the middle of the nineteenth century American physicians depended mainly on crusts for the basis of their vaccine material. Shipped on ivory points, smeared between glass plates, or soaked into thread, it arrived in a dry form that resisted deterioration better than liquid lymph.[65]

This deviation from the classic Jennerian technique of lymph extraction troubled some physicians. In 1865, Joseph M. Toner regretted that "in the United States the crust has been almost entirely substituted for the lymph in propagating the disease [vaccinia]."[66] An 1869 report on vaccination in the United States observed that "most physicians find it inconvenient to vaccinate 'from arm to arm,' and therefore use points of ivory or quill, dipped in vaccine lymph and dried; others take a bit of scab—powdered and dissolved in glycerine or water—to insert, instead of fresh lymph."[67] This process could go horribly wrong, as it did for one Massachusetts physician who "had the misfortune to spread phlegmonous erysipelas among the patients he vaccinated, many dying in consequence," when the glycerine he used underwent "some chemical change."[68] In 1880, Henry Hartshorne, the American editor of a highly regarded nineteenth-century medical textbook, remarked that "in the United States, many practitioners have for a long time been in the habit of using the scab, instead of fluid lymph, for vaccination." He noted that American physicians customarily waited for the scab to detach spontaneously nineteen or twenty days after vaccination. Mixed with water to form a paste, physicians would then smear the paste into the vaccination site. The advantage to this method was that vaccine could then be kept and stored "usually for a month or more."[69] Later observers also noted the popularity of crusts. In 1901 the Providence, Rhode Island, health officer Charles Chapin recalled that American physicians tended to favor crusts over lymph: "humanized virus, so-called, was employed partly in the form of dried lymph on quills, partly by arm to arm method, but mostly by triturating and moistening the crusts."[70]

For all of its convenience, vaccine derived from crust often did not work. One 1869 report declared of crust-based vaccine: "Many physicians fail one in three or four times; and it is very much to be regretted that so many are content with imperfect results."[71] The newly formed Boston Board of Health certainly could attest to this problem when it termed "successful" only little more than half of the vaccinations performed during the 1872 smallpox epidemic.[72] Crust vaccine also led to more complications. Joseph Toner cited ignorant or careless physicians for using the entire crust when only "the central part of it is fit for use, as the lower layer and edge contains . . . foreign matters" that may "excite . . . a pustular inflammation of considerable severity" but still not produce a real vaccination. Yet Toner acknowledged that American physicians believed the convenience of this method outweighed its disadvantages: "If it were not for the difficulty of preserving or obtaining the fluid lymph when wanted, the crusts, I am quite confident, never would be used by the profession."[73]

Although Toner urged the medical profession to use only fresh lymph, reliance on crusts continued until last third of the nineteenth century, and it may have contributed substantially to public disdain for vaccination. At the beginning of the Civil War, the Union army used lymph in the "form of crusts of uncertain age and source, obtained in northern cities."[74] One Framingham, Massachusetts, physician remembered that he had had "to make a single vaccine crust and half of another answer for the vaccination of 700 soldiers."[75] George Winterburn recalled that the New York City health department had a long-established practice of requiring parents to bring their vaccinated children to the Essex Market Dispensary "on the twenty-first day after vaccination" in order for the physicians to scrape off their scabs for use in future vaccine preparations: "The scabs were then taken off and dropped into an open-mouthed, glass fruit jar. A sufficient quantity of water was added from time to time to soften these scabs into a paste, and into this filthy mixture the quills were dipped, then dried, then sold with the official aroma of true Jennerian cow-pox." Winterburn asserted that "many accidents have arisen from the use of impure vaccine, but vaccinists as a rule have been loath to admit the facts, fearing to prejudice the public mind against the whole matter."[76] In 1913, looking back on this practice, the medical professor George Dock observed that it "must have been unsatisfactory," since the scabs came from "a stage of the lesion when specific activity is less and contamination greater than in earlier phases."[77]

Vaccination Techniques

Physicians used a wide variety of techniques and instruments in vaccination. Some made just one puncture, others a couple of scratch lines, still others thoroughly abraded the skin. In 1865, Joseph Toner recommended "an ordinary thumb lancet, introducing the point quite flatly under the scarfskin of the arm, though so superficially as to scarcely draw blood."[78] Edward Seaton observed that British vaccinators used a variety of methods. Sometimes they made "a number of minute superficial punctures . . . with the point of a lancet," and then spread the lymph over the area. Or they rubbed the lymph on first, "then ripping up the cuticle with the point of the lancet." Others made three or four scratches with a needle and then rubbed the lymph on the skin. Many English vaccinators favored "abrading the cuticle by number of fine parallel scratches . . . or by further cross-scratch" until blood oozed, which they "then rapidly wiped away with the finger" and then "plastered on" the lymph. Seaton felt that abrasion gave the best vaccination mark and was "eminently more successful than puncture when dry lymph has to be employed."[79] By the end of the nineteenth century, vaccinators used instruments ranging from lancets, needles, scarifiers, and rakes to "Rose's vaccinator," an "ingenious little instrument" that delivered vaccine via five little needles in a circular cap.[80]

Nineteenth-century physicians differed about how much vaccinators should abrade the skin. Edward Seaton believed that all sorts of methods could give good results if done properly, that is, if the vaccinator inserted good lymph at just the right depth. Nevertheless, he felt that many practitioners failed to get it right, and he saw many cases of smallpox occurring in supposedly well-vaccinated persons.[81] George Winterburn observed New York vaccinators using a "thin bladed and very sharp lancet" to make "a number of scratches, about half an inch long . . . just deep enough to draw a little blood."[82] He thought that if any erred in their technique it was by making the cuts too shallow. Yet, in 1894, the Massachusetts Board of Health recommended that practitioners "scarify or lightly abrade the surface in at least two places about an inch apart, until the scarified spots appear slightly red and moist, but not enough to draw blood."[83] Disagreement about the proper depth continued to perplex vaccinators. In 1902 George Dock complained: "In this country most of the training seems to be derived from the publications of vaccine makers, and it is instructive to see that they recommend . . . extensive scraping or scarification, so deep that a scab forms before the virus begins to act. Such a wound must favor the development of accidental infections."[84] Even as late as the 1960s, the smallpox expert Cyril Dixon noted the difficulty he encountered in getting "unbiased, accurate observations on different techniques carried out under identical conditions."[85]

Physicians disagreed about how many insertions to place in order to ensure a good "take." In 1866, Joseph Toner observed that American practitioners "seldom produce more than one vesicle," when "in Europe, the opinion prevails very generally that one vaccine vesicle cannot be relied upon as affording complete protection against variola," and he thus called for a new standard of six insertions.[86] Edward Seaton maintained that at least five were needed when using the puncture method.[87] Nevertheless, patients' complaints at the extensive discomfort and scarring produced by multiple insertions prompted many American physicians to rely on just one insertion. At a 1901 American Public Health Association meeting, the physician and vaccine producer W. F. Elgin declared that in the United States, "they use a single insertion. . . . I have seen incisions that would almost cover a silver dollar. Now, we recommend using the pin point incision."[88] At the same meeting, the Boston health department chairman Samuel Durgin declared, "I tell my students that I do not believe in one puncture. I believe that not less than three punctures for the primary vaccination and two for the revaccination are doing more and better service than the one puncture."[89] Yet in 1902, another physician cautioned that "two vaccinations made at different times, protect better against smallpox than one vaccination consisting of several insertions."[90] A Cambridge physician also warned against placing the insertions too close together because "if placed too near one another they are liable to coalesce and form a single large vesicle, which is more likely to be injured than several small ones."[91]

Physicians also argued about whether or not to take any extraordinary measures to protect the vaccination site from contact with dirt or germs. Some contended that vaccinations should be left alone to dry in the air, with no need of a dressing.[92] The proprietors of the New England Vaccine Company warned that "dressings, like poultices, oil, tallow, vaseline or water, tending to soften the capsule of the pustule, should never be applied to an unbroken vesicle."[93] The Cambridge city bacteriologist and physician Eugene Darling declared that "shields as permanent dressings are to be condemned, without exception," especially "the transparent celluloid ones, which have been used so widely."[94] The Kentucky State Board of Health secretary Joseph N. McCormack, "the most influential political leader of the profession in the Progressive Era," contended that "protectors and dressings . . . in my experience do more harm than good."[95] Yet many practitioners did not heed this advice. Surgical suppliers like Codman & Shurtleff of Boston advertised vaccination shields along with lancets and vaccine lymph, in a leading 1890s public health journal no less.[96] One Philadelphia physician tacitly implied the continued popularity of shields when he asserted in 1901 that the "worst arms seen by me during this season were on those who had put on 'shields' early and worn them continuously."[97] In 1901, an Ohio physician swore by placing a "pad additionally supported with light bandage" over the vaccination, and he instructed practitioners to "keep the wound protected at all times."[98] A Texas surgeon advised his colleagues "to apply a rather thick pledget of sterile cotton, cover it with gauze or muslin and fasten it in place with narrow strips of adhesive plaster."[99] Physicians still used shields in the early twentieth century, and medical journals published new shield designs.[100] One, for instance, complained in 1902 of "repeated and increasing trouble with irritated, inflamed and infected arms, due to the existing forms of vaccination shield," but then proceeded to argue for his new shield design, declaring that "a shield may be a source of comfort, protection, and satisfaction."[101] Both *American Medicine* and the *Journal of the American Medical Association* published an engraving of his shield, an acknowledgment that many medical practitioners believed in the need to protect a vaccination despite expert opinion to the contrary.

Incompetence plagued nineteenth-century vaccinations. According to George Dock, many laypersons with little or no training took up the business of vaccinating in early nineteenth-century England.[102] By the early twentieth century, few medical students received instruction in vaccination either, leaving a young practitioner to learn about it on his or her own. One Canadian physician remarked before a 1901 American Public Health Association meeting that "it is a matter of notoriety that no teaching, or almost none, is given at our medical schools on the principles and methods of vaccination."[103] Heman Spalding, chief medical inspector for the Chicago health department, complained: "there are doctors, and good ones, too, who have had so little experience with vaccination that they do not know what constitutes a successful vaccination."[104] In 1902, the American surgeon Ernest Mellish agreed that "until very recently" vaccination "was not taught in our medical schools, and young practitioners were left to learn from experience and analogy how to protect their patients from trouble due to vaccination." He figured that inept treatment of vaccinations "contributes a considerable amount of ammunition to the antivaccinationists."[105] A 1902 American Public Health Association report on vaccine also noted "a general absence of teaching, in our schools of medicine, of the principles and practices of vaccination," and it cited "neglect on the part of the operator . . . to prepare the arm properly" and "to protect the wound," as well as "improper method of inoculation," as chief causes for "complaints, especially from the profession, of abnormal results in vaccination."[106] Indeed, a 1905 smallpox outbreak developed into an epidemic in Argyle, Minnesota, because "a local practitioner did not understand the use of the capillary tubes of vaccine virus, and attempted to force the virus through the needle, which he supposed was hollow."[107]

By the end of the century, the teachings of bacteriology had permeated medical thinking and American physicians attributed many vaccination complications to poor aseptic practice. An Ohio physician lamented in 1902 that the incompetence of some of his colleagues led to severe results for their patients. "We frequently hear of Mr. A or Mrs. B having a terribly bad arm, expecting to lose it, etc. Trace this case to the beginning and you will find that the operation was carelessly done, a dirty and sweated sleeve pushed up, the virus carelessly smeared on and the sleeve drawn over it, or if a pad is used, it will be fixed so as to come off the first evening, the patient having no instructions as to how to keep the wound. Then examine the arm carefully and you will find genuine blood poisoning is what is doing the mischief."[108] Eugene Darling noted before a 1902 Massachusetts Medical Society meeting that "physicians should always give detailed instructions to the patient" in caring for their vaccinations, but "this precaution is often neglected by the busy practitioner, or the instructions given are so general as to be of little value."[109] One of his colleagues, John H. McCollom, agreed: "I think the majority of sore arms are due not so much to the carelessness of the individual, as to the physician in not giving sufficient directions."[110] George Dock also criticized practitioners for casually assuming the infallibility of their vaccinations: "If the operation fails the patient is often told he is immune to smallpox; if on the other hand he has a phelgmon he is comforted by being reminded how severely he would have had smallpox had he not been vaccinated."[111]

Many physicians called for a surgical approach by thoroughly washing arms and sterilizing instruments before vaccination. Some even adopted the practice of swabbing the vacinee's arm "with a solution of carbolic acid" or "corrosive sublimate, that being the latest favorite among germicides," which unfortunately left traces on the skin that killed vaccinia virus.[112] In 1897, the proprietors of the New England Vaccine Company worried about the possibility of inducing infections, advising that "the vaccinator should always avoid all forms of vaccinating instruments, or any instrument which is designed for successive cases." They noted that "many operators" used a new "common sewing needle . . . one for each subject," but they suggested "nothing so clean and convenient for the purpose of scarifying as the ivory point" if "not applied to more than one person."[113] In 1902 one Pennsylvania physician, however, swore by his spring lancet, "which leaves no open wound for the introduction germs," claiming "the puncture made by the lancet is barely discernible, and leaves no abraded surface for any sort of exterior infection." He called abrasion an "erroneous technique . . . producing a good culture-medium for germs not intended."[114]

Another common problem revolved around the proper site for a vaccination. Many physicians noted that women preferred not to have a readily visible scar on an arm, and vaccinations—especially the ones with multiple insertions that coalesced into a huge sore—could leave ugly cicatrixes. Yet vaccinations on the legs or other sites ordinarily covered by clothing tended to develop more complications. In 1886, George Winterburn observed "many mothers objecting to having a girl's arm scarred," insisting that the doctor vaccinate on the "inner surface of the thigh several inches below the groin."[115] William Osler remarked that "mothers 'in society' prefer to have girl babies vaccinated on the leg."[116] One medical journal editor agreed: "in deference to the wishes of some mothers and out of regard for the sensibilities of esthetic young women, girls are not rarely vaccinated on the thigh."[117] Many physicians readily obliged, as did one practitioner who considered "it best, if the patient be a female, to vaccinate upon the antero-external aspect of the lower fifth of the thigh; if a right-handed male, the operation should be performed upon the antero-internal portion of the middle third of the left arm."[118] Nevertheless, although Ernest Mellish acknowledged that "women and girls often wish to avoid having a scar on the arm," he warned that "wounds on the leg do not heal as readily as those on the arm," explaining, "I have seen very severe vaccination sores on the lower extremities, even when carefully treated." Noting a report of at least one death from the infection of such a vaccination, he counseled practitioners not to give in to patient whims, emphasizing in italics: "*Do not vaccinate on the lower extremities.*"[119] The New England Vaccine Company also cautioned against "the too common practice of vaccinating the lower limbs," declaring that "vaccinations upon the leg below the knee have often produced serious results."[120] Still John William Moore advised physicians in 1898 that "from an aesthetic point of view, care should be taken to vaccinate girls at some place where the scars will be as far as possible hidden by the future evening dress."[121] And Brouardel agreed that some mothers wanted their daughters vaccinated on the thigh or calf, and "this wish may be respected without any harm." He warned physicians, however, "to cover the points of inoculation with a good dressing and to impress upon the mother" the need to leave it alone.[122] Eugene Darling also believed "there is no objection to vaccinating on the leg in the case of girls . . . but in this location the after-treatment requires somewhat greater care."[123] Women clearly had a great deal of influence in this matter, and physicians attended to their concerns over the possibility of unsightly scars even if it brought their patients a higher risk of infection.

So many elements had to work together to ensure a successful vaccination. In 1886, George Winterburn cautioned that "'vaccination is not a thing to be trifled with, or to be made light of; it is not to be undertaken thoughtlessly, or without due consideration of the condition of the patient, his mode of life, and the circumstances of season and place.'"[124] Physicians had to select good lymph from healthy donors, they had to master the technique of abrading the skin to the correct depth, they had to ensure that the person vaccinated had no health conditions that might jeopardize the process, and they had to follow the progress of vesicle formation to ensure no adverse complications ensued. No one in the nineteenth century took vaccination for granted as a simple, foolproof procedure.

Syphilis and the Transition to Bovine Lymph

Physicians reluctantly and slowly acknowledged the possibility that humanized lymph could transmit syphilis, although widely known outbreaks of it appeared in Italy in 1814, 1821, 1841, 1856, and 1861. In the notorious 1861 Rivalta incident, forty-six children developed syphilis in a vaccination chain originating from the arm of one syphilitic child. These reports did not immediately provoke any changes, however. In 1866, Edward Cator Seaton questioned the Italian physicians' competence and criticized their reports as unreliable. He proposed that the initial vaccinator probably mistook a syphilitic sore for a vesicle, and he declared that "it is quite an open question whether the children were not carelessly syphilized instead of being vaccinated."[125] British medical experts like Seaton claimed that they could avoid syphilis transmission by first carefully selecting lymph "only from the healthiest children, from the most perfect and regular vesicles at the proper period of their course," taking care to extract only "pure, unmixed vaccine lymph, free from the slightest stain of blood."[126] They believed blood, not clear lymph, transmitted syphilis. Thus only careless vaccinators ran the risk of inoculating syphilis with the vaccination.

The British medical community remained skeptical of this possibility until one of their own, the surgeon Jonathan Hutchinson, documented six cases of syphilis transmission by vaccination in patients he treated in the 1870s.[127] Even so, the public vaccinator Robert Cory decided to show that a properly done vaccination could not transmit syphilis by experimenting on himself. From 1877 to 1881 he vaccinated himself four times with lymph extracted from syphilitic infants. The first three vaccinations were fine, but after the last one Cory developed unmistakable symptoms of syphilis.[128] Only then did medical practitioners in the English-speaking world acknowledge the possibility of syphilis transmission via arm-to-arm vaccinations.[129] Nevertheless, British public vaccinators, confident in their technique, backed by government and law, put off changing over to a new form of vaccine until the later 1880s.[130]

Hutchinson's findings reverberated among American physicians accustomed already to obtaining their vaccine lymph in both dry and liquid form from bovine and human sources. In the crowded American medical marketplace, they could not afford to dismiss their patients' anxieties, and thus more quickly accepted the possibility that vaccination might transmit syphilis and other diseases. In 1879, George Winterburn treated a recently vaccinated family in which all the children showed signs of syphilis infection. He refused to entertain the possibility that their widowed mother had acquired the disease through sexual contact because "although very poor, they were neat."[131] Vaccination thus seemed to him the most likely culprit. As a sexually transmitted disease, syphilis evoked intense fear and embarrassment in nineteenth-century society. The idea that children might get it from their vaccinations horrified Victorian-era parents and physicians, and antivaccinationists played on that terror by emphasizing its likelihood in their writings. In 1902, John McCollom investigated several cases of syphilis supposedly acquired from vaccination, determining that it "was used as a cloak to cover this condition." He blamed antivaccination propaganda: "It is so tempting for parents to lay the results of their own iniquities upon vaccination, especially when they are encouraged so to do by shameless agitators."[132]

Still, some experts believed that physicians could avoid any danger of syphilis infection by paying close attention to donors. In 1865, Joseph Toner recommended state control of vaccine production to resolve this issue, asserting that "government should assume to furnish the profession, for the good of her citizens, with pure liquid vaccine lymph."[133] In 1892, William Osler warned practitioners still using humanized lymph to avoid any problems by carefully selecting the donor child, choosing one "healthy, strong, and known to be of good stock, free from tuberculous or syphilitic taint."[134] As late as 1894, the Massachusetts State Board of Health also cautioned physicians never to take lymph "from cases of revaccination, but invariably from a primary case and from an infant in good health and of healthy parentage."[135]

Physicians on both sides of the Atlantic saw that vaccination was in trouble and knew they had to deal with the problem of syphilis transmission. Eliminating humanized lymph provided a solution—and a commercial opportunity. As early as 1842, the Italian physician Pietro Negri successfully propagated vaccine lymph from vesicles inoculated on successive calves in the process of retrovaccination used to refresh vaccine lymph. Bovine lymph possessed two distinct advantages: First, "it absolutely eliminates the possibility of the transmission of syphilis," but perhaps more important, one animal could produce at least a hundred vesicles, becoming essentially a biological vaccine factory.[136] One medical journal editor contrasted the certainties bovine lymph afforded against the risks associated with collecting human lymph and maintaining a sufficient supply of human lymph. "The advantages of having young and healthy animals under control, each of whom will yield sufficient vaccine material for the vaccination of several thousand people, is apparent when compared with the uncertain mode of depending upon the appearance of a mother with the vaccinated infant at the precise day for taking the lymph, and also frequently with a decided unwillingness to allow the child's arm to be disturbed by the irritation consequent upon taking a large supply from a more or less scanty vesicle."[137] Easily controlled, cows afforded vaccinators the convenience of timing lymph extraction precisely.[138] Cows also could not complain, but human mothers and infants tended to object if a physician pinched or scraped an arm too vigorously. Even more important, bovine lymph turned smallpox vaccine into a commodity, opening up the possibility of large-scale production and commercialization of vaccine free from the taint of syphilis.

With these incentives, bovine lymph began to replace humanized lymph in the last quarter of the nineteenth century. As one medical journal editor observed later, "notwithstanding the fact that such transference of other diseases was an occurrence of the rarest kind, the popular demand for a change was sufficient to bring about the gradual introduction of lymph from the calf or heifer."[139] Bovine lymph caught on quickly in the United States—the Union army turned to bovine lymph in 1865.[140] The Massachusetts State Board of

Health noted both humanized and bovine lymph in use during the 1872 epidemic.[141] In 1873, for instance, a Chicago vaccine firm added bovine lymph to its line because of "the increased and widely extending demand for non-humanized vaccine virus," although it continued to offer humanized lymph "through HEALTHY CHILDREN, furnished to us by family physicians of undoubted reliability."[142] In the mid 1880s, George Winterburn declared that "arm-to-arm vaccination has almost ceased in New York."[143] By the 1890s, the Massachusetts State Board of Health advised physicians to "use bovine lymph preferably."[144] The Providence health officer Charles Chapin later recalled that bovine lymph "rapidly became popular and almost entirely displaced the humanized form" largely because "of popular prejudice" against humanized lymph. It gained such wide distribution after 1875 that "almost all the vaccine virus employed in this country was bovine virus furnished on ivory points."[145]

The transition from humanized lymph to bovine lymph in the 1870s commercialized vaccine virus production in American medicine. Previously, any physician could keep up his or her own supply of vaccine by continuously recycling vaccine material in arm-to-arm vaccination and thus had personal knowledge about its freshness and the health of the donor. Winterburn observed that humanized lymph gave physicians greater control of the process: "when the doctor thus had a whole series of vaccinations under direct purview, he was enabled to judge of the quality of the vaccine he was using."[146] By the 1870s, as more physicians accepted the possibility of syphilis transmission from humanized lymph, they turned to bovine lymph produced on vaccine farms. Whether produced from privately owned or public facilities, vaccine lymph became an important medical commodity. Vaccine farms could produce vaccine lymph on a scale impossible with human donors, thus industrializing a hitherto voluntary, personal procedure. No single medical or governmental authority existed to enforce or even encourage the development of any standards of quality control. Commercial vaccine establishments used a wide variety of methods. The New England Vaccine Company acknowledged these disparities. "The technique of bovine vaccination by different operators varies to such an extent, in so many essential features, that space will not admit of descriptions in detail. There is a wide difference of opinions as to the age of the animals best adapted for the cultivation of vaccine lymph, some propagators choosing nursing calves, others yearlings, and many, mature young heifers, preferably from two to four years old. . . . Ideas also vary as to the proper period for opening the vaccine vesicles. Lymph collected from vesicles in their earlier stages is usually considered more reliable, provided no vesicle be opened prior to the fifth day. The period of maturity may vary in different animals, many vesicles not maturing until the sixth day, or one hundred and forty-four hours after the vaccination of the animal."[147]

Previously physicians could exert some control by transferring lymph themselves from person to person. But now they had to buy their vaccine as "an article of commerce" that had "therefore a mercenary element." Winterburn believed that this transition undermined the physician's position when vaccinating his or her patients: "It has assumed a more purely commercial aspect, and the

VACCINE VIRUS.

CODMAN & SHURTLEFF.

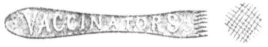

STABLES ESTABLISHED IN 1872.

We continue as for over 20 years to supply animal virus from our own stables from lymph imported by ourselves. The establishment is under the care of a competent physician of long experience in this specialty.
We warrant our virus, giving a fresh supply in failures reported within twenty days.
All Virus is put up in strong air-tight sealed packages.

FROM THE HEIFER.

10 LARGE IVORY POINTS, well charged on both sides, - Net, $1.00
   Orders filled, post-paid, on receipt of price.
SCARIFYING VACCINATOR, Steel, Nickel-plated, (see cut) - - - .25
VACCINATION SHIELD, to protect the limb from the clothes, - - 25
   Orders by Mail or Telegraph answered by return train. Liberal discount on large supplies for Cities, Towns and Institutions.

CODMAN & SHURTLEFF, SUPERIOR SURGICAL INSTRUMENTS.
13 and 15 Tremont Street, Boston, Mass.

Figure 2.2. Codman & Shurtleff advertisement. Note the image of their "scarifying vaccinator." *Journal of the Massachusetts Association of Boards of Health* 7 (1896).

family doctor is simply a 'middleman,' between the vaccine dealer and the vaccinated."[148] In 1894, Samuel W. Abbott complained about this situation to other health officers. "If we could do away entirely with the selling of vaccine lymph, and have it issued directly from a station, as it is in many foreign countries, directly to the physician who uses it, coming from a source that he knows he can rely upon as to the date it is taken from the animal, and not simply the date that it is sold to him,—as I have known here in Boston,—then we should have something that would be of value."[149] Joseph N. McCormick felt that commercial production subverted vaccination: "The propaganda for bovine virus has always been largely a commercial one, and the sore arms and severe constitutional disturbance following its use is responsible for much of the growing prejudice against vaccination."[150]

Some American physicians cashed in on the demand for bovine lymph, creating quite large business concerns out of their vaccine establishments. Henry Austin Martin introduced his special strain of lymph cultivated from the Beaugency cowpox strain to Boston in 1870. By 1882, he claimed to have vaccinated "at least five thousand animals," inducing in each one "sixty to one hundred, or even more vesicles."[151] In the 1890s, his son Francis C. Martin distinguished their lymph, claiming precedence and superior quality at a competitive price: "In 1870 we introduced into America the practice of Animal Vaccination. Our establishment, continued uninterruptedly since, is by far the oldest, largest and best appointed in the country. Our Virus, hitherto the most expensive, can now be obtained by the profession at as low a price as any other."[152] The Pennsylvania physician H. M. Alexander developed his own bovine vaccine in 1882 and started the Lancaster County Vaccine Farms, which eventually became Wyeth Laboratories.[153] The New England Vaccine Company, owned by the physicians William C. Cutler and J. F. Frisbie, offered "pure and reliable animal vaccine lymph, fresh daily" to Boston physicians who could purchase "by mail or telegraph promptly dispatched" ten double-charged ivory points for one dollar.[154] In another advertisement, the New England Vaccine Company bragged that "Boards of Health of Boston, Baltimore, Montreal, Toronto, and many other cities in the United States and Canada, together with the War Department of the United States," favored their vaccine.[155] And Codman & Shurtleff, "established in 1872," declared their virus "from the heifer" was "put up in strong air-tight sealed packages."[156]

Problems with Bovine Lymph and the Transition to Glycerinated Lymph

Though intended as a technical innovation to make vaccination safer, bovine lymph dried on ivory points could contain impurities that produced severe reactions in vaccinations. Contamination with organisms found around animals, dirt, and dung plagued the process unless the handlers adhered to scrupulous cleanliness at all times. In 1882, the homeopath D. H. Beckwith claimed he had used humanized lymph for twenty years and could not "recall a single case that resulted in any permanent injury." Then like many other physicians he switched to bovine lymph and obtained good results until recently, when many vaccinations failed and some went terribly wrong. One patient's arm became so inflamed, "extending over her chest and the left side of her face," that "she had to carry her arm in a sling, and was confined to her room for three or four days."[157] Running sores, offensive discharges, and bedridden patients followed vaccination after vaccination in Beckwith's Cleveland practice. One of his colleagues remarked in response: "I believe the extraordinary demand for bovine virus created by the systematic and sensational newspaper reports, and the foolish declarations of Boards of Health, led producers of the article to put on the market vast numbers of ivory points and quills which had not a particle of the genuine lymph on them only serum, blood, and possible pus."[158]

In 1882 also, a Georgia physician complained about bovine vaccine procured from the New England Vaccine Company. "The result has been fearful. Nearly every one vaccinated has suffered severely from Erythema or Erysipelas, the arm swollen from shoulder to wrist, and the point of puncture presenting the appearance of a sloughing ulcer, discharging freely sanious pus. Many of the sufferers have been confined to bed, with high fever, from five to ten days, requiring the constant application of poultices to the arm, and a free use of morphia for the relief of pain."[159] The owners of the company apparently responded by implementing strict aseptic protocols by the late 1890s and even advertised the advantages of "pure lymph taken from thoroughly cleansed, open vesicles, and stored by drying upon ivory points" as "the safest, most reliable and convenient form."[160] Yet their procedures did not provide a vaccine free from contamination: a 1901 bacteriological study of dry points counted as many as 801 bacteria colonies for each vaccination from the New England Vaccine Company, although the researcher added that "all of these bacteria are harmless, and exist naturally on or in the skin."[161] Few vaccine establishments produced entirely satisfactory dry points from bovine lymph. In 1902, one surgeon despaired that "I know of only one firm that produced *aseptic* dry vaccine."[162]

In 1891, the British researcher Sir Monkton Cope introduced the practice of adding glycerin as a germicide to bovine lymph to ensure the destruction of extraneous microorganisms that caused various infections.[163] This process worked both on liquid lymph stored in capillary tubes and dried lymph stored on ivory points. The 1901 bacteriological study cited above also counted far fewer microorganisms on tube lymph and glycerinated points, with as little as eight per vaccination in the Slee Company's tube virus and twenty-four per vaccination on H. K. Mulford's glycerinated points.[164] One American surgeon celebrated its powers to ensure safe vaccinations: "Now that we have the sterilized glycerinated lymph, it practically always means carelessness in vaccinating or neglect afterward if infection occurs."[165] Physicians considered liquid glycerinated lymph better than dry points that could preserve all sorts of bacteria along with the vaccinia organism. Many physicians and health departments rapidly adopted this new form of vaccine lymph during the 1890s. One practitioner lauded glycerinated lymph. "I did not see a dangerous infection among the thousands of vaccinations made by myself and my assistants at Chicago, and this was not due to any particular antiseptic precautions. . . . I believe thoroughly in glycerinated lymph. The Chicago Health Department has not used anything else for some time. They also require an examination of the lymph by the city bacteriologist. All danger is avoided in the careful use of such virus."[166]

Despite these advantages, however, glycerin worked slowly but surely to eliminate all the organisms it contacted, including the vaccinia virus. The New England Vaccine Company made much of this distinction, asserting that lymph "cannot be sterilized nor purified by any antiseptic agent, without destroying also the life of the active principle of the lymph." It championed the superiority of dry points produced under strict aseptic conditions, accusing competitors of relying on glycerin to purify vaccines composed of crusts known to contain "the debris of broken-down tissue, cell detritus and an admixture of pus."[167] They argued that such vaccines needed glycerin to kill all the extraneous bacteria, but the glycerin ultimately destroyed the vaccinia too and thus produced ineffective vaccinations.

In 1900, the Philadelphia physician W. F. Elgin noted that "of all biological products," vaccine lymph was "one of the most unstable, often becoming inert without any appreciable cause." He pointed out experiments suggesting vaccine virus's vulnerability to temperature extremes. He cited other researchers who found that vaccine lymph did not survive lengthy storage, that even inert points could still contain active extraneous bacteria, that low temperatures did not kill bacteria but only slightly decreased their growth, whereas "hot and especially variable temperatures speedily injure vaccine."[168] Elgin conducted a series of experiments in 1906 that confirmed his earlier suppositions about how summer heat in a physician's office could rapidly render vaccine lymph useless: "The doctor should not carry it around in his vest pocket nor put it in the table drawer in his office; he should not depend on the druggist to supply him in hot weather, but should order direct from the laboratory, and use the virus as soon as possible."[169] Practitioners and druggists probably found it difficult to store vaccine lymph under such stringent conditions consistently in the nineteenth century.

Although manufacturers added it to ensure purity, glycerin by and of itself did not solve the problem of maintaining both a pure *and* a potent vaccine. Release the vaccine too soon, and sore arms and blood poisoning abound. Hold it too long, and the vaccination does not take. Vaccine needed perfect storage conditions to maintain viability until its end date. There was no way to ensure that manufacturers would place their vaccine on the market at the proper time or that physicians would store it properly. Thus one Washington, DC, public health officer declared to his colleagues in 1902 that he "thought too much reliance had been placed on the alleged antiseptic property of glycerin."[170] Another Ohio physician sternly announced to his colleagues at a medical conference: "*I have no use for sterilized lymph.*" Relating his frustrations with vaccinations he performed using "tubes of glycerinized lymph," he asserted, "I did not get a normal result in a single instance." His final verdict: "Gentlemen, it seems to me that, in our desire to spare our patients the discomfort which attends the normal course of the vaccine disease, we are humbugging them, deceiving ourselves, and furnishing ammunition to the antivaccinationists. We vaccinate our patients with this so-called sterilized lymph, assuring them that with this improved form of virus their arms will not be very sore. If we get no results we assure them that they are immune. Later they may take the smallpox; the antivaccinationists point to the case as evidence that vaccination does not protect, and to our patient the argument is conclusive."[171] Such frustration was widespread by 1902. A Cambridge physician told his colleagues that "many physicians still prefer the old unpurified lymph" because of "the difficulty which some have in making it 'take.'"[172] Vaccine producers touted glycerin as a panacea that would cure all of the ills attributed to vaccination, but glycerination of vaccine lymph in and of itself clearly failed to deliver a consistently safe and potent product.

In 1901, M. J. Rosenau, of the United States Hygienic Laboratory, studied glycerinated lymph in various batches of vaccine that he procured on the open market "from reliable pharmacists." His team of bacteriologists found that nearly every producer had sold severely contaminated glycerinated virus in the fall of 1901, leading Rosenau to comment wryly: "No wonder we get sore arms." He concluded that manufacturers and physicians relied too heavily on the power of glycerin to purify the vaccine virus: "We believe the impurities found in the glycerinated virus upon the market are largely due to an over-confidence in the germicidal value of glycerin; operators become careless of contamination, trusting to the glycerin to purify their product. We know glycerin is too feeble in its properties to purify vaccine matter which has initial contamination such as our work indicates." In the pressure to respond to the 1901 outbreaks, many vaccine manufacturers released their product too early, while it was still "green" and filled with extraneous microorganisms. Thus it was not surprising that many people experienced harsh reactions to their vaccinations in the fall of 1901 and winter of 1902. Rosenau regarded glycerin as a poor antiseptic. It killed bacteria slowly, requiring "11 days to kill streptococci, and 20 days to kill diphtheria bacilli." It could not kill microorganisms that existed as spores at all; "in fact, it is a preservative of such infections as tetanus, malignant edema, and the like."[173] Unfortunately it also affected the vaccinia organism; virus treated with glycerin thus had a limited shelf life. Rosenau expanded on this research, publishing a comprehensive report a year later that vindicated glycerinated virus when used at the proper time in its lifespan. Nevertheless, he reiterated his earlier warnings of misplaced confidence in the power of glycerin to purify contaminated vaccine virus.[174]

Physicians in Massachusetts used a number of different vaccines manufactured by private laboratories or farms. Hygienic conditions at these concerns could vary considerably. With no overriding authority to hold these businesses to high standards of preparation or storage, bad or outdated batches inevitably wound up on druggists' shelves. In 1894, Samuel W. Abbott, secretary of the Massachusetts State Board of Health, complained that his department had no way to guarantee high production standards or freshness in the lymph that physicians purchased: "in many cases we know nothing about the mode of obtaining it."[175] Although a state law decreed that "all vaccine institutions in the Commonwealth shall be under the supervision of the state board of health," unfortunately it gave the health department no authority to force producers to comply with its standards.[176] By 1902 vaccine production still remained in the hands of commercial producers despite years of extensive lobbying for state control on the part of health officials and physicians from all over the state. Henry P. Walcott, chairman of the Massachusetts State Board of Health, enumerated how the possibilities for contamination mounted at every step of the process. Firms that looked after profits rather than the public interest could not be trusted. "In the first place, you have got to get a healthy calf; in the next place, you have got to get a set of clean men to do your work; and in the next place, the last place, you have got to remove it absolutely from the temptations of commerce. There must be no temptation whatever to keep a product that is inert or a product that has been improperly prepared. . . . There is no step of the process that can be safely left without constant and accurate supervision."[177] Lacking any outside authority to certify purity and quality, both private physicians and health boards were at the mercy of a chain of producers, middlemen, and advertisers—sometimes with disastrous results for their patients.

Different producers used various methods to obtain lymph. Some used calves, others heifers. Some allowed the animals to cycle through the process just once, others used them many times. Some scraped off the entire scab, crust and lymph together, others were careful to extract only the lymph. A nineteen-year veteran of the Pennsylvania Board of Health complained in 1901 about the differences among the various vaccine producers: "One large and successful producer cleans away the scab and uses only the lymph which oozes from the cleaned surface. He vaccinates the calves with the same material. Another producer says the lymph is absolutely inert, and he uses the scab, in which, he says, the vaccine is all stored. . . . Other producers remove the scab and utilize the soft tissue under the scab, which they scrape off with a spoon. Still others use a peculiar product which is found neither in the scab, the lymph, nor yet in the soft tissues. Now certainly one of these sources must be the correct one, and we should have the matter authoritatively settled."[178] Everyone had an opinion as to which was the best method, but no one had definitive proof. Despite many recent advances in the microscopic understanding of disease organisms, vaccinia and variola viruses remained elusive to microscopic observation. Theobald Smith, a Massachusetts State Board of Health pathologist, believed that ignorance about the nature of the vaccinia and variola at the microscopic level encouraged too many different approaches to vaccine production: "The micro-organisms of variola and vaccinia have not yet been recognized by the microscope, and their presence can be determined only by their effects. This gap in our knowledge is largely responsible for the divergencies in the preparation of vaccine witnessed today."[179] Since no one had yet even seen the vaccinia virus with a microscope, no one could examine a given sample of vaccine to determine its potency. Walcott told a reporter in 1902 that no one could test vaccine lymph for efficacy before use: "There is absolutely nothing in the ivory points to show where the lymph on them comes from. I cannot analyze it to tell whether it is good or bad. If I put it into a man's arm and no harm results I know it is good; if, on the other hand, he has erysipelas, I know it is bad."[180] Individual physicians could not easily determine with any absolute certainty what exactly composed the vaccine they purchased. They had to trust a druggist's or purveyor's assurances as to the freshness or quality of any given batch of vaccine.

By 1902, at least one vaccine company with a national market attempted to parlay these concerns into profits by highlighting its hygienic practices as a marketing strategy. With offices located in Philadelphia, New York, and Chicago, H. K. Mulford advertised that "Mulford's Antitoxins & Vaccines are produced under ideal conditions" in a beautiful, full-color electro-tint engraving featuring cattle on a tranquil farm. Black-and-white photos depicted white-coated technicians in sterile laboratories, cows in stables with nary a dropping in sight, and a sterile operating room for lymph extractions. The H. K. Mulford Company declared that its adherence to "rigid cleanliness—absolute asepsis—confirmatory physiologic tests—thorough equipment—ensure the high standard of Mulford's Preparations."[181] The advertisement also included a color illustration of the benign progress of a vaccination using its vaccine.

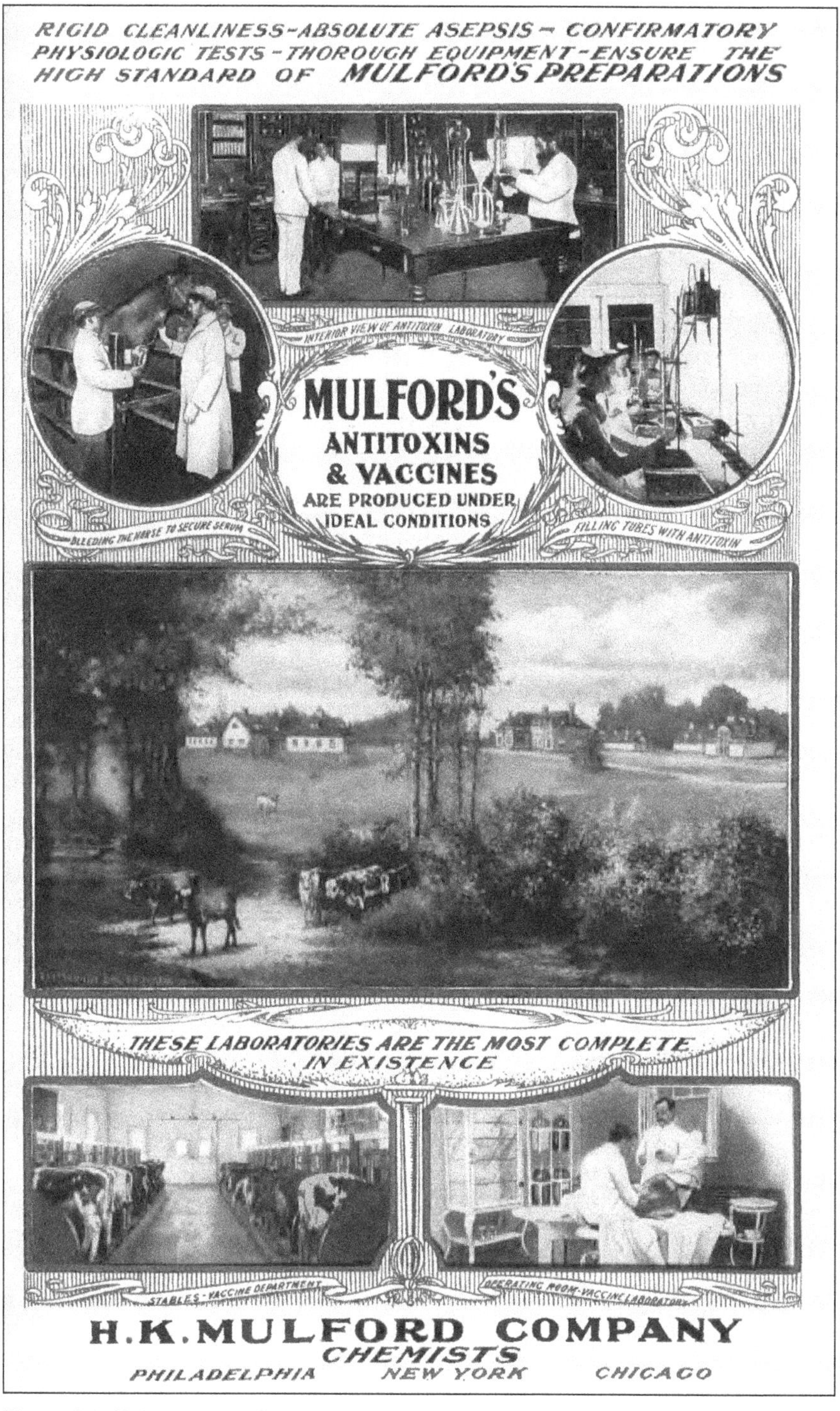

Figure 2.3. H. K. Mulford Company, advertisement. *Cleveland Medical Journal* 1 (1902).

Nevertheless, one *Boston Medical and Surgical Journal* editor observed that commercial competition "occasionally leads producers to unscrupulous methods, not only in the matter of production, but also of advertising their wares." He did not blame commercial vaccine producers entirely: the passage of lymph through many hands contributed substantially to the problem."The physician in general practice, or possibly the agent of a local board of health, obtains his supply of vaccine from a local apothecary, who in turn gets his supply of a wholesale druggist, and he in turn receives it from an agent of some private producer of vaccine. The package of lymph in question is either stamped with a date which represents, not the date of its production, but that of its sale to the final customer; or possibly it is stamped with a date 'Not to be used later than Dec. 25.' The physician uses it on Dec. 10 or 20, and wonders why it fails to 'take.'" Too many practitioners blithely assumed patient insusceptibility from such vaccination failures, he asserted, "not recognizing the fact that the package in question may have been six months old, or may have been subjected to many variable changes of temperature upon the shelves or in the drawers of a local apothecary shop, or in the pockets of a traveling agent." Arguing for government control of the process, he noted how London vaccine stations kept calves on hand from which to draw fresh lymph on the spot.[182]

Physicians were stuck: the individual practitioner, swept up in exigencies of an epidemic, had neither time nor resources to verify the purity and effectiveness of the vaccine he or she purchased. The Toronto health officer Peter Bryce wondered "whether we as users of vaccine, of one form or another, have any guarantee of the honesty and carefulness of the producer."[183] When demand ran high during epidemics, even vaccine producers who tried to maintain high standards found themselves hard pressed to adhere to them. A Texas surgeon warned his colleagues to bear this in mind when selecting vaccine: "If the glycerinated article has not been in the glycerin solution a considerable length of time, pathogenic bacteria or their spores may still be alive and produce unduly severe reaction. This would be more liable to occur when the farms were taxed severely to supply the demand. Then an unreliable firm might send out 'unripe' vaccine."[184] Physicians also were sometimes lax. A St. Paul medical journal pointed out the danger invited by this state of affairs: "The physician who only vaccinates occasionally is too apt to be careless regarding the vaccine which he uses, and the average druggist is not over careful in regard to the vaccine which he dispenses."[185]

The Question of State Control of Vaccine Production

At the turn of the century, as producers vied for their business, physicians debated the merit of various forms of vaccine lymph. Did glycerinated fluid lymph sealed in glass tubes produce fewer ill effects than lymph dried on ivory points? Was a return to humanized lymph a solution to the problem? In a series of papers delivered at the 1900 American Public Health Association meeting, Mexican public health officials argued for humanized lymph, claiming that it conferred permanent immunity against smallpox.[186] One Ohio physician declared at a 1901 American Public Health Association meeting: "Now, if I could always secure good healthy children I would use their virus in preference to much of the virus that we get at the present time. I have used the glycerine tubes for the last few years and get just as many bad sores on the arm as with the points."[187] A few prominent physicians also advocated the use of humanized lymph over glycerinated lymph. Charles Chapin, the great champion of the "new public health," asserted that his Providence, Rhode Island, health department continued to rely on humanized lymph with great success. Providence health authorities had used one strain of humanized lymph since 1856, and kept "careful records of each transfer" since 1868, for a total of 638 transfers. He proudly noted that the Providence lymph still "produces symptoms and a vesicle like those described and figured by Jenner."[188] Joseph N. McCormack also contended that many of the profession's current difficulties with vaccination could be resolved if it would discard glycerinated bovine virus in favor of humanized virus. "After careful observation and a large experience I am convinced that the profession should return to the use of humanized virus, so far as it is possible to do so. This form of virus 'takes' more certainly, produces less local and constitutional disturbance, and appears to give longer and better protection against smallpox. If the virus is obtained from healthy persons known to the physician, no better source for it can be conceived."[189] McCormack believed that business interests rather than the public interest exerted an untoward influence over the profession's vaccination alternatives. By 1902, many medical professionals joined him in his skepticism about continuing to allow commercial interests control over vaccine quality. Editors at the *Journal of the American Medical Association* asserted that government must take some action, even if it meant interfering with private economic interests. "Matters which are of such vital importance to the health of the people are not subjects to be treated carelessly nor only from the viewpoint of commercialism." It declared that "some measures are required to protect the public from improperly prepared vaccine virus," demanding that health authorities inspect vaccine farms and frequently test samples for bacterial content.[190]

Yet in a 1901 study of health departments across the United States, Charles Chapin noted that "in only a few states have state boards of health taken upon themselves to carefully inspect the places where virus is produced, and to test the virus and publish results of their investigations." In 1896, the Pennsylvania State Board of Health "sent a bacteriologist to examine the principal vaccine establishments of the country." Accompanied by a veterinary surgeon, the bacteriologist visited fourteen vaccine producers, making "a most elaborate and complete investigation . . . of the farms and the methods employed, and the condition of the virus produced." Of the total fourteen, he recommended only four. In 1898, Tennessee also sent its inspector to vaccine virus farms in other states—only three achieved a recommendation. The Chicago Board of Health sent its bacteriologist to study "a large number of samples of virus to determine which was most free from extraneous organisms" in 1895. He selected just one as "considerably superior to others."[191] Thus vaccine quality and purity differed enormously among the late-nineteenth-century commercial vaccine establishments, and health departments could do little to rectify these problems other than to recommend one brand over the others.

A 1902 American Public Health Association report on vaccine quality acknowledged that "no practical scheme can be adopted by a state or provincial board of health, under existing legislation, for the supervision of lymph to be used within its jurisdiction." Health departments depended on voluntary efforts of vaccine firms to certify at their own expense "that all lymph sent to such state or province had been tested."[192] In Massachusetts, for instance, state law since 1894 placed all vaccine institutions under the supervision of the state board of health, but in the estimation of Charles Chapin that law had "little value as no penalties are attached."[193] The Board of Health could inspect the premises of vaccine producers in Massachusetts, but it lacked authority to do anything about a purveyor of bad vaccine. And it had no power whatsoever over vaccine it purchased from establishments in other states.

Given the enormous authority each state possessed under its police power to interfere with private enterprise and property to protect public safety, health, welfare, and morality, it seems odd that state legislatures hesitated to strictly regulate the vaccine industry as it developed in the late nineteenth century. George Dock complained about this situation in 1904: "If the general government can furnish pure seed to farmers, and the separate States regulate the sale of oleomargarine, the inspection of oil, etc., or the sale of alcoholics and tobacco, vaccine could easily be put under the public control, provided of course, that the wishes of the people were not thwarted by the unseen but powerful influence of lobbies supported by those who prefer to keep the industry in their own hands."[194] William J. Novak has documented amply the extent to which states legislated on matters of public health and morality with "a plethora of bylaws, ordinances, statutes, and common law restrictions regulating nearly every aspect of early American economy and society, from Sunday observance to the carting of offal."[195] His study ends, however, in 1877, just as the vaccine industry began to develop, as a new idea about government regulation—that of laissez-faire—began to preoccupy American politics and law. As industries like railroads, steel mills, mining, and all sorts of manufacturing concerns grew into giant national corporations in the late nineteenth century, they became a weighty political and financial presence that challenged traditional notions about the propriety of governmental regulation of business. Many cases that reached the United States Supreme Court during this period revolved around the issue of the proper extent of a state's police power to regulate businesses in terms of the Fourteenth Amendment to the federal Constitution. Like other growing industries, vaccine producers also resisted governmental interference with their businesses, unless it suited their individual interests. Larger concerns often supported state regulation if it meant that their smaller rivals would suffer in the process. Big vaccine companies like H. K. Mulford boasted of their strict adherence to the highest technical standards of aseptic cleanliness—standards that smaller operations were hard-pressed to maintain. Thus it tended to support the idea of state and federal regulation.

In 1901 a number of children died from tetanus acquired either after vaccination or inoculation with diphtheria antitoxin in cities in the Midwest and on the East Coast.[196] Although vaccine companies, health officials, physicians, and scientists debated whether or not the vaccine was contaminated, these tragic incidents pushed the idea of federal regulation of vaccine and serum production to the forefront of the nation's political consciousness. In 1902, Congress passed the Biologics Control Act to give the hygienic laboratory of the renamed Public Health and Marine Hospital Service the power to inspect and license vaccine producers.[197]

As Congress deliberated over federal regulation of the vaccine industry in 1901 and 1902, public health officials in Massachusetts sought to resolve their problems by establishing a long-desired state-run vaccine farm. Their campaign struck a nerve in the vaccine and drug industry, which had some very effective lobbyists in the late nineteenth century and a long history of successfully blocking all attempts to bring vaccine production under state supervision.[198] In Boston, for instance, the druggist Henry Canning paid a lobbyist "$1,685.25 in services and expenses in opposing the bill authorizing the State Board of Health to manufacture antitoxin and vaccine virus" in 1902.[199] Canning explained to a local newspaper that vaccines were no different than any other foodstuff or drugs. "Supplying milk, running milk farms, manufacturing ice, constructing ice factories, the establishment of a great laboratory for the production of pure bread, the production of pure flour, the production of drugs and medicines, quinine, and every other drug or medicine which the people need, would be no whit different from the manufacture and distribution of vaccine lymph."[200] Thus state manufacture of vaccine lymph amounted simply to socialism in his view. Even the state health department chairman Walcott demonstrated sensitivity to such concerns when he explained why the state made and distributed antitoxin for free, but not vaccine lymph. "In diphtheria you are dealing with a product which commands a price beyond the possibilities of purchase by the ordinary laboring man. . . . He has got to procure it free of charge from some one, and it is for the benefit of the whole community that he should procure it as soon as possible. By the lives so saved the whole of us are benefited and protected. For that simple reason the Board of Health has never had any question that it was performing a very simple part of its duty in manufacturing this article and distributing it as widely as possible through the agencies of the boards of health throughout the Commonwealth."[201] Walcott saw antitoxin more as a matter of charity performed for the public good than an undue interference in business. Antitoxin additionally was a relatively new product, introduced only in 1894. Commercial interests had not yet invested in production facilities to the degree they had in vaccine lymph, where some private farms had done business for over thirty years by 1902.

Yet in Massachusetts, public health officials and many physicians realized that until government authority could certify and control vaccine purity, suspicion and resistance to vaccination would surely grow. The irony of compelling vaccination without any assurance of control over purity and efficacy was not lost on these physicians and public health officers. The 1901 State Board of Health report noted that supplying vaccine lymph through "agents, middlemen, or wholesale dealers" led to "invariable delays," which allowed "the product to become more or less inert and finally absolutely worthless." It complained that "*the date when the lymph was produced is not made known to the purchaser.* This practice furnishes an opportunity for fraud."[202] Theobald Smith declared: "The State insists upon vaccinal protection, and justly so; but under existing conditions it can do little or nothing towards assuming any responsibility for the quality of the vaccine used."[203] Another physician, A. E. Miller of Needham, Massachusetts, complained at a 1902 meeting of public health officers: "We have a law that compels—at least, that is being tested somewhat now—people to be vaccinated; and these people, if they are compelled to be vaccinated, ought to know that they are to be vaccinated with something that is furnished by the State Board, and is the purest article that can possibly be had."[204] Even worse, many now questioned the efficacy of vaccine lymph available to them in 1901–2. One Cambridge resident lambasted that city's board of health for using ineffective lymph in its vaccination campaign. "If it becomes necessary for the board of health to send out another army of vaccination doctors, perhaps it will see that the same doctors are supplied with the best of vaccine virus, and not the second-hand stuff they have been using during the last scare. Buy from reliable people; see that you get the right goods and your vaccination crusade will be a success and a blessing, and 19 out of 20 cases will be effectual. As it is under present regime, two cases took out of 50."[205] The North Cambridge physician Edmond H. Stevens told colleagues that he had extremely disappointing results from vaccine points purchased during the summer of 1902: "In not one instance have I had a successful vaccination."[206]

Such concerns led the Boston health department chairman Samuel Durgin to petition the Massachusetts state legislature for funds to establish a state vaccine farm, taking the lead from state public health officials like Henry Walcott, who hesitated because he worried about unduly interfering with private enterprise.[207] Yet the Public Health Committee stalled the bill, putting it off for the next session. At a meeting with other Massachusetts public health officials, Durgin blamed his failure on "four or five" druggists sitting on the eleven-member committee who continually thwarted his attempts to get state funding for vaccine production.[208] Even the discovery of a cow "far gone with tuberculosis" that "had furnished nobody knows how many hundreds of vaccine points used for vaccine lymph" did little to sway the committee, provoking one newspaper editor to wonder "why the state vaccine bill is to be killed at the secret order of the druggists."[209] Durgin did not give up, continuing his advocacy to convince legislators to finally authorize state lymph production in 1903 despite the opposition of "a corps of agents" working for vaccine producers.[210]

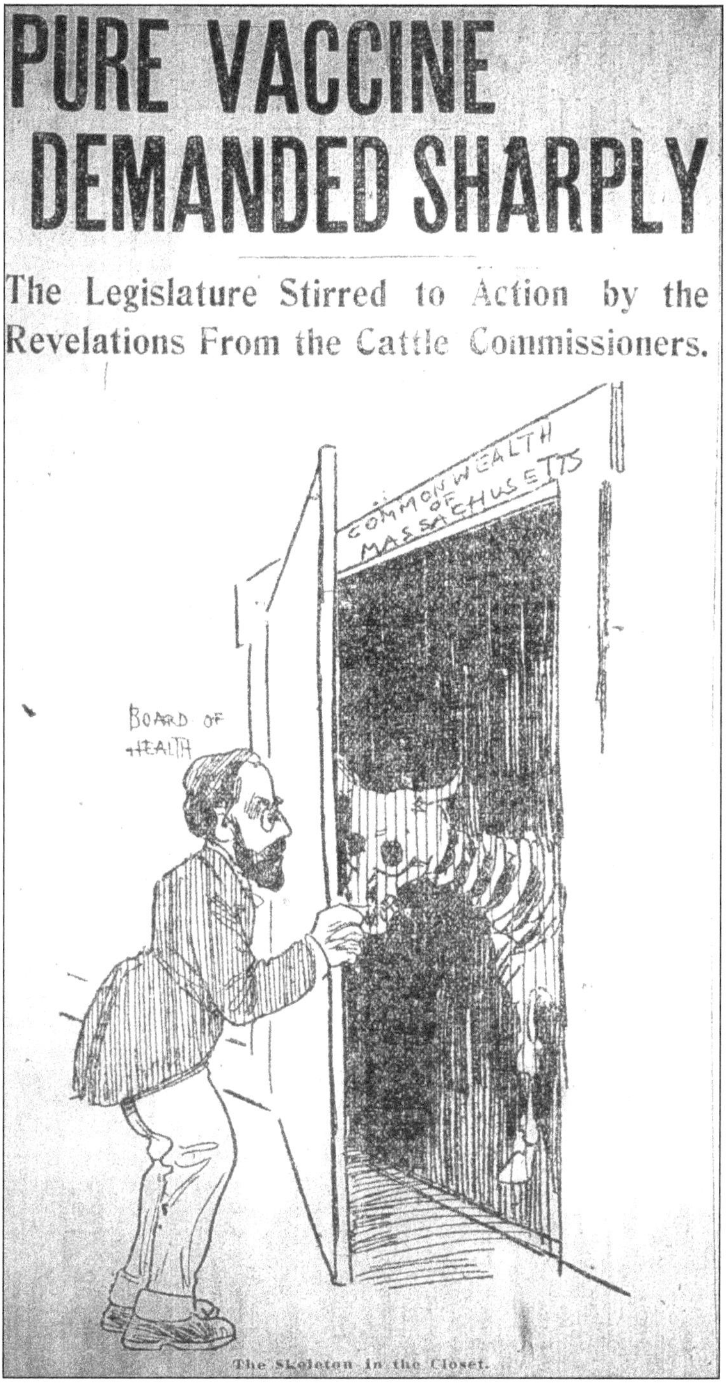
PURE VACCINE DEMANDED SHARPLY

The Legislature Stirred to Action by the Revelations From the Cattle Commissioners.

Figure 2.4. Cartoon referring to tuberculosis in vaccine-farm cows. *Boston Evening Record*, 26 April 1902, 1.

For all the good intentions of public health officials like Samuel Durgin, who saw this legislation as "quieting the fears of our people," his campaign for a state-run vaccine facility might have had the unintended consequence of raising suspicions about the purity of the commercially produced vaccine used by his department.[211] That is exactly what happened as smallpox cases began to mount in 1901 and 1902 in Boston and Cambridge. When local health authorities emphasized vaccination as the bulwark of their control strategy, public anxiety about it led many citizens to avoid or even refuse it.

By the turn of the century, vaccination had been used to prevent smallpox for over one hundred years and vaccine production had become a major industry. But the history of this "boon to humanity" is complicated by the American devotion to free enterprise. Boston health department officials tread cautiously in the area of offering free vaccinations for fear of impinging on private medical practices. Development of untoward effects after vaccination encouraged technological innovations that in turn created a commercial opportunity to make a lot of money from vaccine production. Yet each change in production methods designed to resolve one problem only led to others. By the late nineteenth century, as public health took on the trappings of a profession that manifested objectivity and scientific expertise rather than political cronyism, the new profession led the call for state regulation that could assure vaccine quality. Progressive-era public health professionals who sought to exert their scientific expertise to promote state control of vaccine production ran right up against the burgeoning free market in biologic and pharmaceutical products. Even physicians who supported vaccination quarreled about its safety and effectiveness. And vaccination had a history of transmitting disease and infections that did not instill much confidence. People faced with laws that compelled vaccination with no guarantee of its safety were stuck in the middle. What could they do?

Chapter Three

The 1901–2 Smallpox Epidemic in Boston and Cambridge

By December 1901 smallpox had settled into Boston, eluding health department efforts to control its spread. The health department chairman Samuel Durgin tried to alleviate public anxiety by referring to the epidemic as a "flurry of small-pox," as if it were no more than a minor snowstorm that would soon pass. Yet he had to admit that this epidemic presented a unique challenge: "The prevalence of the disease is not subsiding and is not likely to for a while yet. People are not yet sufficiently vaccinated. The ambulant and unrecognized cases are spread-ing the disease, and have been doing it to an extent which has never before obtained in my experience." Additionally, ignorance of the need to revaccinate only worsened the situation. Too many people and their physicians assumed that a primary vaccination early in life would provide adequate protection many years later. Although he might have blamed himself and his own department for failing to promote vaccination sufficiently, he chose instead to direct the blame more amorphously: "With regard to Boston, I am sorry to say that she has been caught in a poorly-vaccinated condition. We went through the city in the win-ter of 1872 and 1873 and gave thorough vaccination. Since that time we have experienced an unusual freedom from smallpox, much indifference and some misguided objection to vaccination, and are, in consequence, easy victims to smallpox." As the memory of smallpox receded over time, Boston residents had forgotten about the need for vaccination. Durgin also blamed this avoidance of vaccination on Boston's antivaccinationists. In his view, they frightened people with their pamphlets and lectures, "trying to prejudice the public mind against vaccination."[1] By directing attention away from himself and his department, Durgin displayed the deft hand of a seasoned veteran of municipal politics. He understood that this epidemic's stubborn persistence would attract criticism of his performance as a public health leader, but he knew how to weather such storms after a nearly thirty-year career in Boston's tumultuous civic affairs.

In 1901, Durgin was sixty-two years old and nationally acknowledged as a lead-ing public health officer. He possessed impeccable academic and social creden-tials. Born in Maine to a farming family that could trace its ancestry back to the colonial period, he attended first Dartmouth College and then Harvard Medical School. Upon graduation in 1864, he joined the Union army as an assistant surgeon in the First Massachusetts Calvary. Serving at the front in Petersburg and Richmond, he was present at Appomattox Court House for the surrender of Robert E. Lee. After the war, he practiced medicine in Boston's West End until he landed a job as port physician in 1867.

At the time, the Health Committee of Boston's City Council administered all of the city's health regulations. The severe smallpox epidemic of 1872, however, exposed the committee's inability to deal adequately with the crisis, as well as many other sanitary issues.[2] Only the port physician Durgin, "generally lauded for the care which he gave to the smallpox patients at Gallop's Island," continued to stand high in public esteem as pressure mounted for reform of Boston's public health system.[3] Recognizing his efforts and medical expertise, Boston's aldermen appointed him to a newly formed independent board of health in 1873.

Joined by an attorney and a retired businessman, Durgin immediately stood out as the only medical professional on the board. In 1876, Mayor Frederick O. Prince appointed him its chairman.[4] To the mayor's dismay, Durgin refused to give political cronies health department sinecures, preferring instead merit-based hires. Although the mayor attempted to oust him, the Boston medical establishment came out in full force to support his continued tenure, urging medical men to vote against Prince in the next election. Mayor Prince lost that election, while Durgin, clearly the popular choice of elite Boston physicians, remained chairman until his retirement in 1912.[5]

During his tenure as Boston's chief health officer, Samuel Durgin attained national prominence as a leader in public health. Writing just a few years after Durgin's retirement, one commentator remarked that "Dr. Durgin's influence was much wider than his own city," that Durgin's "high scientific attainments and his successful public health administration gave him a national reputation."[6] As his initial differences with Boston's Mayor Prince indicate, he insisted on running his department as a nonpartisan independent bureaucracy, an innovation in municipal government at a time when most city departments routinely hired on the basis of political favoritism. Durgin also advocated the "new public health," which incorporated germ theory into public health practice, redirecting health department efforts away from general environmental sanitation to a bacteriological understanding of disease transmission that emphasized controlling individuals as carriers of disease.[7] Charles V. Chapin, an iconic new public health leader, hailed him as one of the "best sanitary officials" in the United States.[8] In every way, Durgin represented the ideal Progressive-era health officer, an incorruptible medical expert who ran his department according to the best science of the day.

A member of the upper echelon of Boston society, Durgin was the fourth highest paid health officer in the United States.[9] He resided in the socially distinguished Back Bay district, an area of Boston noted for "broad thoroughfares and imposing architecture" and for its beautiful public garden, "the gem of the city parks."[10] Durgin and his wife, Mary Bradford Davis, had two children; she attended Trinity Church on Copley Square, an Episcopalian cathedral described as "the finest church edifice in New England," whose parish was "exceedingly wealthy."[11] In 1885 he joined the Harvard Medical School faculty as a lecturer on hygiene, a prestigious position that he held for many years. He was also an active member of the American Public Health Association, the Massachusetts Medical Society, the Boston Society for Medical Improvement, and the Joseph Webb Lodge of Masons—groups that counted among their members many prominent practitioners and citizens.[12] In 1890, he helped create the Massachusetts Association of Boards of Health. Serving as its vice president for many years, he ran the organization and built it into a distinguished association of health officials. By the turn of the century, it had grown into a national public health organization, boasting a membership of leaders in the "new public health" from many states and cities.[13] The Association's journal acquired a national reputation for the quality of its reports and papers; in 1911 it became the official organ of the American Public Health Association.[14]

Durgin managed to survive hostile mayors and partisan politics to direct successfully one of the first truly independent boards of health in a major American city for thirty-six years. Intimately involved in running the Massachusetts Association of Boards of Health and editing its journal, he was aware of his stature among his peers and took pains to maintain it. In 1940, Charles-Edward A. Winslow recalled Durgin's consciousness of his authority at annual meetings of the Association. "Durgin, however, scarcely missed a meeting and was the usual presiding officer. He was small, prim and precise, with a curious trick of rocking up and down slightly on the balls of his feet. He was a trifle pompous, with a keen sense of the importance of his position in the community and, though known as 'Sammy' in third-party conversation, no one took any liberties with Dr. Durgin to his face."[15] Durgin took his power and responsibilities as Boston's chief health officer seriously, and he happily reminded everyone of their extent. At a legislative hearing on an antivaccination bill, he responded to a heckler who had challenged his decision to release a ship early from quarantine: "I hold the public health of Boston in one hand and its commerce in the other."[16] He clearly saw his duties as crucial to the life of the city, and he wielded his authority with confidence.

By 1902 Durgin was a self-assured veteran of Boston politics and a respected public health expert. During his tenure, he had watched his city double in population to become a metropolis of over half a million. He had built his department up from scratch into an exemplary city health agency. As Boston's port physician from 1867 to 1873, he had witnessed the devastation one severe smallpox epidemic wrought on a poorly vaccinated population in 1872. He had a national reputation as an effective public health official to uphold. As the first smallpox cases began to show up in the summer of 1901, Durgin acted with confidence in his department's ability to contain an epidemic. Despite many setbacks and some criticism in the months to come, he never once wavered in his conviction that he had pursued the correct strategy to control the epidemic.

Boston and Cambridge in 1901

By 1901, Boston had expanded considerably beyond its original boundaries. In the last half of the nineteenth century, Boston changed from a tidy city of merchants to a great sprawling manufacturing metropolis. As factories and other businesses sought space for their physical plants, the city pushed further outward into the countryside and nearby villages. From 1870 to 1900, successive waves of immigration, economic boom and bust, and the development of a streetcar and subway system encouraged people and businesses to move from the original city to surrounding villages and finally into the outermost suburbs. In this process, many affluent long-settled residents fled cramped inner districts for roomy suburban living, ringing the original town in distinct districts representing successive layers of socioeconomic status. Their former homes became lodging houses crammed with roomers in the South End and West End. Some of the districts adjacent to the core of Boston, like Back Bay and Beacon Hill, remained wealthy enclaves, but other inner sections, like Roxbury, East Boston, South Boston, inner Dorchester, and Charlestown, were now inhabited mostly by working families rising out of poverty to lower-middle-class life. By 1900, the socially ambitious, well-to-do families had moved to outer suburbs like Hyde Park, Newton, West Roxbury, and Milton. Boston became "an inner city of work and low income housing, and an outer city of middle- and upper-income residences." A network of streetcars and railroads connecting the outlying suburbs to the inner districts allowed Boston to grow from a city bound by a two-mile radius (the limits of a pedestrian city) to an industrial and suburban metropolis radiating ten miles out from the original center.[17]

Cambridge also expanded into districts radiating from the town originally settled around Harvard University in the 1630s. Cambridgeport and East Cambridge, on the tidal flats of the Charles River, grew as industrial suburbs of Boston in the nineteenth century with that city's rise as a manufacturing center. By 1901, Cambridgeport contained half the total population of Cambridge and served both as a residential and an industrial suburb. Most of its residents were semi-skilled workers, clerks, and small tradespeople, with a smattering of professionals and domestic workers—in short, "a stronghold of the great and powerful social grouping known as the 'middle class,'" according to a social analysis written around 1907.[18]

Although smallpox cropped up all over greater Boston and Cambridge in 1901 and 1902, most of the cases occurred in Roxbury, East Boston, South Boston, Dorchester, East Cambridge, and Cambridgeport. Known at the time for their concentrations of first- and second-generation immigrants, in these districts families struggled to rise from poverty to middle-class life. Social theorists of the time referred to these areas as the "zone of emergence," and they were the subject of much study and comment in the early twentieth century. Tenements, lodging houses, and duplexes prevailed in these sections, but they also contained some single-family homes and cottages. Evoking "the atmosphere of small separate cities . . . with their own banks, department stores, small shops," each district had its own distinctive character.[19] Irish Catholic politicians dominated East Boston, South Boston, and Roxbury, whereas middle-class Protestant politicians ran Dorchester and Cambridgeport.

The Boston Smallpox Epidemic

Smallpox first appeared in Boston in May 1901 among the employees of a large factory. The Board of Health responded promptly to find and isolate all the cases within forty-eight hours. The health department physician Thomas B. Shea later bragged that smallpox "has not been a very great surprise to us. It was foreseen and prepared for by officials in our department."[20] When other outbreaks occurred in the city over the course of that summer, "all known cases were quickly picked up . . . and all necessary precautions put in use."[21] As cases cropped up, the Board of Health removed the afflicted to a detention house, vaccinated the people living in the surrounding neighborhood, and placed contacts of the patients under medical observation for about two weeks. This approach was somewhat novel at the time. Many other communities in Massachusetts and other states usually established quarantines at the homes of smallpox patients, marking them with a red flag and posting police to guard every exit from the premises at considerable cost. Yet in Boston, economics seemed to dictate another course: "Boston health authorities reason that almost equally good results may be obtained without incurring such enormous expenses, as there is absolutely no possibility for the disease to spread from one person to another before it has caused symptoms to appear on the skin, and every patient will be severely ill with headache and backache about three days before there is any eruption whatever."[22] The onset of these symptoms theoretically provided a three-day window of opportunity to isolate a smallpox case and vaccinate contacts. Thus the health department could utilize vaccination and observation as a cheaper, less restrictive method than quarantine to contain outbreaks. Health department physicians visited persons who had been exposed to smallpox "every day, or every second day, until the period of incubation has passed." Durgin assured a nervous public that even though such exposed individuals moved freely about the city, "the board keeps track of such persons during these days of observation and detains them as soon as they begin to feel the headache."[23] Such was his confidence in the health department physicians' diagnostic acumen that he believed they could catch every case before the three-day window expired.

Throughout the summer of 1901, the health department deliberately kept a low profile about the smallpox outbreaks, "for the purpose of preventing an unwarranted scare among the residents of the localities in which the cases were discovered."[24] That policy was probably wise, for residents could not obtain free vaccinations from the city during July and August anyway, since the vaccination office was closed for that period.[25] From the health department's perspective, as long as it could contain the outbreaks with prompt isolation and vaccination of the exposed, unnecessary publicity would only hinder rather than help them.

News reports of the first tragic death of a smallpox victim changed that policy overnight. On 18 August, a Sunday afternoon, a desperate father sought medical care for his sick infant, pushing his baby "along the public thoroughfares from his home to the City Hospital in a baby carriage." Although the father (identified just by his surname, McKenna) "did not know the nature of the child's disease," Boston City Hospital physicians realized immediately that the baby had smallpox. They hustled the child into an ambulance to the Swett Street detention house, but the baby never made it, dying en route. Health department authorities discovered to their chagrin that the parents first had taken their baby to a dispensary where physicians had diagnosed the infant's illness as measles. The ramifications of this fact were not lost on a reporter who cautioned that "hundreds of people were undoubtedly exposed to the danger of catching the disease" in the course of the McKenna baby's trips in search of medical care.[26]

Health officials then moved swiftly to isolate the rest of the McKenna family—father, mother, a twenty-month-old girl, and a four-year-old boy—on Gallop's Island, the city's quarantine station. They also vaccinated about eight hundred persons who lived near the McKennas. Although the board of health initially reassured the public that "no spread of the disease is feared," new cases soon appeared in Roxbury, where the McKennas resided. Worse, not all of these cases traced back to the McKennas. The Boston health department now had no idea from whom the cases had spread, and it now openly urged "all persons who have not been vaccinated, especially those living in the vicinity of Cabot street, to be vaccinated at once." Although the health department still emphasized vaccination of known contacts, by advising general vaccination now it sent the message that smallpox threatened to spill out into other areas of Boston. Hoping to reach more people, the health department set up a free vaccination clinic at the Hammond Street Schoolhouse in Roxbury open to all comers during evening hours of six to nine for the convenience of working people. So popular was the clinic that it averaged four hundred vaccinations per night in its first week, with nearly six hundred attending on the evening of 5 September.[27]

As the number of cases increased, Roxbury residents became increasingly anxious that the board had not done enough to suppress the epidemic. Two called on Durgin to register their complaints. Representative James A. Watson of Ward 18 protested "that strenuous methods be resorted to, with a departure from the present system." He complained that dispensary physicians had misdiagnosed many smallpox cases as measles, allowing the patients to leave and mingle with the general public. Most disturbing in his view, the health department had neither disinfected nor quarantined the dispensaries. Watson thought it scandalous that though they had been exposed to smallpox, "the physicians in charge were going in and out, and treating other patients steadily." Durgin tried to distance his department from these dispensaries, calling them "fake" because they were privately owned businesses as opposed to those run as charities.[28] Physicians who staffed commercial dispensaries usually lacked the social connections and academic background necessary to obtain prestigious appointments at volunteer (charitable) hospitals and dispensaries. Durgin probably felt safe insinuating they had less medical expertise. Representative Watson wanted the health department to quarantine smallpox contacts rather than simply observe them. When he challenged Durgin's handling of the epidemic, he gave voice to a common skepticism of the health department's ability to track and isolate exposed people before they could infect others. Durgin assured Watson that his department removed the sick and disinfected routinely, "without any delay," but he still insisted that immediate vaccination of contacts rather than quarantine was the most effective way to control smallpox.

Watson also wanted the schools closed "until smallpox had been stamped out," a sentiment echoed by another caller, A. P. Frederickson, a Roxbury landlord. Durgin worried about the threat unvaccinated persons, especially children, posed to the city, but he did not think that closing the schools would resolve the problem. It did not help that a 1901 inspection found one in fifteen Boston schoolchildren had never been vaccinated, despite ordinances requiring vaccination for admission.[29] Even those already vaccinated might be susceptible if their immunity had lapsed since their last vaccination. Durgin, however, asserted that school should remain open because there physicians "could more easily ascertain just what school children have been vaccinated." Frederickson disagreed, telling him that "people were very much alarmed at the situation, and were fearful that if the children went to school, they would be infected." He planned on keeping his own daughter at home for the duration.[30] Unimpressed by Durgin's tactics, eighteen local physicians and 265 parents signed a petition asking for school closures. The superintendent of schools, Edwin P. Seaver, ignored Durgin and temporarily closed five schools in the vicinity.[31]

Given the level of knowledge about smallpox at the time, citizens' protests were not unreasonable. A South Framingham physician, L. M. Palmer, complained at a July 1902 meeting of public health officials: "I think we don't know absolutely yet where small-pox comes from or how far it may be carried. We know only in a measure."[32] Even the *Evening Transcript* commented on the lack of scientific certainty about smallpox. "No bacterial study of the disease is being made at any of the local laboratories, largely because of the difficulty which all bacteriologists have experienced in their efforts to determine the etiology of this malady. While they all seem to agree that it is caused by an organism, no one has thus far been able to isolate that creature and say whether it is an animal or a vegetable organism of the bacteria breed."[33] From the perspective of a public that had come to admire and depend on laboratory science as the highest source of medical knowledge about infectious diseases, such news proved unsettling. If medical experts could not see or experiment on smallpox germs, how could the public trust their judgment? In a way, critics of the health department's policies simply turned the much vaunted achievements of microbiology on their head by calling into question the board of health's preference for vaccination over other sanitary measures when there was not a shred of evidence derived from laboratory observation to back it up. Granted, the health officers proffered statistics that showed how effectively vaccination controlled smallpox outbreaks, but those statistics were also the source of much contention between pro and antivaccinationists.

Not all physicians and health officials shared the Boston Board of Health's acclaim for vaccination "as the best of all the means for combating this disease and preventing its further spread."[34] Some physicians and boards of health in other towns, not trusting vaccination alone, took elaborate precautions to prevent the transmission of smallpox after they had visited a smallpox victim. One newspaper described the routine followed by the physician P. F. Gahan when he visited Miranda Mason, an eighteen-year-old Nova Scotian, currently the sole occupant of Medford's drafty, bat-infested pesthouse. "On each of these visits, Dr. Gahan steps into an outhouse, near the pest house, and changes all his clothes. Then he goes in to see the patient. Coming out, he strips in the outhouse, bathes in an antiseptic wash, puts on his street clothes, leaving the pest house suit behind, and drives home. He has given up his private practice and is virtually in quarantine at his house, although not actually so."[35] Such a lack of confidence in the power of vaccination from a medical man must have made more than a few people nervous about the Boston health department's methods of epidemic control. At least one eminent Boston practitioner worried that vaccination alone might not prevent the transmission of smallpox. The president of the Massachusetts Medical Society, Dr. Francis Draper, admitted that after visiting a smallpox patient, "he would take a long walk in the open air and change his clothing before going among persons." Although Draper added that he knew of no case where a person not ill with smallpox had transmitted it to a third party, he still recommended such measures "in the interest of safety and precaution."[36]

Public health officials in other states did not consider such precautions at all excessive, but instead simply a responsible approach to infectious disease. Durgin had faced his peers' wrath a few years previously in this matter when he proclaimed at an American Public Health Association meeting that the clothing of a well person was "a very small factor" in the transmission of smallpox.[37] One Minnesota health officer countered Durgin's assertion by decrying the habit of too easily trusting in vaccination alone to prevent the transmission of smallpox: "The way some physicians go about amongst infectious diseases, without taking proper precautions, is a disgrace to the medical profession. . . . Many of us can cite instances in which physicians have undoubtedly conveyed the germs of contagious or infectious diseases to healthy people."[38] These physicians were not clinging to old-fashioned notions about disease transmission: a recent medical textbook warned that smallpox "clings to articles of furniture or of dress, which in this way become fomites or carriers of infection. It may be conveyed through the medium of a person not himself ill of it."[39]

During a 1902 legislative hearing on vaccination, the Harvard professor and physician Reginald H. Fitz shocked the audience with his casual disdain for public safety, remarking that the only safeguard he undertook after visiting a smallpox patient was to "walk a long distance in the open air." When his appalled interrogators asked whether he posed a threat to people he might then meet on the streets, he declared, "I walk through unfrequented streets and so don't meet many."[40] Fitz sincerely believed that vaccination rendered his person immune to smallpox and thus incapable of transmitting it to others.

Thomas B. Shea, chief medical officer of the Boston Board of Health, likewise admitted that he had traveled in "a crowded railroad car after attending a case of smallpox without a change of clothing." When asked "if he was not a menace to the people in the train?" Shea retorted that "he did not think it possible for a third person to carry smallpox." Yet when quizzed further about whether he would allow others "to leave the house as you did, without taking any precautions to protect the people," Shea declared, "No, sir: I would not. The Board of Health has confidence in its physicians and does not think they need to take the same precautions as are required of others."[41]

Although these physicians believed that a vaccinated person could not transmit the disease by carrying the germs on his or her person, other medical authorities and public opinion differed. Many more believed that physicians ought to carry out at least a modicum of disinfection prior to going out among the general populace. Shea's indifference to public anxiety about contagion provoked his skeptical audience to react "with shouts of derisive laughter."[42] The idea that health department physicians somehow possessed an innate ability to stop the transmission of germs without taking any steps to clean themselves or their clothing simply offended common sense. Health department officials might have faith that vaccination alone would stop smallpox transmission, but the general public and other physicians did not necessarily share it.

At least one elected official questioned the wisdom of relying so heavily on vaccination. In Cambridge, Mayor John H. H. McNamee personally confronted his health board, complaining "that they have neither quarantined houses where smallpox cases have been found, nor taken other means to warn citizens of the danger of going to such houses."[43] Even the State Board of Health agreed that the Cambridge health department quarantine protocol lacked sufficient rigor.[44] An editorial congratulating the mayor indicated public support for a return to strict quarantine practices. "There are strong differences of opinion regarding the best methods of dealing with the disease. Some have insisted that when a smallpox patient is taken from a house, it should be quarantined, with all its inmates . . . the mayor will try to secure an adoption of the quarantine plan, and in this he will have the support of conservative citizens. It may not be necessary to go thus far, but in such an emergency it is better to err by doing too much than by doing too little. Public sentiment favors extreme measures for the protection of the people."[45] Despite this pressure from the mayor, the newspaper, and many citizens, Cambridge Board of Health Chairman E. Edwin Spencer persisted in allowing exposed persons their freedom after vaccination.[46]

Other Massachusetts towns remained unconvinced that vaccination and isolation of the sick alone would suffice. Salem continued to quarantine people who had been exposed to smallpox cases, even when a two-week quarantine of eighty people severely stretched the town's budget.[47] The Wakefield Board of Health vaccinated but then quarantined for two weeks ten people who had lived in the same rooming house as a smallpox victim.[48] Malden quarantined the mother and sister of a man who had died from "smallpox in the most malignant form."[49] When the notorious antivaccinationist Dr. Immanuel Pfeiffer fell ill with smallpox in Bedford, the town selectmen quarantined the entire household for the duration of his illness even though everyone submitted immediately to vaccination.[50] Many Massachusetts towns and villages apparently felt more comfortable with sticking to traditional measures of smallpox control. One newspaper noted how their response differed from that of the Boston health department. "In other Massachusetts cities quarantine regulations are established at the house where smallpox is discovered. The house itself is usually designated by a red flag placed in front of it, with police officers detailed at every exit to prevent the people inside from coming out, as well as to warn outsiders from going in. Such regulations are maintained for about a fortnight at considerable expense to the community."[51] Traditional public health measures like the closure of public schools, fumigation, and quarantine seemed more certain to many physicians and public officials to limit the spread of smallpox. It seemed foolish to discard them, especially when so many of the smallpox cases seemed to show up in vaccinated persons, albeit in people vaccinated some time ago. For instance, when the Newton Board of Health abandoned quarantine, "the board was blamed somewhat when the public learned that the quarantine of suspects had been discontinued."[52]

Public health officials discussing various containment strategies at a professional meeting in early 1902 revealed some significant differences over the propriety of quarantine. One experienced public health officer cautioned that the vagaries by which smallpox traveled from person to person created quite a quandary. Gardner T. Swartz of the vaunted Providence, Rhode Island, health department warned his colleagues that people who had been exposed to a smallpox patient in the process of desquamation (the shedding of dried up pustules) "should be quarantined, no matter if they are vaccinated, until the vaccination takes in a thorough way or until the fourteen days are past."[53] Yet other Massachusetts health authorities disagreed. James C. Coffey of the Worcester Board of Health declared that his city merely vaccinated "everybody who has been exposed" and then relied on daily visits from a medical inspector for a two-week period to ensure that no one had fallen ill. "That is all. We don't lock anybody up. We don't put any policeman at the door. We let them go and come." Coffey acknowledged that this approach "has got to be, of course, modified by circumstances." "It may be that you would have a case of small-pox among a lot of Italian laborers, upon whom you could not depend. Then, of course, you would have to adopt different methods. But, as a rule, among the settled persons in the community, you will find—or at least we have found—that the method is efficacious; and we have had no difficulty in stamping out the disease."[54] The question of quarantine and vaccination thus involved social, economic, and cultural considerations. Health authorities recommended quarantine for immigrants or itinerant workers, but allowed "the settled persons in the community" their freedom.

Seen in this light, we could interpret the decision to rely solely on vaccination as a sign of a more tolerant, open attitude toward those individuals otherwise marginalized as untrustworthy because they were nonwhite, poor, foreign born, or uneducated. Indeed, many leading physicians of the Boston medical establishment overwhelmingly supported vaccination over sanitation and quarantine. Later in 1902, at another meeting of public health officials, one of Durgin's colleagues asked about his approach to smallpox as compared with other Massachusetts towns. He replied bluntly, "We don't quarantine families for smallpox in Boston." Yet in Boston, which contained the overwhelming majority of smallpox cases, financial considerations probably weighed just as heavily on health officials' minds. James Coffey rose to support Durgin: "We do as they do in Boston. . . . There is no expense attached to it; and, consequently, there are no bills to be paid."[55] Quarantines were outrageously expensive. Health departments that relied on vaccination alone could hold themselves up as paragons of efficiency and fiscal responsibility.

Vaccination represented modernity and progress because it fit well with germ theory's emphasis on the role individuals played in disease transmission, whereas sanitary campaigns to rid streets of filth seemed antiquated because they represented older modes of medical thinking that attributed disease transmission to miasma. Vaccination plugged in easily to the new paradigm, obviating the need for elaborate hygienic regimens or expensive draconian quarantines of those exposed to smallpox victims. Vaccination thus promoted efficiency and economy in public health work. Yet such ideas proved unsettling to a public conditioned to think of disease control in terms of cleaning up filth or disinfecting to kill germs. Chairman Durgin's refusal to quarantine particularly violated the common sense of many people. Parents wanted to keep their children home from school. People questioned allowing those exposed to smallpox (albeit vaccinated) their freedom. They wondered why the city had not engaged in a massive clean-up campaign according to well-known dictates of sanitation. One concerned Dorchester resident even wrote to the *Boston Globe*, wondering why the Board of Health "so grossly neglected sanitary precautions in her section of the city."[56]

By the end of October new cases of smallpox had appeared in "nearly every section of the city."[57] Alarmingly, some of the new cases "had already suffered weeks without any knowledge of the matter having come to the attention of the Board of Health." Many of the afflicted persons did not realize they even had smallpox, but "undoubtedly carried it to friends and associates with whom they have been at liberty to mingle."[58] Durgin later recalled that the mildness of the smallpox attacks contributed substantially to its spread in the first months of the epidemic. "Early in the season there were quite a large number of those extremely mild cases. They appeared more like chicken-pox; and many were overlooked by the attending physicians on that account, and some were overlooked by even the patient himself. I saw quite a few who were at work, feeling as healthy as ever."[59] Smallpox victims too often either recovered without a physician's care or postponed consulting their doctor, providing ample opportunities for passing on their infection to others, as in the instance of a man living in Egleston Square who transmitted his mild smallpox to his wife. The husband "recovered without the service of a physician, so that the presence of the disease did not become known to the neighbors before his wife contracted it."[60] A few weeks later, Boston health inspectors found twelve men sick with smallpox "laboring with their sleeves rolled up in close contact with all the other employees" in a factory that employed two thousand workers.[61] Durgin complained that such behavior nullified his department's efforts to contain the epidemic: "We are not notified as a rule until the afflicted person has been suffering for many days, and others have come in contact with the germs. In most cases we cannot ascertain just who has been exposed to contagion, and therefore, we are powerless."[62] Few of Boston's citizens had seen or experienced smallpox personally since the last great epidemic of 1871–73. Those who had lived through that epidemic remembered a dire, loathsome disease that routinely killed almost a third of its victims.[63] This disease more often resembled an irritating but bearable affliction like chickenpox.

Problems with Smallpox Diagnosis

By 1901 few physicians had appreciable clinical experience with smallpox. As one Rhode Island physician put it, "the physician in general practice is seldom called upon to treat a case of smallpox."[64] The *Boston Medical and Surgical Journal* lamented the ignorance of many doctors: "A majority of the medical profession, at the present time, have never had an opportunity to become familiar with the disease." The relative absence of smallpox also led to complacency about vaccination, preventing "younger members of the profession . . . from recognizing the importance of, or learning the reasons for employing vaccination as a measure of prevention."[65] The physician Charles Good declared that smallpox "coming . . . with the stealth of a thief in the night . . . found many members of the medical profession napping." He argued that professional ignorance of proper vaccination technique and smallpox diagnosis, exacerbated by reports about vaccinia complications, led to a "tendency to increase the public alarm, and at the same time diminish the confidence of the public in the medical profession and in their colaborers, the vaccine manufacturers."[66] Frederick Dillingham, a New York City public health official, deplored the confusion. "The outbreak of smallpox all over the country during the past four years has been the cause of a great deal of controversy among physicians: many failing to recognize the true nature of the disease made diagnoses of varicella, eczema, vaccinia, Cuban itch, pseudo smallpox, Philippine rash, etc., and consequently observed none of the necessary precautions for preventing the spread of the malady."[67] Having no prior experience with smallpox in such a mild form, physicians at first believed it to be a new disease of foreign origin, and they had difficulty in correlating its signs and symptoms with those of classic smallpox. We now know this particular pandemic featured the first appearance of variola minor, a milder form of smallpox with a death rate of 2 to 6 percent among the unvaccinated. It broke out initially in the continental United States in 1896 and slowly spread throughout the country.[68] When a dread disease like smallpox appeared in such a substantially altered form, lay people understandably misinterpreted their symptoms. Physicians' diagnostic errors, however, particularly frustrated public health authorities like Samuel Durgin, who grumbled at "lax" physicians causing "an unnecessary delay in notifying our office."[69]

Medical journals featured many articles about this mild smallpox and how to distinguish its most telling diagnostic signs.[70] Some writers disputed whether or not this disease was smallpox at all, or some new ailment.[71] The American Medical Association even sponsored a special symposium on small-pox at its June 1901 annual meeting to help rectify medical uncertainty about diagnosis.[72] Despite these efforts and even though the city and state health departments provided resident experts who willingly traveled to confirm small-pox diagnoses, Boston physicians seemed reluctant to call on their assistance in doubtful cases. Durgin complained that too many cases slipped through the health department net because "in many instances no suspicions on the part of the family or patient or physician have been aroused."[73] One case that particu-larly infuriated Durgin involved a man "with a profuse eruption of small-pox from head to feet" who lived in a "well-filled tenement house." His clergyman reported the smallpox case to the health department, even though a physician had attended him previously. When the physician finally got around to calling in the case, Durgin indignantly informed him "of the regrets of the health department that it is obliged to depend on the clergy instead of the profession to diagnosticate and report smallpox."[74]

Physicians' failure to recognize and then immediately notify the Board of Health about smallpox victims accounted for much of its spread. In 1901, the Massachusetts State Board of Health sent medical inspectors to investigate 107 cases of suspected smallpox. They found case after case in which smallpox symptoms had gone unrecognized and transmitted the disease in more severe form to others. In one instance, a physician failed to recognize his own case and infected the wife of a man he treated for fractured ribs.[75] Likewise, many peo-ple ill with smallpox continued to go about their daily business ignorant of the true nature of their malady, inexorably exposing all and sundry to the disease. Durgin sourly acknowledged this fact as he tried to explain his department's failure to gain control over the epidemic. "Cases thus go on through a large part or their entire course, with exposure of a large number of people, to the cases on the street, at hospital clinics, in the street cars, in the work shops, or in the home of the patient, and no information of the case may reach the Board of Health until some subsequent case happens to be severe enough in character, or typical enough in appearance to reach the Board of Health. In this way the dis-ease is spread, defying measurably the most extensive expert and vigorous mea-sures that this department can exercise."[76] To his chagrin, smallpox continued to spread in the Boston area. He begged both the public and their physicians to report any uncertain case: "All we ask is that every suspicious case shall be at once reported to us, that we may make an investigation."[77]

Reluctance to report suspicions of smallpox possibly also derived from aver-sion to Boston's Smallpox Hospital. One antivaccinationist medical editor sympathized with hapless smallpox victims forced into isolation hospitals by health officials: "Smallpox patients are treated so cruelly, with so little regard for their physical necessities, that any one who suspects that he has smallpox tries to escape the vigilance of the health authorities. This leads them to expose the public in their efforts to keep hidden."[78] Up until the late nineteenth century, hospitals generally took in only those too poor to afford home care. Surgeries were commonly performed in the patient's home or the physician's office. Before the advent of organized nursing and the application of asepsis in surgery and wound treatment, hospitals were dangerous places. Hospital patients so routinely acquired deadly infections that physicians even had a name for the syndrome, "hospitalism." People with any means at all received care at home from their relatives, physicians, and hired nurses. Throughout the nineteenth century, only the destitute applied for hospital care. Thus sick people preferred to avoid hospitals, and hospitals avoided people with infectious diseases like smallpox. Instead, cities, towns, and villages set up special places for the infectious sick—pesthouses—usually a building (sometimes the jail or poorhouse) commandeered or erected quickly for the epidemic, although occasionally a city might build one to have on hand. Bereft of the comfort of home and family during a frightening illness, many people only reluctantly went to the pesthouse. In an 1894 smallpox epidemic in Milwaukee, for instance, riots broke out when health authorities attempted remove sick children to the local pesthouse there.[79]

By 1900 advances in surgery and nursing care had re-created the hospital as a site for advanced treatment in an aseptic setting, but some people may have been slow to change their attitudes, especially in regard to pesthouses.[80] Deplored as "an isolated, shabby structure with dreary environments," the city pesthouse rarely attained high standards of staffing and equipment.[81] One Boston newspaper condemned the health department for sending smallpox victims to a poorly equipped hospital reached only by an arduous trip in frigid weather. "Small-pox patients have been treated worse than brutes. It seems to be a crime to have the disease and no mercy has been given. When the true history of the pest-house on Galloupe's Island is made public it will shock the people of Boston. The Board of Health mismanaged the thing from the start. . . . Shovel the patients in there and get them out of the way is the only thing they care about. . . . The Galloupe Island business is a disgrace to the city."[82] Medical leaders regarded popular prejudice against the pesthouse as a major problem in the campaign to suppress contagious diseases. Smallpox victims did not go willingly to the local pesthouse—they were sent there. Patients with mild cases proved especially resistant to the idea that they must go into strict isolation. One Boston physician complained, "it is difficult at any time to convince them that they have a disease which is a menace to the public."[83] Well aware of this reluctance to enter the pesthouse, Durgin remarked in a Massachusetts Medical Society meeting: "Many persons in the community think that when one enters the pest house it means 'good-bye forever.' Great dread is associated with that word. . . . I believe we should do everything in our power to overcome this natural dread by calling it a hospital, and making the people feel that every comfort will be provided for the sick person."[84] Seeking to dispel this dread, Durgin assured Boston citizens that their city's isolation hospitals "are well fitted and possess all the means for the comforts and wellbeing of the patients."[85]

Another case of misdiagnosis marked a second turning point in the health department's vaccination strategy in mid-November. City Councilman George A. Flynn of Ward 17 contracted smallpox, but even though he saw a physician for his illness, the doctor did not recognize it as smallpox. Flynn, not feeling terribly sick, went about the business of campaigning in his ward, thus exposing many people to smallpox, albeit unintentionally. Tragically, though he experienced only mild symptoms, he infected his wife, and she came down with a virulent, ultimately fatal case of smallpox. Her physician recognized the nature of her illness, but did not immediately report it either, leaving the occupants of her house "at liberty to mingle with the other people in the district, some of them attending church." News of her condition, however, quickly circulated and many voters avoided the campaign caucus meeting "because of a fear of coming into contact with infected persons."[86]

Since Flynn had been "in and about the City Hall" during his illness, "there was a great rush to physicians by usually dignified city officials" who feared for their health.[87] Certainly many must have wondered about the vaccination status of their elected officials, if exposure to Councilman Lynn had caused such a panic. The Board of Health may have wondered also: it now intensified its vaccination campaign, calling for general vaccination throughout the city in recognition that "its [smallpox] general prevalence is likely to infect public conveyances and meeting-places."[88] No longer could Durgin claim to trace the origin of every case of smallpox; nor was the disease confined to the tenements and lodging houses. If prominent citizens like the Flynns could get it, anyone, anywhere could too. Tracing contacts, vaccinating neighbors, and disinfecting victims' homes could not control the epidemic when physicians would not report or could not recognize cases. Durgin had to admit that this epidemic threatened to run away from him. He had to fall back on emphasizing general vaccination in order to stop the chain of transmission. He had to compel everyone to get vaccinated. Given the situation, it was his only hope to regain control.

The Boston Vaccination Campaign

Health department efforts to control the epidemic must have seemed ineffectual to many onlookers as the numbers of cases mounted monthly, from "12 in August, to 30 in September, to 49 in October, to 195 in November, to 201 in December."[89] Faced with outbreaks of smallpox in the suburbs of Brookline, Newton, Lynn, and Hyde Park, Durgin resorted to stronger measures. On Saturday, 16 November, he assembled ten physicians, ten health department inspectors, and fifteen policemen, divided them into "virus squads," and sent them to make "a tour of the public licensed lodging-houses" that night in the "crowded tenement district, where most of the people display total ignorance as to the purposes of vaccination." Most of the people accepted the vaccination offered by the squads: out of 1,091 persons visited, only 14 refused vaccination. Although one newspaper asserted that "there were no clubs pulled by policemen in order to induce persons to be vaccinated," several incidents in which homeless men were forcibly vaccinated belied that claim.[90] Undoubtedly the simple presence of a club-wielding policeman added some extra element of coercion beyond that of simple persuasion.

Many people seemed to have mixed feelings about vaccination. A *Boston Post* editor wondered whether the city had given way to undue panic over smallpox. While declaring it "the obvious duty . . . on the part of citizens generally who have not been recently vaccinated to protect themselves without delay by that slight operation," the editor derided the notion that Boston was in the grip of an epidemic. "One case of the disease among every 10,000 inhabitants cannot by any stretch of sensational imagining be made to appear as an epidemic."[91] Reporting on crowds gathered in various venues throughout Boston to receive their vaccinations, the *Evening Transcript* declared that "vaccination has become almost a fad in the city." Yet it observed that many of the recipients seemed to need extra persuasion to get their vaccinations. "Some submit to the treatment from actual fear, others because of choice, preferring it to the possibility of a greater evil, still others because of compulsion from the Board of Health or from employers who insist on it as one of the conditions for employment, and there are thousands of men, women and children who accept it at this time because so many others do and because it costs them nothing."[92]

As smallpox cases mounted in late November, the health department opened twenty-six free vaccination stations at schools scattered throughout Boston, with hours convenient for working people, from seven to nine in the evening, Monday through Saturday. On Sundays, the stations were open from two to four in the afternoon.[93] On 19 November, the Board of Health reported that it had distributed thirty thousand vaccine points to its physicians. The *Evening Transcript* guessed that physicians in private practice probably "have vaccinated as many as the Board of Health," but presented no evidence to back up the speculation.[94]

Yet this initial enthusiasm slacked off considerably by early December, and Durgin expressed concern to the *Boston Post* about the lack of interest in vaccination: "There are, without doubt, more than 200,000 people in Boston today, who, though many of them have at some time in their lives been vaccinated, are today, not fully immune, and who should, without delay, be vaccinated or revaccinated for self-protection and as a plain duty to the community."[95] Public nonchalance and procrastination about vaccination pushed Durgin to take extreme measures. On 26 December 1901, he announced a general vaccination order for all of Boston's inhabitants as state law permitted, sending physicians by January 1902 "into portions of the city where most needed to give free vaccinations in the homes and places of business, and to take the names of those who refused to be vaccinated."[96] As we shall see, Bostonians did not accord them an enthusiastic reception.

Smallpox in Cambridge

Smallpox came slightly later to the city of Cambridge, Boston's neighbor just across the Charles River. The first cases appeared in October 1901, but with a far lighter impact.[97] By 18 January 1902, Cambridge had had only 20 cases with 4 deaths, compared with 681 cases and 108 deaths in Boston. Even taking its smaller population into account, if smallpox had hit it as hard as Boston, it would have experienced nearly five times as many cases in the same period.[98]

Cambridge had its own mayor, city council, and health department. Like Boston, the chairman of its Board of Health was a physician, E. Edwin Spencer, but there the resemblance ends, for Spencer had a different social outlook, medical training, and professional manner from that of Durgin. In 1902 Spencer was sixty-nine years old, suffering from heart disease that would kill him a year later.[99] Spencer's academic credentials were not as illustrious as Durgin's Dartmouth and Harvard degrees. To begin with, Spencer was trained as an eclectic physician and he retained eclecticism as his professional identity. He first attended the Eclectic Medical Institute of Cincinnati, Ohio, graduating with high honors in 1856. Originating in the late 1820s, eclectic medicine rejected the bloodletting and chemically based drugs of the regular (allopathic) school, using instead botanically based therapeutics. Eclectics also tended to be more open to adopting various therapeutic approaches. As Ron Numbers noted, "they borrowed from just about every system available, including homeopathy, hydropathy, phrenology—even allopathy." Eclectics studied anatomy, obstetrics, and surgery—the same courses as those offered in regular medical schools, and by the turn of the century represented "about one-tenth of the medical profession."[100]

After his graduation Spencer moved to Winchedon, Massachusetts, to work in the office of his brother-in-law, a physician, while he attended another eclectic medical school, Worcester Medical College, graduating in 1859.[101] Spencer turned down a professorship at the Eclectic Medical Institute, moving to Cambridge in 1873 to take over a retiring physician's practice. He began his association with the Cambridge health department a few years later as city physician. In 1891, the mayor of Cambridge appointed him to the Board of Health, and in 1893 he was elected its chairman. Unlike Durgin, who was quite well paid, Spencer received no compensation for his office and had to depend on his practice and position as a state pension examiner to make a living. Spencer participated in several medical organizations, playing an especially prominent role in the Massachusetts Eclectic Medical Society as a charter member, president, and then treasurer for the last fifteen years. He belonged also to the National Eclectic Medical Society, the Massachusetts Association of Boards of Health, the Boston district Medical Association, serving as its president, and the Cambridge Art Circle, leading its literature section. Spencer was politically active, "a staunch Democrat" who had once run for office, "and was at all times a loyal member of the party."[102] Despite his political affiliation, he apparently left politics aside in his job as head of the Cambridge health department. The editor of the *Cambridge*

Chronicle remembered him as "a Democrat, but not a politician. He has been appointed repeatedly by Non-partisan mayors."[103]

Despite his financial dependence on the proceeds of his practice, Spencer had a reputation for "unfailing charity" in treating the poor for free.[104] A fellow Board of Health member and close friend, the attorney William Rodman Peabody, recalled that Spencer took a broad view of public health. "Dr. Spencer carried with him into his work on the board of health an overflowing sympathy for the sick and unfortunate. He gave a liberal interpretation to the word health, feeling that it was his duty not only to guard those who were unable to protect themselves from actual disease but also to make their life more comfortable and better worth the living. The poor, he believed, should so far as practicable breathe as clean air and sleep as undisturbed sleep and eat as pure food as the rich, and he taught that the best care obtainable for the sick was an economy for the city as compared with any system of niggardly saving, since it resulted in a more speedy recovery of the patient and gave to the community a more productive citizen."[105] Spencer saw his mission as a public health officer not only as that of a guardian against the invasion of microbes but also as an advocate for better food, housing, and working conditions. All who knew him remarked on his grace under pressure, especially the criticism he faced for his decision to forgo strict quarantines during the smallpox epidemic. William Peabody admired Spencer's fortitude: "When he knew he was right, public criticism was apparently a matter of indifference to him."[106]

Despite his awareness of his own health problems, Spencer gave his time unflinchingly during the smallpox epidemic, going out at all hours to examine and attend smallpox victims.[107] He paid a high price for his adherence to duty. Reluctant to patronize a physician so continuously exposed to smallpox, his patients fell away, resulting in the "practical annihilation of his private practice." Spencer took on smallpox in Cambridge as a personal battle in which he paid, at least in the eyes of his contemporaries, the ultimate price of first his practice and then his life. Whether his heart condition would have killed him anyway does not really matter. His friends and colleagues believed without a doubt that his zeal to do his duty, the stress of dealing with the epidemic, and the consequent loss of his practice were the true culprits. For instance, Peabody declared of Spencer: "He did the duty which was set before him but he had to give his life to do it. No soldier ever saw death more clearly or advanced to meet it more unhesitatingly."[108] Unlike Durgin, Spencer had no local fiefdom or national reputation to protect: he had only his duty as he saw it, a duty "he discharged unflinchingly and well."[109]

At the beginning of 1902, E. Edwin Spencer could count his city lucky to have relatively few smallpox victims to care for. Despite his pleas over the years, the town council had refused to appropriate funds for a permanent isolation hospital, and thus had no place to house smallpox patients once the epidemic hit.[110] The city had to rent a house on New Street for $3,500 in the fall of 1901, and it took over neighboring dwellings as the patient load increased until it occupied the entire street. It then cordoned off the street and restricted travel in its vicinity.[111] For the most part, Spencer followed the same tactics that Durgin used in Boston. He removed the sick to the isolation hospital, vaccinated, then inspected the exposed daily during the incubation period and disinfected the premises occupied by the infected. He opened up free vaccination stations in October 1901 and maintained them until August 1902.[112]

Like Durgin, Spencer did not quarantine well persons, except for a few cases, declaring, "quarantine maintained by force is not only extremely expensive and oppressive but is inefficient, inoperative, and even dangerous." Spencer believed that quarantines were dangerous because people often fled at the slightest hint it might be enforced: "In a thickly settled district persons who are unwilling to be restrained usually can escape by window or roof and disappear, or else, at the first rumor of small-pox, people scatter from the house before the arrival of the authorities and are, therefore, lost before they can be vaccinated and often before their identity is known."[113] Like Durgin, Spencer relied on vaccination as his main line of defense. Even in the face of intense criticism, he refused to quarantine healthy vaccinated persons who had been exposed to smallpox cases. Spencer remained convinced that vaccination, not quarantine, could provide the only real security from smallpox: "The safety of the community lies in vaccination and to accomplish satisfactory vaccination of the inhabitants of the city the board of health needs the co-operation of the people."[114] If exposed individuals fled from health department vaccinators because they feared incarceration for weeks, he would never get control of the epidemic. Spencer truly believed that cooperation rather than coercion was the key to obtaining compliance in vaccination.

Spencer did not immediately follow suit with a vaccination order for his city. With only 15 cases cropping up in 1901 in his jurisdiction compared with 514 cases in Boston, he did not see the need to demand general compulsory vaccination immediately even though traffic between the two cities flowed so constantly that they functioned virtually as one entity.[115] His reliance on free voluntary vaccination—offered at stations located in each section of the city—met with but a lukewarm response from Cambridge's nearly one hundred thousand residents. The East Cambridge station performed 2,258 vaccinations and the Cambridgeport station gave out 2,054, but the stations located in Old Cambridge and North Cambridge attracted only 843 and 638 takers, respectively.[116] Only after late February returns showed an ominous growth in smallpox cases did he issue a formal vaccination order on 27 February 1902.[117]

Although most of these new cases were concentrated primarily in two wards, Spencer took a more evenhanded approach than Durgin to his vaccination sweeps. Whereas Durgin had targeted only certain sections of Boston (claiming that he just attacked smallpox where it lived), Spencer attempted to contact every household in the city, including the students at Harvard.[118] His vaccination sweep sent a corps of seventeen physicians beginning on 7 March 1902, ostensibly "to make a house-to-house canvas and vaccinate everybody."[119] A second sweep of the city issued after smallpox resurged in late June. Unfortunately, although vaccinators supposedly visited every Cambridge household and vaccinated "all inhabitants whom they could find," the number they actually vaccinated turned out to be less than one-quarter of the city's population—exactly 21,685 persons out of a total population of 96,334, just a little more than a fifth of the total population.[120] Additionally, when the health department chairman Spencer surveyed the city's private physicians, he found that they had performed 25,990 vaccinations, to cover just a little over a quarter of the total population. These vaccinations taken with those from the free vaccination stations (5,793 in 1901 and 2,745 in 1902) amounted to 56,213, meaning that only 58 percent of the people received vaccinations between October 1901 and December 1902.[121] Put another way, 42 percent somehow avoided vaccination. Like Boston, Cambridge also seemed to have a problem with public enthusiasm for vaccination in 1902.

Although both cities preferred and argued for vaccination as the most efficient and least disruptive public health strategy, the epidemic moved too quickly for it to work to limit the outbreak. The new mild type of smallpox confused physicians and lay people alike. Individuals sick or convalescing still went to work, church, or school. They moved about the cities on public transportation, carrying on their daily business of shopping and visiting. Physicians too often only belatedly realized they were dealing with smallpox among their patients, and the health departments did not receive notification of smallpox cases quickly enough to stop transmission to new victims. Despite their efforts to offer and later demand vaccination, not enough people were vaccinated quickly enough to contain the epidemic.

Even though both the Boston and Cambridge health departments had worked with the utmost speed to deliver vaccinations to the people, it became apparent as they conducted their vaccination operations that many people were avoiding them. Uncertainty about the safety of vaccination had built up over the course of the nineteenth century—anxiety prompted in part by the antivaccination movement. Now the residents of Boston and Cambridge, conscious of the controversy, questioned whether the vaccinations on offer were safe to use. They procrastinated on the issue, further impeding efforts to vaccinate the population sufficiently to stop the spread of smallpox.

Chapter Four

The Hazards of Vaccination in 1901–2

In early 1902, with smallpox cases cropping up in the hundreds through-out Boston, a health department physician called at a Beacon Hill lodging house. His job seemed simple: the Board of Health had ordered everyone not vaccinated in the last five years to get it done and it sent out squads of doctors, door-to-door, to make sure that each resident complied. The physician even had the backing of a Massachusetts state law that decreed jail time or a fine for those who refused. Yet a reporter who followed this physician on his rounds discovered that the task was anything but simple. The individuals he encountered used all sorts of wily tactics to avoid inspection of their vaccination scars. They blatantly lied or adroitly manipulated the hapless doctor to escape vaccination.

Two female tenants invoked the privilege of gender to avoid exposing their flesh to a strange man's scrutiny. One young woman declared: "Why doctor, you see I've got on a tight-fitting sleeve, and I can't roll it up." Another lady stammered modestly that her vaccination was on her leg and she simply "looked out the window while the physician beat a hasty retreat down the hall." Other tenants worked as a sort of tag team. One man swore he had been vaccinated four years ago, exclaiming: "and I was sick for two weeks!" But when the doctor tried to look at the man's vaccination scar, a boy distracted him "with questions on all sorts of subjects, much to the relief of the man who had been carrying his scar for at least 15 years." The ease of their evasions led the reporter to conclude: "enforcement of compulsory vaccination is not as strict as it might be in many cases."[1]

These people were not antivaccinationists. They did not argue about vaccination or civil liberty—they just seemed wary, seeking instead to misdirect or put off the doctors. Physicians in other states also reported a common distaste for vaccination. Frederick Dillingham, the assistant sanitary superintendent of the New York City Department of Health, observed that when the Girl's High School of Brooklyn ordered its pupils to produce their vaccination certificates or face expulsion, the two thousand students raised "such a storm of excited protest" that it rescinded the order.[2] The Pennsylvania physician William R. Fisher noticed how parents procrastinated over vaccination: "Vaccination is apt to be looked upon as a trying ordeal at best and it is natural that parents should feel that once is better than twice, and put off the operation until the time when the law makes it obligatory."[3] People postponed vaccinating their children in the first place, and then few routinely sought revaccination even though medical authorities repeatedly proclaimed that one vaccination was not sufficient for a lifetime's protection against smallpox. As we have seen in earlier chapters, vaccination had developed a reputation for trouble and complications over the course of the nineteenth century. No one regarded this simple medical operation as trivial or entirely benign. Ordinary people weighed the risks of vaccination and only reluctantly accepted it as a necessary evil forced on them by their employers or the law.

Vaccination Rates in 1901–2

At the turn of the century, no one could say with any certainty just how many people experienced bad outcomes from vaccinations, or even how many people were vaccinated. Although public health authorities had recognized the value of vaccination for at least a century, no state or federal agency compiled data on vaccinations. In 1902, one prominent Boston physician attempted to rectify this situation and correct public misapprehension about the dangers of vaccination. John H. McCollom sent out a questionnaire on vaccination to 2,700 members of the Massachusetts Medical Society and got 1,859 responses. An overwhelming number of physicians—1,701—had never observed any vaccination complication in their careers. The remaining physicians reported relatively small numbers of problems—35 deaths, 68 "moderately severe effects, in which individuals were unable to attend to business for four or five weeks," and 54 cases of serious infections.[4] McCollom attributed much of the current furor over vaccination to guilt-ridden parents seeking to cast blame on anyone but themselves. "Many of the alleged injurious effects after careful investigation have been proved to have no connection with vaccination either directly or indirectly, but have been shown to be due to carelessness on the part of the individual."[5] McCollom's logic dished out cold comfort to those pondering the risks of vaccination, and it insulted grieving parents who probably thought they had done their best to care for their children. Such statistics lacked meaning in the face of singular tragedy to those who had witnessed, experienced, or heard of bad effects from vaccination.

A significant number of people in Boston avoided vaccinating their children despite reassurances from physicians like McCollom. The slight possibility of severe consequences acquired great weight in the calculus of risk when they considered vaccination. Massachusetts had compulsory vaccination since 1855. It possessed a highly regarded public health system at both the state and municipal level staffed by leading health officers. By law, public schools required either vaccination or a physician's certificate attesting to a child's unfitness for vaccination for admission. Yet as smallpox cases mounted throughout the city in

1901, investigations of Boston schoolchildren revealed that at least 1 in 15 pupils went unvaccinated.[6] That is, out of 90,144 pupils aged five to fifteen, around 6.7 percent were not vaccinated.[7] Certain locations had even higher percentages. Master Young of the Prince School testified in 1902 that "many of his pupils had certificates of exemption from vaccination." Master Mead of the Chapman School in East Boston, with a student population of 1,200, had nearly 20 percent unvaccinated.[8] The Boston health department chief Samuel H. Durgin was appalled that so many children had escaped vaccination despite the laws requiring it. "The vaccination of school children is a matter that has been overlooked with almost provoking carelessness. We had no idea conditions were so lax until we began to investigate these cases. In nearly every case we found that the victim had not been vaccinated. Frequently we found whole families where not a single member had been vaccinated. Occasionally we were informed that a child had been vaccinated, but that it did not 'take,' but there was no attempt at revaccination."[9] He even found a young man who had lost an eye after his bout with smallpox. Never vaccinated, he still attended school, passing "through all the grades of the East Boston public schools."[10] He complained that few parents sought another vaccination for their adolescent children and adults almost never got one for themselves voluntarily, creating a population "in a receptive condition for the disease."[11]

From the beginning of 1901 through January 1902, the Boston Board of Health gave 180,000 free vaccinations, and Durgin estimated that private physicians and "railroad companies, mercantile and other establishments" accounted for another 300,000 vaccinations.[12] Yet these numbers amounted to only 84.4 percent of the city's 574,642 inhabitants.[13] This means that over 15 percent of the population (and maybe even more) had managed to evade vaccination even after the 1901 general vaccination order. Perhaps some had received a vaccination in the last five years and thus did not need one, but it seems unlikely given the scenario of vaccination neglect that Durgin presented in his 1901 *Annual Report*. As we have seen in the preceding chapter, Durgin's counterpart across the Charles River, E. Edwin Spencer, chairman of the Cambridge Board of Health, found even worse results for his city, with a vaccination rate of less than 60 percent of the population.[14] It seems that a significant proportion of both Boston and Cambridge residents avoided vaccination, even in the face of an epidemic.

Problems with Vaccination in 1901–2

Some experienced vaccinators argued that ideally vaccination should cause no problems. Theresa Bannan, a public vaccinator in Syracuse, New York, asserted that "with *proper* vaccine, the course is mild in all cases." Vesicles formed four to six days after the operation, coalescing into a pustule with a surrounding area of redness (the aerola), which should enlarge only to a diameter of one to three inches. The pustule dried up into a scab that fell off in two or three weeks. Fever was "usual from the eighth to the tenth day" after vaccination, but "other consti-tutional disturbances are slight or absent." Infants and young children seemed to deal with vaccination best, "giving no signs of discomfort."[15]

Yet many lay people and even physicians may not have known what to expect in the course of a normal vaccination. Samuel Durgin complained that both physicians and lay people misunderstood vaccination when they blithely assumed that the mere act of abrading the skin assured protection against smallpox. "There is one grievous mistake concerning vaccination which ought to be corrected, namely, many people suppose that scarification upon the arm or attempt at vaccination, means what is professionally and legally known and understood to be vaccination, and I am sorry to say that many physicians certify to the vaccination of children immediately after the operation or attempt at vac-cination has been performed, while the patient may be and oftentimes has been absolutely without vaccination."[16] In other words, too many physicians failed to ensure their vaccinations took. Patients believed they had received a vaccination simply because a trusted doctor had performed an operation on them. If they then contracted smallpox, they blamed vaccination as useless rather than ques-tion their physician's competence.

Many people also believed that vaccination necessarily induced soreness and swelling. The *St. Paul Medical Journal* observed, "some physicians, and the major-ity of the laity, seem to think that vaccination which has not produced a very painful arm or leg, has not been successful."[17] Durgin attempted to rectify such misapprehensions by explaining that "many people believe if they get a big arm the vaccination is correspondingly good. This should be regarded as an error." He warned that "aseptic conditions are as necessary in this little operation as in any other operation in minor surgery." Although a patient could experience "constitutional disturbances, local swelling of the arm, and glandular tender-ness," he or she should not suffer the sort of inflammation that would accom-pany blood poisoning.[18]

Apparently Durgin's remarks did not filter through to the general public, for many people in Boston and Cambridge routinely expected severe discomfort and temporary disability from vaccination. When Major Taylor, the great cham-pion of American and European cycling, postponed his return to the American professional racing circuit because of his recent vaccination, the *Boston Post* agreed "this of course made it impossible for him to ride until he had recovered from the effects of his inoculation." The paper even speculated that Taylor had deliberately gotten vaccinated in order to have an excuse not to ride "so that he could rest a few weeks before taking up racing."[19] If an elite athlete expected that vaccination would seriously impede his performance, what did more ordi-nary citizens anticipate? Vaccination also afflicted international celebrities. The famous British actress Lillie Langtry had to abandon the stage in 1901 because her vaccination "flew to her throat, producing acute inflammation of the vocal chords." Another actress, Ada Reeve, suffered for six months from a bad arm after her vaccination.[20] A limerick entitled "The Vaccinated" hinted at the pain from a normal vaccination.

Oft daily those you meet abroad
Halt in your path with grave alarm:
Their stern expressions plainly say,
"Sir, don't you dare to bump my arm!"[21]

Another poem, "A Vaccine Point," also inferred that people expected to suffer greatly from their vaccinations, though that was nothing compared with the scarring left by a bout with smallpox.

At the hearing just given, one point was omitted
Though doctor against doctor in combat was pitted;
For while the good people who calmly submitted
To free vaccination are much to be pitied,
That those who prefer the disease to the cure
Will also be pitted is equally sure.[22]

Some manufacturers evidently thought suffering from vaccination presented a sales opportunity. The Howard Health Company promised that its product would "mitigate" vaccination's "action in your system, or modify it to a degree that you will not become poisoned in blood by the VILE VIRUS."[23] One advertisement for an antiseptic wash, Cabot's Sulpho-Napthol, proclaimed its usefulness "For Vaccinated Arms. . . . To relieve that itching."[24]

City employees were not exactly enthusiastic about the prospect of inflamed, painful arms. On 26 November, Boston Mayor Thomas N. Hart formally advised all municipal departments to vaccinate their employees.[25] The Boston Police Department initially hesitated to compel vaccination because many patrolmen objected that "sore arms" would interfere with the performance of their duties.[26] The *Transcript* reported that detectives and clerical workers at police headquarters submitted only because they felt pressured to do so. Though the police commissioner recommended rather than ordered vaccination, these employees understood it as an order, "and very few, if any, care to go contrary to their wishes."[27] When Postmaster Hibbard ordered a general vaccination for all employees, one newspaper proclaimed: "All will have sore arms."[28] These city workers accepted vaccination as a necessary evil, apparently expecting that even if vaccination proceeded according to normal parameters, it involved considerable discomfort and impaired their ability to work. They were not antivaccinationists but they feared vaccination and submitted only reluctantly to it.

Many other Bostonians also demonstrated an aversion to vaccination. When the firm of J. A. Dreyfus & Sons ordered its female employees to vaccinate, they refused en masse. Not until Carl Dreyfus "bared his own arm, displaying a fresh scarification," could he convince the reluctant women to go along with the plan.[29] These women hesitated when vaccination could protect them from a disfiguring and possibly deadly disease because they feared vaccination might be worse. Again, they were not antivaccinationists but they certainly put off vaccination until their boss told them they had to do it.

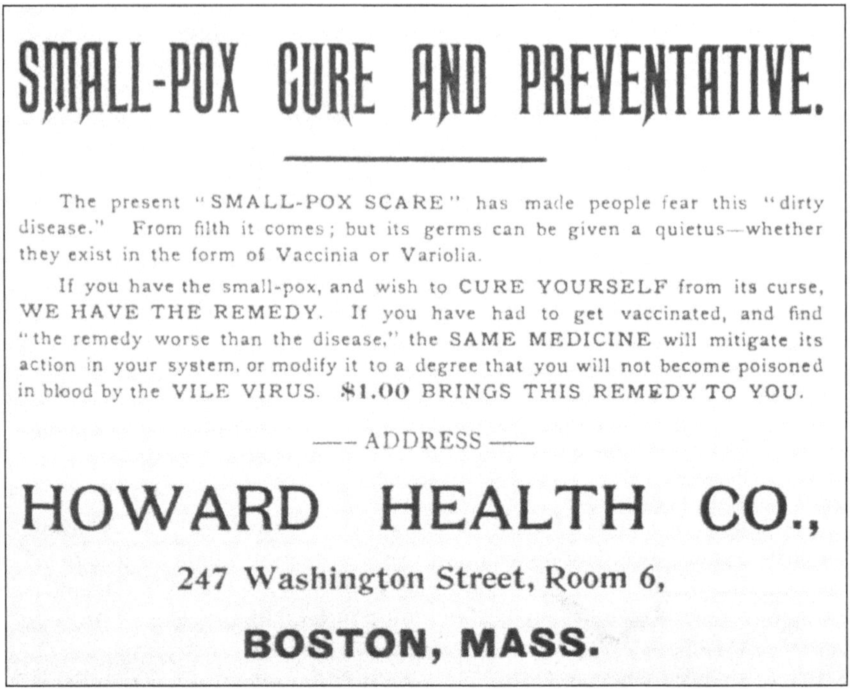

SMALL-POX CURE AND PREVENTATIVE.

The present "SMALL-POX SCARE" has made people fear this "dirty disease." From filth it comes; but its germs can be given a quietus—whether they exist in the form of Vaccinia or Variolia.

If you have the small-pox, and wish to CURE YOURSELF from its curse, WE HAVE THE REMEDY. If you have had to get vaccinated, and find "the remedy worse than the disease," the SAME MEDICINE will mitigate its action in your system, or modify it to a degree that you will not become poisoned in blood by the VILE VIRUS. $1.00 BRINGS THIS REMEDY TO YOU.

—— ADDRESS ——

HOWARD HEALTH CO.,

247 Washington Street, Room 6,

BOSTON, MASS.

Figure 4.1. Advertisement for Howard Health Company. *Our Home Rights* 1 (November 1901): 45.

Anecdotes about vaccination complications abounded throughout the Northeast and Midwest during 1901 and 1902. A Camden, New Jersey, physician, for instance, reported that "a fairly large proportion of arms inoculated developed intense sores, requiring from eight to ten weeks to heal completely."[30] In New York State, the physician Theresa Bannon also experienced considerable difficulties with at least one brand of vaccine virus she used in 1902. "Constitutional effects were marked—high fever for several days, loss of appetite, nausea, and vomiting was the constant report confirmed by the pale faces of the children; the arms were painful, the areola was extensive, often reaching the elbow and wrist; the pustule was small and shallow, the scab thin, often undermined or but partially covering the ulcer beneath. . . . That such virus does much to injure the cause of vaccination is to be expected. Physicians are helplessly in the hands of the producers with their commercial spirit."[31] Some vaccinations had even resulted in death. After her vaccination in early 1901 "at school by the Health Department physician," a fifteen-year-old Chicago girl succumbed to an illness that physicians initially thought to be appendicitis. When the celebrated surgeon Christian Fenger opened up her abdomen, however, he found the appendix "free and uninvolved." The girl died the next day, and an autopsy showed that the vaccination on her leg had induced peritonitis.[32]

After the death of his son from the effects of vaccination, the mayor of Gas City, Indiana, rescinded the town's school vaccination orders.[33] Other parents filed wrongful death suits against vaccinating physicians. In Philadelphia, Mrs. Bridget Nugent obtained a judgment of $1,000 against the physician Harvey M. Righter, alleging that his contaminated vaccine lymph had caused her six-year-old son to contract a fatal case of impetigo contagiosa. Although the judge advised the jury to believe the physician's account over that of the victim's mother, it still returned a verdict for the plaintiff, indicating that, in this instance at least, public patience with vaccination had worn thin.[34] Such tragedies may not have convinced people that vaccination was wrong per se, but they may have made many apprehensive about the quality of the lymph then in use. One Boston physician so distrusted the purity of his vaccine that when forced by law to vaccinate, he advised a patient to swab her family's vaccinations with rubbing alcohol to sterilize the area, even though that action thus rendered the vaccination ineffective.[35]

The Boston dermatologist Harvey P. Towle reported treating five patients who experienced rather frightening skin eruptions after their vaccinations in the winter of 1901–2. A two-year-old boy in his care developed red patches all over his body six days after his vaccination and could not stand, for "any movement of the knees called forth a cry of pain." Itchy sores erupted all over the back, chest, abdomen, and forehead of a six-year-old girl eight days after her vaccination. An adult woman experienced itching and swelling of her arm and knees after her vaccination. Vaccination apparently revived an old case of psoriasis in one other adult patient, and it caused lesions to appear on old eczema sites on the body of a four-year-old boy.[36] The antivaccinationist editor Joseph M. Greene howled derisively at Towle's puzzlement over the lack of medical research on these reactions: "Dr. Towle will have no difficulty in finding the right 'references' if he goes to proper quarters."[37]

Greene's ridicule stemmed from the fact that he and other antivaccinationists had been publishing accounts of bad effects from vaccination for over a year by late 1902. Beginning in October 1901, Immanuel Pfeiffer, Boston's most outspoken antivaccinationist physician, visited two families, the Shores and the Leavitts, who resided in the same rooming house. The Shores informed him that two weeks after their infant daughter's vaccination in August 1901, "large sores commenced to appear on the back of the head and afterwards on the face." The Leavitts then showed him their daughter, vaccinated nearly two years ago, but now "almost rotten with eczema for twenty months; its ears nearly came off; the body is now like raw beef." Pfeiffer documented their plight as "The Fruit of Vaccination" in the pages of his magazine, *Our Home Rights*, and included a photograph of the afflicted baby, Annie Shore, her face and head covered with lesions. Pfeiffer claimed both sets of parents told him that "there were many similar cases."[38] Joseph Greene later noted of Annie Shore that "the child for months presented a pitiful appearance, its face being covered with large scabbed sores which seem to resist all attempts at healing."[39]

The cases of eight-month-old Annie Shore and two-year-old Jennie Leavitt circulated widely in the antivaccination press. Greene featured the story with a photograph of Annie Shore on the cover of *The Animals' Defender*, the organ of the New England Anti-vivisection Society, and he later sent it on to a Minneapolis antivaccination journal, *The Liberator*, in 1903.[40] Ultimately the osteopath Reuben Swinburne Clymer also documented the Shore and Leavitt cases in his 1904 antivaccination book, *Vaccination Brought Home to You.*[41]

Aware that medical critics would treat this information with skepticism, these antivaccination writers provided facts that any Bostonian could easily check to bolster its credibility. They gave out full names, addresses, hospitals, and attending physicians' identities in their case studies. To prove the veracity of his account, for instance, Greene included Annie Shore's father's name, Abraham Shore, as well as the date and the hospital site of her vaccination in his account.[42] Pfeiffer and Greene both provided the address of the rooming house in which both families lodged, 10 Billerica St.[43] Greene even added an observation about the Shore family's appearance: "The parents are fine looking and healthy people, and their home is neat, clean, and well-kept."[44] Thus he assured his readers that he personally had seen that the hygienic Shores were innocent parties in their daughter's travail.

Greene also organized heart-wrenching testimony of several parents and their children before the Massachusetts state legislature's Joint Committee on Public Health in early 1902. Among them was a little child whose "face was one mass of sores," probably Annie Shore. Several physicians and parents testified to the harm wrought by vaccination. Dr. Cutting of Newtonville told how he watched two vaccinated children die of blood poisoning "as a result of vaccination." Mrs. Smith of Winthrop produced her teenage son, who had been vaccinated at five, "and had ever since then been deprived of the use of his arm." One father, Fred W. Hatch, declared that "vaccination was against all common sense" after describing how his daughter became afflicted with eczema after her vaccination.[45]

Immanuel Pfeiffer zealously recounted cases of vaccination injury in his magazine, inspiring readers to dread vaccination even if they had not personally witnessed such effects. "We are daily visited by many people who have been vaccinated to their sorrow, suffering from swollen, sore arms and in other ways. They all declare that they will never again submit to such stupid, barbaric treatment. Some are very emphatic in their expression and speak of revolvers and shot-guns should they ever be approached by a vaccinator. We hear of many fatal results and where we can get the facts, we gladly give them to our readers."[46] He also published letters occasionally from individuals who had witnessed bad effects from vaccinations in Boston. For example, when the Parker House hotel and restaurant vaccinated its 350 employees, Thomas B. Lohan reported terrible reactions: "Quite a few are out sick from the effects . . . and the majority have swollen arms. The swelling extends to the fingers in some cases and also takes effect under the armpits and on the side; while large festering sores some of them three inches in diameter act as a monument to the spot where the deadly virus had been injected."[47] A Boston elevated railway worker likewise told

Pfeiffer of arms so swollen after vaccination that "some of the men have gone to the hospital, and one man will probably have to have his arm amputated."[48]

Yet it was Joseph Green, more than any other antivaccinationist, who made the case against vaccination for the Boston public. Working as a one-man clearinghouse of vaccination tragedy, he related every case of vaccination injury in graphic detail by collecting and publishing affidavits of "vaccination disasters" in *The Animals' Defender*.[49] Eventually he shared these testimonials with Lora Little, editor of *The Liberator*. Even though provaccination medical authorities at the time may have regarded these testimonials with skepticism, the people afflicted certainly believed wholeheartedly that vaccination had caused their troubles, as did their families, friends, neighbors, and sometimes even their physicians. Historians who dismiss these stories as irrational ravings risk buying into the rhetoric of provaccinationists who occasionally indulged in a bit of tinkering with the facts to suit their beliefs, as we shall see below in the case of tetanus after vaccination. Both sides manipulated data to suit their agendas and ignored inconvenient facts when it suited them.

Many of these cases involved young adults who fell so ill from the effects of their vaccination that they could not work for considerable lengths of time. For instance, when his employer asked nineteen-year-old Stanley Hollis to get vaccinated in December 1901, he complied. Unfortunately, even though "one of the most respected physicians of Brookline" performed the vaccination, Hollis nearly died from complications. "In about a week the arm began to swell until it reached the proportions of a large man's thigh. . . . It then turned black. Ten days after vaccination the lad began bleeding at the nose and mouth, and for two days and nights masses of mucous clotted blood and pus were pulled from his mouth, the poison of which caused his lips to swell to double the normal size. The odor was frightful and "all the rags had to be burned." The amount of blood lost was between two and three pailfuls. Meanwhile three eminent doctors (two of Boston) held consultations and "gave no encouragement" for life. The lad, being young and of great vitality, survived, after 7 weeks of suffering and a loss of 30 lbs. weight."[50] Greene enumerated case after case. Zoeth Rich, an employee of the Turner Center Cream Company of Boston, received his vaccination in late November 1901, but his arm swelled badly, erupted in blisters, eventually turned black, "and now is withered." He had to quit his job and move back home with his parents.[51] The mailman Samuel Vaughan "was laid up for six weeks from blood poisoning" after his vaccination.[52] A police officer in Winthrop, John McCarron, also suffered from blood poisoning after his vaccination, to such an extent that "two doctors have advised amputation of the arm to save McCarron's life."[53] Benjamin F. Thurston, a motorman for the Boston Elevated Railway Company, fell ill with blood poisoning after vaccination in November 1901, "and since that time has been unable to do any work."[54] A furnace tender at the Gurney iron foundry, Joseph Sullivan, became paralyzed on his left side after his vaccination.[55] Miss G. Williams, long employed by the Waltham Watch Company, "did not desire" her vaccination, but "the edict went forth that the employees must be 'vaccinated or leave.'" She fell so ill that she could not work for fourteen weeks: "her limbs swelled to twice their size and her sufferings were terrible." Greene reported that her physician "acknowledged it was caused by vaccination."[56]

Bostonians knew about cases of vaccination injury. Family, coworkers, friends, neighbors, and acquaintances gossiped about such sufferings. One Boston newspaper editor acknowledged, "probably there are few of us who have not known in our personal experience instances of life-long injury, and even death, directly and confessedly due to the introduction of poison into the system by vaccination."[57] Joseph Greene declared that one of the largest employers, the Boston Elevated Railway Company, had "numerous instances of terrible blood-poisoning" among its workers.[58] Indeed, the *Boston Post* reported that several business owners made a point of testifying before the state legislature's Public Health Committee that none of their workers had been permanently injured by vaccination primarily to counter such stories. None of them, however, owned the businesses that employed the men and women in Greene's affidavits.[59]

Stories about vaccination problems in other sections of the country also profoundly affected Bostonians' perceptions of vaccination. Cleveland received national attention for its health officer's dramatic resolution of its vaccination troubles. During the summer of 1901, complaints about severe reactions were so pervasive that the health officer Martin Friedrich halted public vaccination until he could obtain pure virus. Of the incident, he laconically recalled: "Last year the virus took altogether too well. Fully one-fourth developed sepsis." Friedrich encountered utterly repugnant epilogues to some vaccinations. "The arms swelled clear to the elbow; yes, clear to the wrist-joint, with high fever and enlargement of the axillary glands; pieces of flesh as big as a dollar and twice as thick would drop right out, leaving ugly suppurating wounds, which to heal took from six weeks to three months. I had to dress a little girl's arm for 15 weeks before it got well. This is not vaccinia, it is sepsis pure and simple, and such a vaccination does not protect against smallpox."

Public confidence in vaccination plummeted in the face of such results, according to Friedrich. A number of times, he witnessed people washing their arms immediately after their vaccinations "to prevent them from getting sore." He later remarked that he could not in good conscience advise vaccination when it produced such terrifying results. "A man would have to have a heart of stone if he would not melt at the sight of the misery which vaccination with impure virus produces. Visit a happy family with your impure virus and make your appearance, at the same house, two weeks later, and you will be horror-stricken with the change that has taken place. Instead of a smile they will receive you with a curse. The father has been thrown out of employment on account of a sore arm, every child is crying with pain, shrieking as soon as they see you come, the mother frantic with fear that next week the family is going to starve, that some child may lose an arm or even its life, and you stand there and witness the tears and cries and pains and misery of which you have been the cause. The man who can stand all that is no man." Under such circumstances, Friedrich asserted that compulsory vaccination would never work in Cleveland because "vaccination is so unpopular that it would prove a dead letter." He found that problems with bad reactions had so severely undermined public confidence in his health department that it could not adequately perform its function. People "became antagonistic instead of working in harmony with us, and hid cases and helped their neighbors hide them, jumped quarantine whenever there was a chance." Friedrich claimed that he had received a "score of letters . . . from all over the country" confirming "that others are having exactly the same experience."[60]

Bostonians heard a lot about Friedrich's solution to vaccination problems in early 1902.[61] The local antivaccinationist physician Charles E. Page summarized Friedrich's experience in testimony before the Joint Committee on Public Health in late January 1902, and the *Boston Evening Record* also published one of Page's letters on Friedrich. In language that must have had particular resonance for city dwellers disgusted with filth and overcrowding, Page described how Friedrich abandoned enforced vaccination and instead "sent an army of inspectors throughout the tenement districts with the power to cleanse."[62] Where vaccination did nothing to change the physical appearance of a city, cleaning it up made sense to many accustomed to thinking of disease as borne by filth and stench. Residents could see, touch, and smell the transformation wrought by a thorough cleansing—a much more satisfying experience than standing in line for vaccinations. Such an experience also had great resonance in an age when municipal reform commonly applied metaphors of cleansing to describe citizens taking back control of corrupt city governments.

A few months later, *The Arena*, a widely read Boston magazine, featured an account of Friedrich's abandonment of compulsory vaccination in favor of disinfection and strict quarantine. Its editor, Benjamin Orange Flower, championed social and political reform, declaring that *The Arena* had a "settled policy . . . to keep abreast of the best progressive thought of the period." Flower celebrated Friedrich's stand as an act of scientific rationalism and political courage that expressed the highest goals of municipal reform. "It would be difficult to overestimate the importance of Dr. Friedrich's victory. He has opened the way for the stamping out of this scourge without running the risk of sowing the seeds of disease or corrupting the blood and endangering the life of the people. His method is strictly scientific and in perfect alignment with twentieth-century thought, and, if promptly acted upon by other municipalities, not only will smallpox be controlled, but there will be a marked diminution in the ravages of other 'germ diseases.'"[63] Flower's article depicted Friedrich as a fearless and incorruptible health officer who would rather risk censure from his peers than bring harm to the health of citizens he had pledged to protect. Though Flower never mentioned the Boston health department's general vaccination order or its chairman, Samuel H. Durgin, perceptive readers could easily infer an unflattering contrast with Friedrich. Flower's warm characterization of Friedrich thus worked as an oblique criticism of Durgin's management of the smallpox epidemic. Learning about Cleveland's success possibly led many to question the wisdom of the Boston and Cambridge health departments' reliance on vaccination over quarantine and stricter sanitation.

Tetanus after Vaccination

If some Bostonians proved reluctant to vaccinate, they had even more reason to fear it in the late summer and fall of 1901 as several Northeastern and Midwestern cities experienced a sharp rise in tetanus cases, outbreaks widely reported as linked to vaccination. Medical experts were puzzled: most textbooks never even mentioned tetanus as a complication of vaccination.[64] An editorial in the *Journal of the American Medical Association* agreed that "the cases of tetanus following [vaccination], so far as known in medical literature, could almost be counted on the ten fingers up to the past year."[65]

No one could deny that instances of tetanus subsequent to vaccination had jumped alarmingly, with forty-five authenticated cases reported for 1901 alone, when previously medical literature had documented only seventeen cases altogether over the last sixty-one years. Such a sharp rise demanded attention and an explanation: these vaccination cases stuck out compared with the incidence of tetanus generally, which had actually declined a bit in these cities. Additionally, these outbreaks occurred only in North America—European countries experienced no increases in this complication. These facts convinced at least one medical expert that "some exceptional condition existed that changed an unimportant and infrequent complication into a very important and frequent one."[66]

In Cleveland, Ohio, four cases of tetanus after vaccination in September added to the health officer Friedrich's woes. Although he still supported vaccination, he later explained that the rash of bad reactions followed by these tetanus cases forced him "to the conclusion that the lymph we used contained more than vaccine, and that vaccination had become a drawback in the fight with smallpox, so I dropped it."[67] In an interview, Friedrich recalled how personal experience with a tetanus victim had forced his decision. "I am a firm supporter of vaccination, but I would rather have one hundred cases of smallpox than one case of lockjaw, for I could do something for smallpox patients but lockjaw is fatal. Some of the virus we get from manufacturers is impure. Nothing is more terrible than a case of tetanus. I remained night and day with a poor girl, who had it, at the City Hospital, but nothing could save her."[68] Eventually, Americans learned of many such cases. To Cleveland's four cases were added eleven in Camden, New Jersey, five in Atlantic City, New Jersey, and twenty-five in Philadelphia from October through December 1901.[69] One medical journal declared: "all over the country are heard more or less positively-expressed suspicions of the purity of much of the vaccine virus at present on the market."[70] For instance, even though a Philadelphia coroner had testified that he did not believe vaccine virus could have caused the tetanus death of six-year-old Maria McGinley, a jury still returned a verdict of traumatic tetanus after vaccination in July 1901.[71] In Florida, Benjamin Higgins sued the city of Jacksonville for $10,000 damages after his wife died from tetanus after her vaccination by the city physician.[72] Additionally, in October and November 1901, at least ten children in St. Louis, Missouri, died from tetanus after inoculation with diphtheria antitoxin. News that a coroner's jury had found positive evidence of tetanus toxin contamination in the St. Louis antitoxin, antitoxin produced by the bacteriologic division of that city's board of health, added to public anxiety about the safety of smallpox vaccine.[73] Anxiety even spread to areas with no reported tetanus cases. In mid-November, parents of four thousand New York City schoolchildren, spurred by reports of seven deaths among the Camden tetanus victims, met to protest vaccination in their schools.[74] The New York County Medical Association consequently felt impelled to investigate the health department's antitoxin and vaccine virus production, despite the absence of any reported cases in their city.[75]

The fact that only a few children developed tetanus in the course of thousands of vaccinations did little to quell public outcry for some positive assurance of vaccine purity. Boston newspapers reported on the Camden and Philadelphia tetanus cases, and one editorial thundered: "To vaccinate a child with infected lymph is a species of murder."[76] In deciding whether to vaccinate their children, parents now had to make a terrible choice, to weigh the slight risk of tetanus attendant upon vaccination against that of contracting smallpox. With no immunization against tetanus yet developed, and the only available treatment a moderately successful antitoxin serum, most physicians agreed that cases of traumatic tetanus usually terminated in an agonizing death.[77] As one medical journal editor sympathized, parents now faced a horrible dilemma: "Smallpox, however possible, is but a possibility, and dreaded principally because of the disfigurement; the present epidemic is a mild one, and at its worst, smallpox has none of the terrors of lockjaw. Parents will choose the lesser evil and refuse to allow their children to be vaccinated."[78] Robert Willson, a Philadelphia physician who had treated many tetanus victims, affirmed that possible contamination of vaccine virus posed a great problem for medicine: "no question of modern medicine has appealed with more urgency to both physician and patient."[79]

George M. Gould, the editor of the Philadelphia-based *American Medicine*, noted that antivaccinationists quickly incorporated the tetanus cases into their arguments. "The tetanus complication in vaccine and diphtheria inoculations is arousing the hopes of the antimedicals of the whole world, and they are filling their own periodicals and all others to which they can gain admission with screams of 'medical murder,' etc. . . . It would be a terrible public calamity if because of some minor error we should be stampeded by fright and ignorant prejudice into forgetfulness of our foremost duty of safeguarding the public health." Gould worried that these tetanus cases had heightened public anxiety over vaccination at the worst possible time. Antivaccinationist literature, in his opinion, just exacerbated that fear, fomenting panic that could have lasting repercussions for public health. To repair public trust in vaccination, he called for its suspension in places where tetanus cases had occurred, pending an "immediate and thorough" investigation.[80] A week later, Gould despaired that the tetanus cases may have caused real damage to the public's acceptance of vaccination: "Meanwhile the profession has lost much hard-gained ground in the cause of vaccination and we must fight the wearisome battle harder than ever, else in a few years the scourge will sweep across the country in virulent form, and the pitted and the blind will haunt us to our graves."[81] Public health officials had to act quickly to restore confidence in the safety of vaccinations. Thus various health departments throughout the region launched special inquiries into the purity of vaccine lymph.

The conclusions of some official investigations, however, did little to satisfy a skeptical public. The Camden Board of Health, for instance, found "absolutely no evidence to show the vaccine used was contaminated."[82] And a committee of the Medical Society of the State of New Jersey reported that its investigation found no fault with vaccinators' technique, only that "certain atmospheric conditions, for example, a long period of dry weather and high winds, explained the outbreak."[83] Yet Rueben Swinburne Clymer, a Pennsylvania antivaccinationist physician, disparaged official explanations that cited exceptionally dusty conditions as the cause for the increased tetanus cases: "It strikes one as very singular that the germs in the street dust of Camden, Philadelphia and St. Louis selected only persons who had been vaccinated; and very wonderful that the germs crawled up shirt sleeves and crowded under the bandages and plasters covering the vaccinated portions of the victims' arms."[84] If tetanus germs were so prevalent in the air, then why were there not more tetanus cases generally? Months later an editorial in the *Journal of the American Medical Association* complained this continuing discrepancy "is a question that disturbs the laity and helps the antivaccination cause."[85]

Most physicians also refused to believe that either the vaccine or their technique could have caused tetanus. Instead they blamed patients' and their families' carelessness and ignorance. In 1901, the Pennsylvania State Board of Health adopted a resolution that faulted victims rather than physicians: "It has yet to be shown that vaccine virus ever contains or becomes contaminated with the germ of tetanus; when such an occurrence takes place it is because, owing to the carelessness, usually on the part of the person vaccinated, the germs of tetanus gain access to the wound on the arm as they may to any other wound, abrasion or scratch upon the surface."[86] The Vermont physician Lyman Allen also blamed tetanus victims for insufficient care of their vaccination wounds: "the laity seem to think that the ulcer of vaccination is different from other ulcerations, and that it should be left unprotected and untreated."[87] When four-year-old "Della B." contracted tetanus after vaccination in early spring of 1901, the family doctor Willis S. Cooke absolved himself and the vaccine of any responsibility for her illness. "The vaccine was, without doubt, above suspicion, and I do not think my method of application was at fault, because I have always felt that surgical cleanliness was as essential in this as in any other operation, and have acted accordingly. . . . The child was sent into the country shortly after the wound was made, and, the weather being warm, was allowed to play out of doors. Dust and dirt carrying the germs settled on the legs and perspiration washed it into the sore."[88] Since he had vaccinated the older sister at the same time with no untoward result, Cooke felt reasonably sure that the vaccine itself could not have introduced tetanus germs, although he placed a protective shield over the sore. He blamed the girl's father not only for sending her away to the country and thus exposing her to barnyard dirt, but also for failing to bring her back for an examination a week after the vaccination.

Similarly, the Philadelphia physician Robert N. Willson, reporting on a case of tetanus after vaccination, refused to accuse the vaccinating physician directly, though he criticized the common practice of placing a celluloid shield over the vaccination. Although the shield was intended to protect the sore, instead the covering sealed it and thus provided, he thought, the perfect anaerobic environment for tetanus germs. Rather than condemn any colleague, however, he decried the public for its ignorance about germs and looked to the father of the vaccinated toddler for the source of infection. "Irritation by shirt and sleeve and a popular prejudice against cleansing even a healing vaccine sore, combined, as is usually the case, to invite any and every possible source of infection to contribute its willing mite or magnificence to the ruin of the unlucky subject. . . . My own case could not but have been repeatedly exposed to contact with the person of the father [a coachman], and thus to the bacilli that caused the disease."[89]

In another article looking at over fifty cases of tetanus, Willson concluded in each case that interference with the vaccination sore seemed the most likely explanation for the tetanus infections. One involved a ten-year-old boy who liked "to finger the wound and exhibit it to his playmates" and "to pound his arm violently with his fist, apparently to show them that it did not hurt." Willson argued that the tetanus bacillus is "always found in the dirt of the street," and since many of the tetanus cases occurred just as the scab fell off, about twenty days after the vaccination, tetanus had to come from secondary infection of the vaccine site, not from the vaccine.[90] Some conscientious parents of tetanus victims may have regarded such explanations as self-serving and conflicting. What were they to do? Lock their children up? Bind their arms and legs? Use a shield or leave it off? Clean the sore or leave it alone?

The physician Joseph McFarland, professor of pathology and bacteriology at the Medico-Chirurgical College at Philadelphia, reached a different conclusion. McFarland, formerly employed by the H. K. Mulford Company, one of the biggest vaccine producers, had recently taken a position with Parke-Davis, a rival pharmaceutical company.[91] In early 1902, he analyzed the relationship between tetanus cases and brands of vaccine virus used, including that of his former employer. He originally thought he would find nothing wrong and hoped this would enhance the reputation of vaccination. He lamented that the Camden cases "have been so exploited in the newspapers, and have been made the subject of so many editorials and comments in the medical press, that they will, no doubt, form the starting point of numerous future attacks against vaccination."[92] Yet in an early paper, McFarland arrived at the disquieting conclusion that "there is a very intimate relationship between vaccine virus and tetanus, and that at times tetanus bacilli are contained in the virus."[93] In his published article, he found that with the exception of one person, all the tetanus victims had been vaccinated with a certain brand of virus, which he identified only as "virus E," a product of one of the "largest manufacturers." Even worse, this type of vaccine, the "supposedly best and most refined preparation," was glycerinated lymph.[94] Although McFarland did not name that manufacturer in his published article, it was his old employer, H. K. Mulford. Quick to jump on any opportunity to secure an advantage, Mulford's longtime rival H. M. Alexander used the opportunity to indict glycerinated lymph while proclaiming the safety of its dry points in a heated public relations battle.[95] The ensuing dispute only added to public qualms about the safety of vaccination and impelled Congress to pass the 1902 Biologics Control Act to provide for limited federal oversight of vaccine production.

A year later, Milton J. Rosenau of the United States Public Health and Marine Hospital Service's hygienic laboratory confirmed that "tetanus spores may live a long time in vaccine virus," finding them "alive and virulent" for nearly a year both on dry points and in glycerinated lymph. Although the spores lost virulence over time and did not produce tetanus when injected into mice, they "may be revived into active virulent cultures by growing in fresh bouillon under favorable conditions."[96] Thus although Rosenau did not directly link contaminated vaccine virus to the tetanus outbreaks, his study indicated its possibility given the right circumstances.

Cases of tetanus after vaccination appeared in Boston and Cambridge as well. In late December 1901, the *Boston Journal* reported the tetanus death of five-year-old Annie Caswell of Cambridge. Vaccinated on 17 December by Dr. Charles Dudley, Annie developed symptoms of lockjaw nine days later. Although "every precaution was taken" in the aftercare of her vaccination, and Dr. C. T. Weeks administered antitetanus serum, she died two days after the onset of symptoms.[97] A Cambridge newspaper reported that her attending physicians "believe that the vaccine used might have been impure or that some foreign substance may have gotten into the sore and caused lockjaw." Her death certificate listed tetanus as the principal cause of death, with vaccination as the contributing cause.[98] Later in early 1902, her mother testified about her daughter's agonizing death before the Massachusetts Legislature's Joint Public Health Committee.[99] Nineteen-year-old Christina Jorgensen, daughter of the captain of the Nantucket shoals lightship, also died of tetanus a few weeks after her vaccination of 4 December 1901.[100] Several Boston newspapers recounted her father's dramatic efforts to reach her through rough seas after learning by telegraph of his daughter's dire condition.[101]

Joseph Greene collected stories of tetanus deaths from all over the United States, reporting on the lockjaw cases in Cleveland, Ohio, just weeks after they occurred.[102] Writing of the tetanus death of a Philadelphia girl, he noted that "her crazed father threatened to shoot the doctor who performed the operation."[103] In various issues of *The Animals' Defender*, Greene repeatedly raised the issue of tetanus as well as other complications after vaccination, giving names, addresses, and dates for specific afflicted individuals.[104] He listed victims like "the little daughter of Victor Jarrett, 35 Hancock St., Boston," a child who "was healthy and strong" at the time of her vaccination, yet succumbed to tetanus shortly afterward.[105] He quoted parents like "Mrs. Brower of 217 North Front Street, the mother of one of the victims," who cried, "'Never, never again shall I have one of my children vaccinated.'"[106] Poignant tales of death and suffering after vaccination rapidly spread throughout the Boston area, becoming a common feature in the antivaccination and antivivisection press and pamphlet literature.

Other sources indicate that people in the Boston and Cambridge area particularly feared tetanus contamination. In early 1902, Harvard president Charles W. Eliot complained to the press that antivaccinationists stirred up anxiety about vaccination: "The antivaccinationists try to scare us by telling of horrible and loathsome diseases caused by vaccination. They point to cases of lockjaw."[107] A few months earlier, a Boston physician tried to alleviate qualms about the safety of the city's vaccine virus. Noting that many Bostonians retained "a prejudice against free vaccination, because some people have an idea that the vaccination is not always good," George W. Galvin offered free vaccinations to all Emergency Hospital certificate holders, declaring their apprehensions about tetanus unfounded. "Much prejudice has been aroused by a few cases of lockjaw reported caused by vaccination, but the danger from such a result is almost absolutely nil. I am positive there is no bad virus on the market, and there is absolutely no danger from lockjaw, if the vaccination is made under proper conditions. That is, there should be absolute cleanliness, and the operation should be made in such a way that there is no danger from contamination by sweat, dirt, cold, etc. Then lockjaw is impossible."[108] Some entrepreneurs in the Boston area believed dread of tetanus after vaccination offered a market niche for their product, antibacterial powder: "It's the only safeguard, and if proper steps are taken there will be no pain, swelling, itching or disagreeable sensations following vaccination or dangers from tetanus (lockjaw), if the scarification is treated with Anti-bacteria Powder."[109] In ads placed prominently on the first page of the *Boston Post* and laid out to look at first glance like Board of Health notices, the Bactil Chemical Company sought to capitalize on disquiet about tetanus and aftereffects of vaccination.[110] Thus tetanus after vaccination, though rare, became an important source of doubt about the safety of the vaccine virus currently on offer.

Doubt about the safety of commercial vaccine afflicted Boston's chief health officer, Samuel Durgin, as well. On 3 December 1901, he announced his intention to petition the legislature for authorization to manufacture vaccine lymph.[111] This was not the first time that Durgin had attempted to convince the Massachusetts legislators of the need for state control of vaccine production. Several years earlier, a similar petition had been "defeated by the active opposition of certain local producers."[112] Now, in the face of a smallpox epidemic, he sought to try again.

Durgin's determination to wrest control of vaccine production from private businesses might have caused thoughtful citizens to wonder about the health department's confidence in the quality of vaccine it currently purchased from those same firms—lymph that it offered free to the public at city vaccination stations. As news of these tetanus cases spread, interest in vaccination waned. By the second week of December, demand for vaccination dropped off so drastically

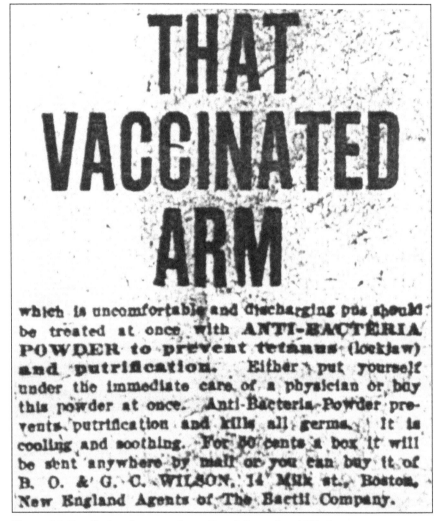

Figure 4.2. Bactil advertisement. *Boston Post*, 2 December 1901, 1.

that Durgin decided to close the free vaccination stations even though he worried that a huge proportion of Boston's inhabitants remained unprotected against smallpox.[113] Then on 26 December, Durgin ordered citywide compulsory vaccination. Publicity about tetanus cases incited public squeamishness about vaccination, and Durgin concluded that only compulsion would resolve the situation. Yet such was his concern for commerce that he deliberately held up the order until after the Christmas season ended, even though he knew any delay meant that the unvaccinated would mix with ambulant and unrecognized smallpox cases in the department stores and streetcars of Boston.[114]

One newspaper editor acknowledged the dampening effect of the Christina Jorgenson and Annie Caswell cases, declaring they "have recalled the New Jersey cases to people's minds, and brought some measure of anxiety home to us."[115] Seeking to assuage these fears, Durgin confidently declared that vaccine lymph itself could not cause tetanus, but rather tetanus resulted from the recipient's poor hygiene. Tetanus deaths thus "need worry nobody. Think of the thousands upon thousands who have rushed to be vaccinated!"[116] Despite Durgin's public confidence in the purity of vaccine lymph, an editorial in the same paper that day, which supported vaccination, admitted that in "one case it is stated that the germ of lockjaw can be laid to the vaccine virus."[117] Such an admission hardly encouraged public confidence in the safety of vaccination. Later, in June 1902, the same newspaper acknowledged this situation in a short editorial note supporting state production of vaccine lymph: "One case of lockjaw in the city itself and one in Belmont, both traced by the attending physicians to the bacillus of lockjaw in the vaccine—have helped greatly to create the present situation. The people saw the results of impure vaccine and dreaded to take the risk."[118] Like the people living in and around Boston, many throughout the Eastern seaboard and the Midwest greatly feared the possibility, however remote, of contracting tetanus after vaccination. A Pennsylvania newspaper editor worried that vaccination thus produced a stark life or death lottery: "What is impure virus? How is it to be distinguished from that which is fit for use? The test seems to be on a level with the old example of the toadstool and mushroom: if it's a mushroom you live and if it's a toadstool you die."[119] When faced with such dire consequences, and having no way to assure the quality of the vaccine, people thus hesitated at the prospect of vaccination. Despite the fact that tetanus afflicted only a handful of thousands vaccinated, fear of that slight possibility made people stop to ponder the risks of vaccination—a dangerous procrastination in the face of smallpox. And the potential for other complications also provoked much stalling over vaccination at that time.

Incidents of vaccination failure, cases of bad effects, injury, and even death after vaccination mounted in the summer and fall of 1901 and continued into 1902. Such cases not only increased public anxiety about vaccination but they also worried health officials sufficiently that they sought to gain control over vaccine production. Taken together, physicians' mistakes in smallpox diagnosis, ignorance of proper vaccination, and problems with inert or contaminated vaccine lymph shook public confidence in the basic safety and efficacy of vaccination and the ability of their physicians to administer it. Accounts of injury and tragedy after vaccination further rattled their nerves. Faced with smallpox so mild, vaccination with all its risks appeared unwarranted. Many simply put it off until either coerced by employers or compelled by law to get it done.

Expectation of severe effects made many people nervous about vaccination. When a motorman on the Brookline division of the Boston elevated railroad came down with smallpox, the company ordered vaccinations for all employees. Although they "submitted patiently," many did so with reservations, according to the *Boston Post*: "There was many a groan and grimace of pain, and many a man who begged for the postponement of the operation in his particular case, but the authorities were inexorable and each and every one was put through the terrible ordeal regardless of 'ill health,' 'sick wife' or 'previous vaccination' subterfuges."[120] Perhaps the reporter was a bit facetious in describing vaccination as a "terrible ordeal," but many of the men evidently would have avoided vaccination if given the choice. Other articles also hint at a general underlying distaste for vaccination among the public. For instance, the *Evening Transcript* explained why businesses preferred to vaccinate their employees on the job rather than leave it up to each individual: "It is easier for them than for the city to overcome the natural public aversion for the operation, and they reach a great many who would never think of going to any of the free vaccination stations opened by the Board of Health, much less think of employing a private physician to inoculate them." By describing the aversion to vaccination as "natural," this writer recognized that people had reason to believe it was a grueling operation. The article also hinted that this "aversion" stemmed from past experience with vaccination by concluding that "as a rule vaccination is done with more care than in former years."[121]

The vast majority of Boston and Cambridge residents may not have directly challenged vaccination, but they certainly seemed skittish about it. Harvard president Charles W. Eliot pointed out that a number of wealthy families avoided vaccinating their children because some of Boston's "best-known homeopathic physicians in the Back Bay" advised against it.[122] Eliot strongly supported vaccination, and he reminded his interviewer not to make too much of these physicians' adherence to homeopathy: the Massachusetts Homeopathic Medical Society had recently passed a resolution supporting vaccination.[123]

Some prominent figures avoided vaccination with sad results. In Weymouth, Massachusetts, Father J. J. Murphy, unvaccinated since childhood, neglected to get vaccinated even though his archbishop advised vaccination. After attending a smallpox patient in his town's pesthouse, he then visited Boston and contracted a mild case of smallpox. Having "no idea of the nature of his affliction," he continued his pastoral work in the community.[124] Father Murphy ignored his archbishop by neglecting to vaccinate and then knowingly exposed himself to smallpox. Weymouth had offered free vaccination to all its citizens for months. Given the health department pleas for vaccination, such inaction suggests that he regarded vaccination as useless or dangerous.

One of Boston's highest city officials also avoided vaccination, with dire results. City Councilman George A. Flynn (featured in the previous chapter) had not bothered to get vaccinated nor thought it necessary to vaccinate his family, even after he sought a physician's care for his smallpox symptoms. As a result, he infected his unvaccinated wife, who contracted it in severe form and died. Although Councilman Flynn "was entirely ignorant of the nature of his malady," the fact that neither he nor his wife sought vaccination at all shows that they did not consider it warranted even during an epidemic.[125] Flynn's family physician, equally ignorant, did not recommend vaccination even as a general precaution. An attitude of wariness toward vaccination appears to underlie this

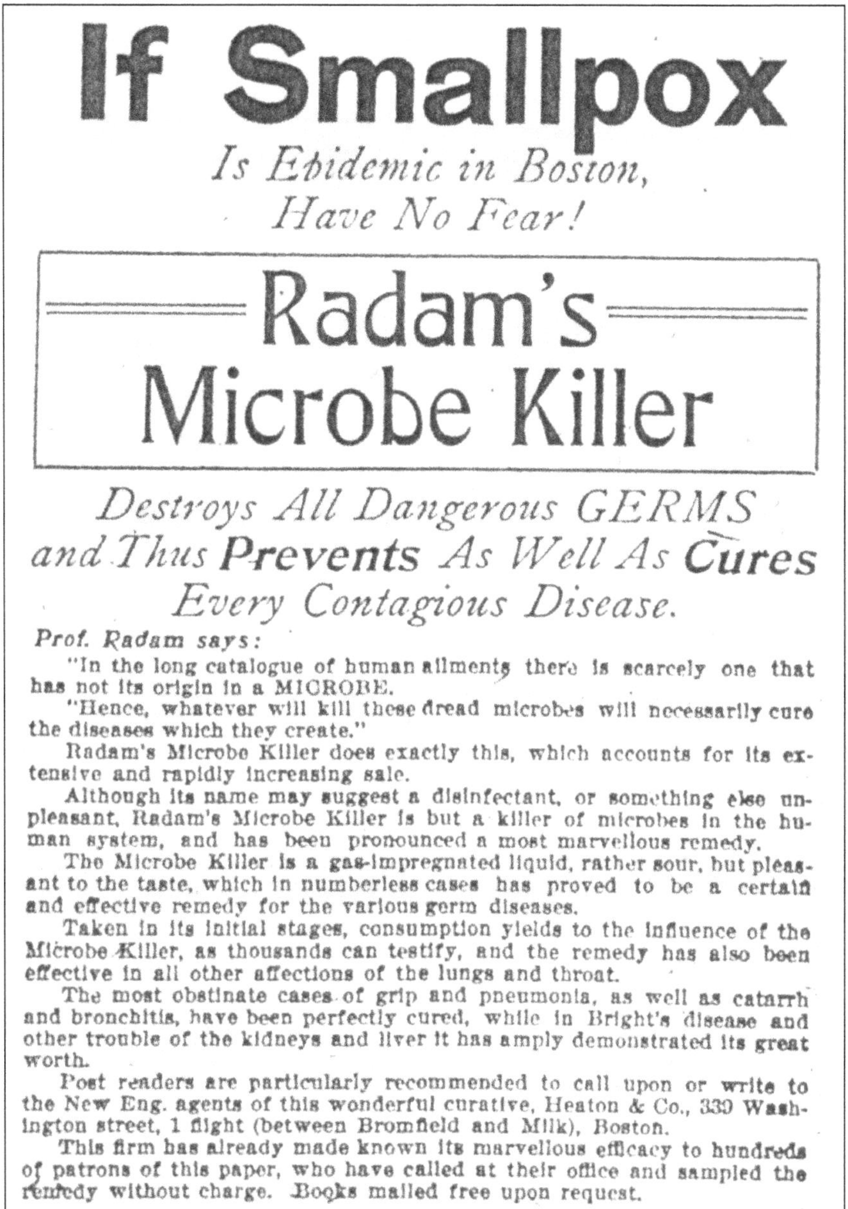

If Smallpox

Is Epidemic in Boston,
Have No Fear!

Radam's
Microbe Killer

Destroys All Dangerous GERMS
and Thus **Prevents** *As Well As* **Cures**
Every Contagious Disease.

Prof. Radam says:

"In the long catalogue of human ailments there is scarcely one that has not its origin in a MICROBE.

"Hence, whatever will kill these dread microbes will necessarily cure the diseases which they create."

Radam's Microbe Killer does exactly this, which accounts for its extensive and rapidly increasing sale.

Although its name may suggest a disinfectant, or something else unpleasant, Radam's Microbe Killer is but a killer of microbes in the human system, and has been pronounced a most marvellous remedy.

The Microbe Killer is a gas-impregnated liquid, rather sour, but pleasant to the taste, which in numberless cases has proved to be a certain and effective remedy for the various germ diseases.

Taken in its initial stages, consumption yields to the influence of the Microbe Killer, as thousands can testify, and the remedy has also been effective in all other affections of the lungs and throat.

The most obstinate cases of grip and pneumonia, as well as catarrh and bronchitis, have been perfectly cured, while in Bright's disease and other trouble of the kidneys and liver it has amply demonstrated its great worth.

Post readers are particularly recommended to call upon or write to the New Eng. agents of this wonderful curative, Heaton & Co., 339 Washington street, 1 flight (between Bromfield and Milk), Boston.

This firm has already made known its marvellous efficacy to hundreds of patrons of this paper, who have called at their office and sampled the remedy without charge. Books mailed free upon request.

Figure 4.3. Radam's Microbe Killer advertisement. *Boston Post*, 4 December 1901, 7.

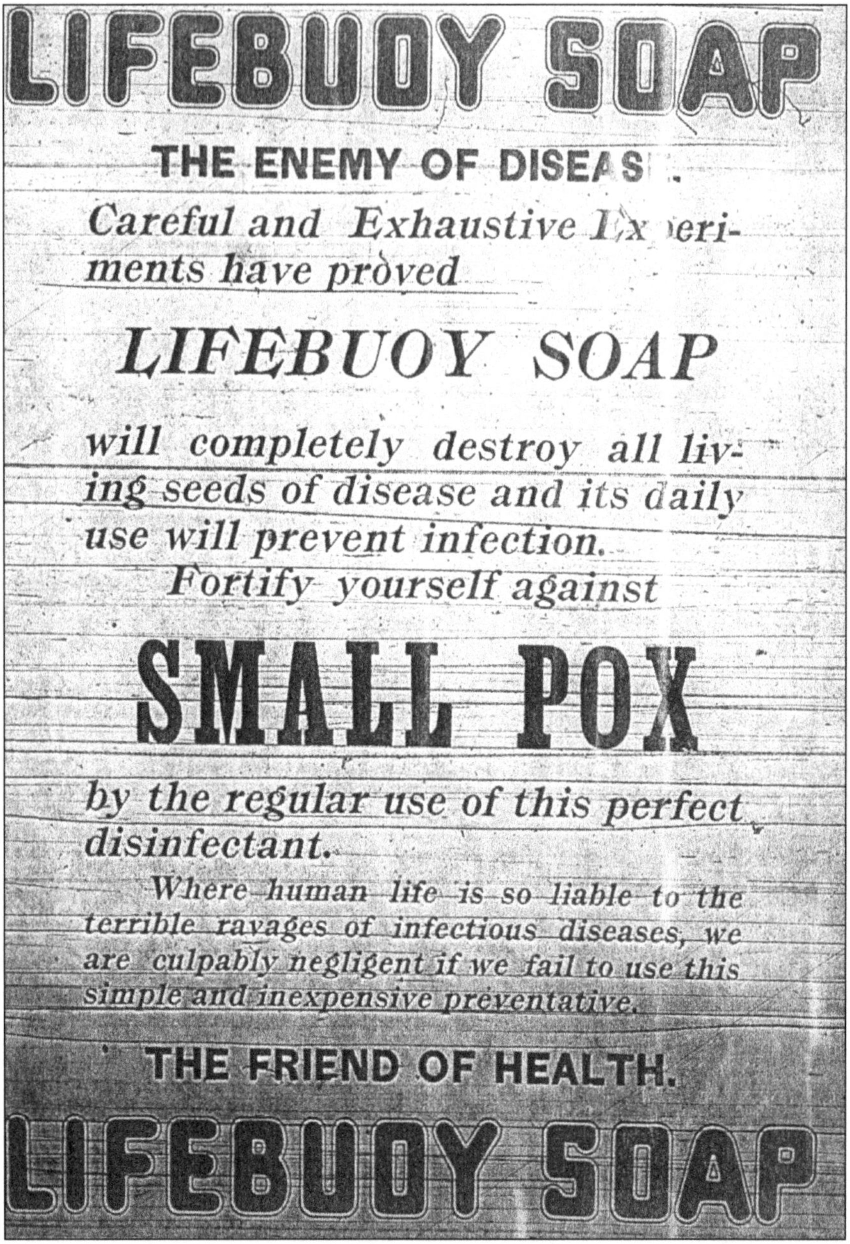

Figure 4.4. Advertisement for Lifebuoy soap. *Cambridge Chronicle*, 28 June 1902, 3.

tragedy—wariness on the Flynns' part as well as that of their family doctor. How else do we explain a public official's failure to obtain vaccinations for himself and his family during an epidemic? How do we explain the physician's failure to advise vaccination? They all feared vaccination more than they did smallpox.

Advertisements indicate that many people sought protection from smallpox through other means and that they suspected vaccination alone did not protect against smallpox. Several manufacturers of medicines, soaps, and disinfectants seemed to believe that a substantial market existed for their products when sold as smallpox preventatives, and their advertisements for various disinfectant liquids, vapors, and pills purporting to kill smallpox germs appeared in Boston and Cambridge newspapers. Radam's Microbe Killer, "a gas-impregnated liquid, rather sour, but pleasant to the taste," promised both to prevent and cure "every contagious disease" in an advertisement entitled "If Smallpox Is Epidemic in Boston, Have No Fear!"[126]

Another notice placed strategically beneath a vaccination station announcement claimed "smallpox germs killed by inhaling" G.G. Disinfectant vapor.[127] Advertised under the heading "Smallpox Prevented," Coomb's Germicide Tablets claimed to render "the blood germ proof, without harm, even to children."[128] And if pills, liquids, and vapors failed to do the trick, washing with Lifebuoy soap might serve to dispel any extra qualms about catching smallpox: "Careful and Exhaustive Experiments have proved LIFEBUOY SOAP will completely destroy all living seeds of disease and its daily use will prevent infection. Fortify yourself against SMALL POX by the regular use of this disinfectant."[129] These advertisers clearly aimed at reaping a profit from anxiety about smallpox with a sales pitch that targeted both people who lacked confidence in their vaccinations and those who had avoided vaccination altogether.

Both physicians and laypersons at the turn of the century understood that vaccination involved a lot more than a simple prick or scrape on an arm. Vaccination was a serious medical procedure that could incapacitate a person for days if not weeks. In 1901-2 it became even more problematic as more vaccinations than ever before went awry. Antivaccinationists quickly publicized every instance of death or injury that seemed to implicate vaccination, causing many in Boston and Cambridge to approach it with a great deal of apprehension. Many thoughtful people stalled as long as possible or avoided it altogether. Rather than accept vaccination as standard state-of-the-art protection against smallpox, many regarded it instead as controversial and argued for alternative preventive strategies. Thus it is not surprising to learn that people generally put off vaccination, submitting to it only because their employers or health department officials backed up by policemen demanded it.

Chapter Five

Massachusetts Antivaccinationists

Problems with contaminated or inert vaccine frustrated many physicians and led to widespread public anxiety about the safety of vaccination in 1901–2. Although many people worried about vaccination and avoided it, only a few actually stepped up to organize antivaccination societies, write about the dangers of vaccination, and lobby their state legislators for repeal of compulsory laws. Those who adopted a public stance against vaccination had varying motivations. Some antivaccinationists emphasized the antidemocratic nature of compulsion and coercion, others resented any state laws or regulations that interfered with private medical judgment about their patients, and still others questioned the propriety of compelling vaccination when the state could not ensure its safety. Many antivaccinationists felt that public health officials and medical societies displayed an unscientific attitude by refusing to acknowledge well-documented problems with vaccination. By the turn of the twentieth century, a loose network of antivaccination activists and physicians came together in Boston to organize formally as the Massachusetts Anti-compulsory Vaccination Society (MACVS).

Antivaccinationists were not cranks, crazy, or the lunatic fringe, despite the derogatory comments of their opponents. The New Englanders attracted to antivaccination tended to be well educated and socially respected by virtue of their lineage at a time when such backgrounds mattered a lot. Some of them were physicians trained at the best schools in the United States and even Europe. It would be a mistake to assume that their rhetoric about civil rights meant that they all opposed state action in public health, social justice, or the economy. These Massachusetts antivaccinationists were not antigovernment libertarians, but instead thoughtful people who posed legitimate questions about state interference in individual health matters, matters that they believed should remain between the patient and his or her doctor. They called for government regulations to ensure better living and working conditions for the poor as well as pure food and water. They supported traditional public health measures by insisting on strict adherence to quarantine, isolation of the sick, street cleaning, and disinfection—all tactics that invaded, disrupted, or damaged businesses, lives, and property. Some of them demanded government regulation of the vaccine market. In this, they looked to the past, to time-honored police power traditions rather than to the new public health that focused on individuals as carriers of disease. They wanted their local governments to do more, not less, to control smallpox. Additionally, many of them thought that AMA support for compulsory vaccination represented one facet of a monopolistic impulse that sought to bring American medicine under the control of a select elite. Their concern for civil liberty in medicine did not mean that they sought to diminish the role of government in their lives. Instead they wanted government to ensure fairness in the medical marketplace as well as respect for their personal health concerns. If any label has to be attached to antivaccination, populism is far more appropriate than libertarianism.

Public Health Authorities and Antivaccination in 1902

In a talk given to an audience of Massachusetts health officers in early 1902, the Boston city physician Thomas B. Shea argued that health officials could not afford to shrug off antivaccinationists as a minor nuisance—they distributed dangerous literature that had convinced people to refuse vaccination even after exposure to smallpox. Shea blamed antivaccinationists for exacerbating the current smallpox epidemic. He recalled meeting a nurse attending a smallpox victim who had never been vaccinated because she did not "believe in it." Despite all his persuasive efforts, she refused vaccination and came down with smallpox. Although she survived, Shea lamented that smallpox had left her "disfigured, utterly useless for her calling," speculating that "she would much prefer to have died rather than to have recovered." He also recalled the case of an unvaccinated young man whose smallpox ended fatally. "Gentlemen, what legacy do you think he left his father? In searching through his effects, a circular issued by our friends, the anti-vaccinationists, was found in his pocket; and his father said that that accounted for his obstinacy in refusing to be vaccinated. His father and the rest of the family had been vaccinated within three months successfully, and this young man refused vaccination; and he paid dearly for his convictions. He went to the hospital, and he died within seventy-two hours."

Shea went on to describe the most horrific case of all: a family (like many in Boston) that put off vaccination as long as possible. The father and mother "were anti-vaccinationists," but they had their two school-age children vaccinated in order to attend public school, yet left their two younger children unvaccinated. When smallpox struck the father, the mother remained so steadfast in her antivaccination convictions that she still refused vaccination for herself and her two unvaccinated children. When she developed smallpox, the health department shipped her off to the isolation hospital and immediately vaccinated the children. One child came down with a mild case, while the other remained well. Both parents unfortunately died, leaving their children orphans and, Shea conjectured, "I suppose wards of the State." In his opinion, tragedies like these could have been prevented. Antivaccinationists had a lot to answer for. "Gentlemen, those are some of the results that we have found in Boston to-day as the result of anti-vaccination. And that is the reason, and the only reason, that small-pox is in Boston to-day and the other cities of this Commonwealth. It is because people refuse vaccination."[1] Shea felt that

Boston's antivaccinationists had raised enough doubt about the efficacy and safety of vaccination to impede health department vaccination efforts. Now they posed an even greater threat: that they might convince the state legislature to abolish compulsory vaccination altogether.

Antivaccinationists particularly frustrated Samuel Holmes Durgin, chairman of the Boston Board of Health. He complained bitterly in his 1902 *Annual Report* that they had sabotaged his vaccination campaign. "A serious drawback to our vaccinal protection against smallpox arises from the fact that Boston is practically a hot-bed of the anti-vaccine heresy, and although the vaccine house is built upon a rock, and is not likely to fall, the noisy storm has frightened many of our people into a dangerous neglect or opposition to vaccinal protection."[2] Germinating in Boston's "hot-bed"—a "hot-bed" is composted earth that promotes rapid growth of seedlings—antivaccination seemed to spring up in full bloom that year. Although Durgin usually adopted an objective stance in his annual reports, antivaccinationatists so frustrated him that he dropped into metaphorical and biblical terms to describe the situation.

In language that equated vaccination with a religion whose creed demanded absolute obedience, Durgin branded antivaccinationists not simply as his adversaries but as heretics, the worst sort of offenders. By declaring that "the vaccine house is built on a rock" he referred to a New Testament conversation between Jesus and his chief disciple, Peter: "You are Peter, the Rock; and on this rock I will build my church, and the powers of death shall never conquer it."[3] By asserting that vaccination stood on a similar unshakeable foundation, the "rock" of scientific medicine, Durgin implied that ignorant laypersons or renegade physicians had no standing to dispute its decisions. Opposition to compulsory vaccination indeed seemed quite heretical to him.

Durgin's outburst against antivaccination demonstrates just how deeply leading medical men like him revered vaccination's iconic status and how embattled they felt about it. Embarrassed as well—Durgin had to admit in his official report that antivaccinationists had stymied his efforts despite his power to leverage considerable legal authority to compel vaccination.[4]

Antivaccination at the Turn of the Century

Since 1855, Massachusetts state law had required parents or guardians to vaccinate their children before the age of two and forbade public schools to admit any unvaccinated pupils. It obliged large mills and factories to vaccinate their operatives and public institutions such as jails, poorhouses, orphanages, and asylums to vaccinate their inmates. It also granted local boards of health the power to order the vaccination and revaccination of all inhabitants during smallpox epidemics.[5] In 1882, the Hyde Park resident Alfred Ellingwood Giles published *The Iniquity of Compulsory Vaccination*, hoping that it would "aid towards the speedy repeal of those insidious ruthless iniquities—the Massachusetts *Compulsory* Vaccination Statutes."[6] Citing British and American medical authorities but also sources like the 1874 *Annual Report of the Massachusetts Board of Health,* Giles argued that they routinely acknowledged vaccination's injurious effects. He likened disputes over various medical theories and practices to quarrels over religion: "All men in Massachusetts have an equal right . . . to their respective religious opinions and practices. Why should they not all have an equal right . . . to their respective medical opinions and practices?" Splintered into sects with their own schools and societies, medicine looked more like a medley of competing religious denominations than a monolithic profession to most Americans. Giles believed that if both state and federal constitutions protected freedom of religious belief and practice, that right should extend to individual health as well. "Surely the Legislature has no rightful power to imperil that good health, by compelling its possessor to submit himself to the disputed theories and experiments of the doctors." Giles noted that physicians disagreed about vaccination: "Some doctors and some people believe that vaccination prevents small-pox; and other doctors and other people, equally intelligent, that it . . . tends to produce small-pox and many other diseases." He argued that in the face of medical controversy over vaccination, legislatures should refrain from making laws that compelled it. "It is not the legitimate business of the Legislature to select, or to favor any one of the many existing medical systems and theories of the doctors, nor is it good policy, to attempt to coerce any one of the inhabitants, much less all the people, to take any particular one's medicines, or to submit to his practices; any more than it is its function to establish a particular religious system, and to compel people's acceptance of it."[7] This point—that states should not make laws forcing people to favor one medical system over another—would remain at the heart of American antivaccinationists' arguments for many years to come.

In 1894, the venerated antislavery activist William Lloyd Garrison, along with other Massachusetts citizens, petitioned for the abolition of compulsory vaccination in three separate bills. Another group petitioned for an amendment to allow unvaccinated children to attend public school.[8] Although these abolition bills each failed to pass out of committee, the legislature substantially altered the vaccination law that year. Another bill sought to strengthen the vaccination law by mandating that all public school pupils must show certificates of vaccination. This effort backfired when the testimony of Boston physician William B. Sanders instead persuaded state legislators to amend it to allow sickly or weak children a reprieve from the requirement.[9] The vague language of the amended law did not explicitly spell out the conditions under which a physician could certify unfitness. Nor did it even require the physician to personally examine the child before issuing a certificate. Thus a registered physician could certify any child—even through the mail—as unfit for vaccination and that child could still attend public school with no questions asked.[10] Antivaccinationist parents enthusiastically took advantage of this amendment to send their unvaccinated children to school, much to the consternation of public health officials.

Inspired perhaps by the new law, the Springfield physician Charles Wardell Amerige compiled thirty-two pages of medical testimony against vaccination in his 1895 pamphlet *Vaccination a Curse.*[11] Amerige may have hoped to generate publicity for his practice and to enhance a less than savory reputation after achieving unwelcome notoriety in 1893, when he was charged with conspiring to commit a healthy patient to an insane asylum at the behest of the man's wife. Over the course of his trial, testimony about his unorthodox medical practice, reliance on mesmerism, and diploma-mill academic credentials damaged his reputation among his peers.[12]

Contending that "it is a mystery why the practice has not been legally forbidden, instead of legally enforced, among a free and enlightened people," Amerige exhorted his readers "to exert every power to save their innocent children from further contamination by vaccination" by repealing the vaccination laws "to protect your children."[13] Citing various medical authorities, he argued that vaccination led to erysipelas, tuberculosis, syphilis, and even tooth decay. Like many antivaccinationists, Amerige supported his polemic against vaccination with quotations and statistics drawn from medical journals and treatises. Most lay and even many medically trained readers could not easily dismiss his evidence. Only physicians with intimate knowledge of the medical texts in question could easily spot quotations taken out of context or question Amerige's interpretations of the data.

Amerige's tract conveniently served to align him with a select group of potential clients seeking exemption certificates for their children and it circulated for years among antivaccinationists. Eight years later, *The Liberator* listed his pamphlet at a price of 10 cents a copy in advertisements for antivaccination literature.[14] It was still circulating thirteen years later when the Boston antivaccinationist and social reformer Aurin F. Hill presented it to the legislature in 1908.[15]

Sometime in the late 1890s, an antivaccination network of writers, physicians, speakers, and editors began to coalesce around Joseph M. Greene of Dorchester, Massachusetts. In 1890, Greene wrote a prizewinning essay against vivisection for a contest sponsored by George Thorndike Angell, president of the American Humane Education Society. Five years later, Greene founded the New England Anti-vivisection Society (NEAVS) with the Boston attorney Philip G. Peabody, who had served as judge in the contest. A number of prominent Bostonians joined NEAVS, including the physician Henry J. Bigelow, the *Boston Evening Transcript* editor in chief Edward Clemont, and the author Abby Morton Diaz.[16] Greene became the corresponding secretary and treasurer for the society and also edited its journal, *The Animals' Defender*. In the late 1890s he became a fixture in Massachusetts medical politics as one of the most visible and vocal antivivisectionists, testifying at State House hearings and excoriating Massachusetts Institute of Technology professor William T. Sedgwick, Harvard president Charles W. Eliot, and professor Henry P. Bowditch for promoting animal experimentation.[17]

Greene used his editorial authority on behalf of antivaccination as well in *The Animals' Defender* and displayed the 1894 exemption law prominently in each issue for the edification of its readers.[18] He exhorted them to "fall back upon the State law as it now stands," declaring, "there are honest and enlightened physicians . . . who would gladly give this testimony in every case."[19] Greene did not rely on words alone—he took an active role in antivaccination by coordinating from his office a network of accommodating physicians who furnished exemption certificates practically on demand. In his 1901 two-page pamphlet *Vaccination Is the Curse of Childhood,* he offered to connect any applicant with "hundreds of physicians in Massachusetts who are well aware of the uselessness and evil effects of vaccination."[20] It circulated widely, much to the annoyance of the Boston health department physician Thomas B. Shea: "We cannot go in any district of this city, we cannot find cases of small-pox, without, inside forty-eight hours, each and every one of the inhabitants having placed in their hands a circular from the Anti-vaccination Society condemning vaccination."[21]

Greene warned parents to protect their children from vaccination at all costs, underlining uncertainties about the origin of vaccine lymph as well as its potential to transmit diseases that were well documented in nineteenth-century medical literature. He pointed out problems with glycerinated lymph and accused local health officials of concealing from the public "numerous cases of serious illness and blood-poisoning, and several deaths" from vaccination. Condemning all serum therapies as a "craze" and a "blood-poisoning campaign," he cautioned, "do not allow your child to be vaccinated," and he denounced compulsory vaccination as "an ATROCIOUS CRIME . . . a *violation of the Constitution of the United States.*" Exhorting parents not to allow school or health authorities to bully them into vaccination, he included the full text of the 1894 exemption law to fortify their resolve.[22]

Greene's publication of *Vaccination Is the Curse of Childhood* shows the emergence of a core community of antivaccination practitioners who would certify any child presented to them as unfit, a community for which he acted as a broker connecting them with interested parents. Harvard president Charles W. Eliot remarked on their influence among Boston's elite families: "I know of one or two of the best-known homeopathic physicians in the Back Bay who are still opposing vaccination very strongly. They have a large practice. I understand that many of the children of the rich families in that section of the city have never been vaccinated because the family physician advised against it."[23] Eliot probably was referring to William B. Sanders, the homeopathic physician who had persuaded the state legislature to amend the vaccination law in 1894. No diploma mill graduate, he had trained at one of the best medical schools in the 1880s.[24] Sanders maintained a flourishing Back Bay practice in exemption certificates throughout the late 1890s, with Greene noting that "numerous pupils of the schools have received certificates from Dr. Sanders."[25] Late in 1901, another antivaccination writer declared that Sanders "and many other physicians in the state, have issued thousands of exemption certificates."[26] This practice especially irritated Samuel H. Durgin, who accused antivaccinationists of using "this law as a convenience to their belief, . . . and they are certifying the most healthy children as unfit subjects for vaccination."[27] As far as he was concerned, antivaccinationists took advantage of the law's vagueness and violated its spirit by enabling healthy individuals to evade vaccination.

"Any medical theory which sets aside the laws of health, and teaches that the spreading of natural or artificial disease can be advantageous to the community, is misleading, mischievous, and opposed to common sense; and any teacher, whatever his assumption of authority, title, or degree, who inculcates such doctrine, is a perverter of common sense, and an enemy of the human race."

VACCINATION
..IS THE..
CURSE OF CHILDHOOD.

IMPORTANT FACTS FOR PARENTS AND GUARDIANS, AND FOR THE PEOPLE.

WHAT IS VACCINE VIRUS?

The virus injected into the human arm for the alleged purpose of preventing small-pox, may be any one, or a combination, of the following *pus products :*
(1) The original Horse-grease Cow-pox of Jenner; (2) A combination of Cow-pox and Small-pox virus; (3) Swine-pox; (4) Horse-pox; (5) Spontaneous Cow-pox; (6) Small-pox matter passed through the cow; (7) Donkey-lymph; (8) Buffalo-lymph; and many more pus products of disease, having passed through various animal and human bodies, and carrying with them the seeds of *erysipelas, scrofula, consumption, eczema, leprosy, syphilis* and other loathsome diseases. No physician can tell you, for a certainty, *what it is* which he advises to have injected into the blood of your child.

What is the New Glycerinated Calf Lymph

so much boasted of, and styled "pure vaccine lymph " ?
It is the vaccine matter described above, mixed with *glycerine,* which is a substance especially adapted for the growth of the seeds of disease. Deadly diseases have been and are transmitted by its use. It has been condemned by expert witnesses before the English Royal Commission of 1889–1896 (Drs. Barlow and Acland); by Sir George Buchanan, M.D., F.R.S., the *Indian Lancet* and many others. There is and can be no such thing as "pure vaccine lymph."

What are the Results of Vaccination?

Disease, constitutional debility, death. Many a sufferer from debility and blood deterioration can trace that condition to vaccination; and many other like sufferers from vaccination are not aware of the real cause of their condition. The cause of such sickness and death is too often *concealed under some other name.*
The people have sifted this matter, and have learned these

Figure 5.1. Front of J. M. Greene's 1901 pamphlet, *Vaccination Is the Curse of Childhood*, No. 15 in Opposition to Vaccination Pamphlets, 1874–1901, Boston Medical Library in Francis A. Countway Library of Medicine, Harvard University.

Facts Concerning Vaccination :

(1) That no number of vaccination "marks" will prevent small-pox; the vaccinated and re-vaccinated in civil life, and in the army, everywhere, have the disease.

(2) That it does not mitigate small-pox; the vaccinated frequently die of the most malignant kind, while the unvaccinated as well as the vaccinated experience the mildest form.

(3) That small-pox vaccination (or "inoculation") gives small-pox instead of preventing it; while Cow-pox vaccination cannot prevent small-pox, since it *bears no relation to that disease.*

(4) That the vaccination imposture is, in times of small-pox "scare," a great source of revenue to doctors, many of whom really believe in a delusion they have not the energy or courage to investigate.

(5) That the inoculation craze is extending to many other diseases, and we are threatened with a general blood-poisoning crusade with the so-called "Antitoxins" of cholera, consumption, "hydrophobia," yellow fever, diphtheria, etc.

(6) That compulsory vaccination, or the forcible implantation of disease into a body, on the theory that it may in the future prevent some other disease, is an ATROCIOUS CRIME, which has no place in the laws of any civilized community and is inherently a *violation of the Constitution of the United States.*

(7) That Sanitation—which means good drainage, good ventilation, pure water and healthy food—is the only preventive of small-pox and other epidemics.

Vaccination Condemned.

When the vaccination theory is carefully and impartially examined, its absurdities and dangers become manifest. The following are a few of the distinguished investigators and experts in the study of epidemic disease who unqualifiedly condemn it: Chas. Creighton, M.D., M.A.; E. M. Crookshank, M.D., M.R.C.S.; R. Hall Bakewell, M.D., M.R.C.S.; Alfred Russel Wallace, LL.D.; Benj. Ward Richardson, M.D., F.R.S.; Wm. Job Collins, M.D., F.R.C.S.; M. R. Leverson, M.A., Ph.D., M.D.; Prof. Ricord, M.D.; McConnell Reed, M.D.; Herbert Spencer.

Do not Allow your Child to be Vaccinated.

In Boston, within the past few months, numerous cases of serious illness and blood-poisoning, and several deaths, have been the result of vaccination. In the fatal cases the real facts are concealed from the public, some disease, WHICH HAS BEEN THE DIRECT RESULT OF VACCINATION, being given as the cause of death.

You say, "My child will not be allowed to attend the public schools of Massachusetts unless vaccinated." *That is a mistake.* The following is from Public Statutes for 1894; Chapter 515, Sect. 2 :

"All children who shall present a certificate, signed by a regular practicing physician, that they are unfit subjects for vaccination, shall not be subject to the provisions of section 9 of chapter 47 of the public statutes, excluding unvaccinated children from public schools, and all children upon such a certificate shall be exempted from the provisions of this act."

There are hundreds of physicians in Massachusetts who are well aware of the uselessness and evil effects of vaccination. Apply to any one of them for a certificate of exemption for your child.

Write to Room 77, No. 1 Beacon St., Boston, for names of such physicians if they are unknown to you.

SAVE THE CHILDREN.

"The first duty of a parent is to *protect his offspring,* and to resist every attack upon their health at any and every cost, no matter from what quarter it may come."

Figure 5.2. Back side of J. M. Greene's 1901 pamphlet, *Vaccination is the Curse of Childhood,* No. 15 in Opposition to Vaccination Pamphlets, 1874–1901, Boston Medical Library in Francis A. Countway Library of Medicine, Harvard University.

The Boston physician Immanuel Pfeiffer also carried on quite a business in issuing unfitness certificates to schoolchildren, according to Durgin, who testified in 1902 that he had "read an advertisement, in which Dr. Pfeiffer offered to grant 'unfit' certificates to any children."[28] Pfeiffer acquired a great deal of notoriety for his opposition to vaccination in the last months of 1901. Taking a leading role in the resistance, he rallied the antivaccinationists in his new magazine, *Our Home Rights,* calling for abolition of the compulsory vaccination law and waging a personal war with Durgin. Pfeiffer impressed Greene, who first met the physician in the summer of 1901. From that point on, the two men cooperated in their antivaccination work. Greene accorded *Our Home Rights* prominent advertising space in each issue of *The Animals' Defender.*[29] Pfeiffer in turn published Greene's accounts of vaccination injuries and deaths in his journal.

Pfeiffer and Greene both recounted stories of public officials who ignored the 1894 exemption law. Pfeiffer accused health officials of overstepping their authority, insisting that they disregarded exemption certificates and vaccinated children against the wishes of their parents.[30] He thundered: "Think of such a brutal violation of a plain law; even those in favor of vaccination must blush, when ignorant, selfish, public servants so far forget what they owe the people."[31] Greene reported that some health and school officials defied the law by refusing to honor exemption certificates and even vaccinated a few children before their parents could stop them. These "infractions, in which public school pupils, holding 'exemption certificates,' have been in some instances forcibly vaccinated in spite of protest, and in others have been forcibly deprived of schooling," angered antivaccinationists during the fall of 1901.[32] School officials sent home children like Marjorie Keating, turned out of her Dorchester school "in tears" despite her exemption certificate. School physicians bullied parents like an Arlington mother who recounted how a school doctor refused her son's certificate and "'allowed herself to be bulldozed into having it done.'" One father, D. W. Logan of Abington, declared they had vaccinated his child in school "without the parent's knowledge."[33] Pfeiffer threatened to sue, and Hyde Park parents later filed one on behalf of two excluded children who possessed valid exemption certificates.[34]

Pfeiffer also eagerly provided certificates of unfitness for vaccination to adults. Even though the 1894 vaccination law did not cover adults, many physicians under contract to vaccinate at businesses and manufacturing plants did not know that. A Boston Elevated Railway Company employee reported that the physician suspended vaccinations when some of the men displayed their certificates.[35] Thomas P. Lohan, a Parker House Hotel worker, bragged that his certificate enabled him alone, out of 350 employees, to avoid vaccination in November 1901. One of Pfeiffer's adult sons similarly evaded vaccination at his employer's establishment, and Pfeiffer boasted that he had "issued certificates to many persons, they have all been accepted."[36]

Unfitness certificates also showed up in communities outside of Boston. The physician N. K. Noyes of Duxbury complained in January 1901, "there is trouble in our section with people who are sending up to Boston, and for a dollar apiece are getting the certificates of disability."[37] A Hyde Park health board member similarly grumbled, "some of the children have certificates from physicians in Boston, which they procured without being seen by the physician in attendance."[38]

Joseph Greene not only served as a broker for this trade in certificates but he also provided an invaluable conduit of information about antivaccination from his Beacon Street office. Featuring both local and national news of antivaccination protests and lawsuits, he ran stories and commentaries about vaccination injuries and deaths. Although he often threaded commentary throughout his coverage, Greene did not rely on generalities alone to make his point. He furnished names, dates, addresses, and sources for his information. For instance, he identified specific victims in lockjaw and blood poisoning cases after vaccination, giving the newspaper and date of the story.[39] He also invited people to contact him, submitting their personal experiences with vaccination injuries and deaths.[40] Greene not only published these stories in *The Animals' Defender* but he also shared them with other antivaccination periodicals like *The Liberator* and *Our Home Rights*.[41] He followed Massachusetts Anti-compulsory Vaccination Society meetings and the progress of its legal appeals against the vaccination laws.[42]

As a leading antivivisectionist, Greene could appeal to a far broader audience than other antivaccinationist writers.[43] Many socially prominent and wealthy people supported humane treatment of animals and regulation of animal experimentation. Greene's editorials thus reached many individuals who would not otherwise read antivaccination literature, and he probably brought together many individuals interested in both causes.[44] Several Boston homeopathic physicians apparently connected through *The Animals' Defender*. James B. Bell, Caroline Eliza Hastings, and Sara Newcomb Merrick pop up again and again in its pages, writing letters or testifying against vaccination and vivisection. Bell, a homeopath and "expert surgeon" who had practiced medicine in Boston for decades, petitioned to abolish the compulsory vaccination law in 1894, but then testified before the state legislature against vivisection in 1901 and later against vaccination in 1902.[45] Hastings also appeared at the same two State House hearings in 1901 and 1902. Merrick wrote letters critical of animal experimentation in 1901 and served as a MACVS officer by 1903.[46]

As pressure to vaccinate mounted in 1901, parental anger at school officials' refusals to honor exemption certificates built up to a boiling point. Employer-mandated vaccination and the post-Christmas general vaccination order compounded their outrage. Thus in early January 1902, concerned citizens organized a new antivaccination society, the Massachusetts Anti-compulsory Vaccination Society (MACVS). At its initial meeting, MACVS elected the stockbroker William Bassett president. Three days later the nominating committee of the society appointed Joshua T. Small of Provincetown and William F. Simpson vice presidents and designated as directors state Representative John. F. Foster, Ezra H. Baker, George H. Goodwin, and Ralph B. Williams.[47] One newspaper editor agreed that health department enforcement of vaccination "awakened and strengthened the protest" and "demand for change in the law has never been so vigorous and emphatic."[48] The new organization conducted regular monthly meetings for at least the next two years and accrued new members as its test cases wound their way through the courts.[49] By 1903, for instance, the labor activist Aurin F. Hill testified against compulsory vaccination and corresponded on behalf of MACVS to solicit funds for Henning Jacobson's Supreme Court appeal. He continued to work for antivaccination throughout the next decade.[50] The patent holder and chemist Charles Asbury Simpson, an 1875 Massachusetts Institute of Technology graduate, also joined.[51] Immanuel Pfeiffer attended meetings and exerted great influence in MACVS. He was on close terms with the society's vice president, Joshua T. Small, who regularly contributed to *Our Home Rights*.[52] Pfeiffer also testified with other society members during legislative hearings on vaccination in 1902. When he suggested the eminent attorney and Democratic Party politician George Fred Williams for MACVS's appeal of the compulsory vaccination statute to the United States Supreme Court, the society assented "with a unanimous vote," indicating that its members trusted Pfeiffer's judgment.[53]

Impelled by concern about the "unwarrantable infringement of personal liberties" and anxiety about the safety of vaccination, MACVS founders decided to emphasize their opposition to legal compulsion by calling their society "anti-compulsory" rather than "antivaccination," a strategic choice perhaps to gain sympathy from those who accepted vaccination but abhorred compulsion.[54] Proclaiming the "crystallization of public sentiment in opposition to the unjust and tyrannical laws enforcing compulsory vaccination" as its highest priority, the society then ranked "diffusion of literature upon the subject" second. Opposition to any new legislation to strengthen compulsory vaccination statutes came third. Last, MACVS promised "to furnish aid and assistance to those who may need it in resistance to the enforcement of compulsory vaccination."[55] The society hoped to attract not only those already opposed to vaccination but also those who supported it yet questioned the propriety of legal compulsion.

Antivaccination and Organized Medicine

Americans at the turn of the century regarded antivaccination as one of the great controversies of their time. One historian of Progressive-era reform movements links antivaccination to "one of America's most democratic political traditions, a populism that has often represented a radical challenge to the authority of economic, political, and cultural elites." In his study of Progressive-era Portland, Oregon, Robert D. Johnston argues that antivaccinationists "went far beyond a simple defensive libertarianism to develop a comprehensive and indeed radical, democratic ideology of health and the body" that he calls "a middle-class populism of the body."[56] Massachusetts antivaccinationists certainly saw themselves as grassroots frontline warriors engaged in a battle for medical freedom against a privileged class of physicians who sought to monopolize the profession.

They regarded contention about vaccination as a scientific dispute so great that it would be tyrannical to allow any one view to predominate by enshrining it in law. Although they argued strenuously against vaccination in all of their literature, compulsory vaccination truly raised their ire.

In a classic 1982 study of the American medical profession, Paul Starr noted how state medical societies and the American Medical Association campaigned vigorously in the early twentieth century to reorganize the profession and reform medical education as a "consolidation of professional authority." They sought to raise the status of orthodox medicine not only by restricting access to the profession but also by basing its cultural authority on exclusive possession of scientific training and knowledge. Starr argued that "knowledge must be transformed into authority, and authority into market power, before gains from scientific advance can be privately appropriated by a profession," and contemporaries who witnessed the AMA's drive for hegemony certainly understood it on those terms.[57] The Boston editor Benjamin Orange Flower, for instance, criticized all "law-bulwarked privilege, possessing monopoly power," that sought "to shackle nonconformist thought . . . and to rob the people of the right and benefit of personally testing the virtue of truth of the newer systems or methods." Flower regarded antivaccination as a "vital question" of his day, a battle "to preserve the rights of the people from the most dangerous monopoly-seeking class in our land to-day."[58] Antivaccinationists fought not only the intrusion of the state in the personal realm of health but also disputed who could claim legitimate scientific authority over medical matters like vaccination. They saw themselves as the vanguard of the free marketplace in ideas and medical practice, fighting to preserve fundamental American values of freedom of thought, speech, association, and enterprise from the predations of an elite group of physicians who sought to hijack American government to serve selfish commercial interests.

With this critical perspective, antivaccinationists tended to raise doubts not only about vaccination but also the whole medical reform and research agenda promoted by elite medical leaders and wealthy corporation owners in the early twentieth century. Whereas the reforming elite argued that closing substandard medical schools and passing medical licensing laws ultimately benefited the public, many antivaccinationists retorted that such reform served only the interest of elite practitioners because it created a medical monopoly that would unfairly enrich them and allow them to control entry into the profession. They argued that selfish physicians and businessmen had overly glorified the successes of germ theory and laboratory science, hyping a few spectacular cures (rabies, diphtheria) while downplaying disastrous failures (tuberculin). "Was there not a time when the would-be leaders of the profession wanted to compel the use of tuberculin? And to-day where is there a remedy so thoroughly discredited as tuberculin? . . . Before we start compelling people to do this and that, we want to be sure we are right."[59] They questioned the value of new serum therapies, the ethics of experimentation on animals, and the "new public health" disregard for time-honored sanitary measures like quarantine and street cleaning. They challenged the idea that a specific disease inevitably followed exposure to a given microbe, instead arguing that healthy bodies naturally resisted infectious diseases (tuberculosis was a leading example, but they also included smallpox). They wondered why business leaders like John D. Rockefeller so readily poured money into research foundations when the laboring poor lacked adequate housing, water, and food. Antivaccinationists thus threatened the entire reform agenda so dear to the AMA at the turn of the century.

The antivaccination community nurtured a group of lay and medical writers who expressed a different vision of health, one based on the idea of creating health from within through proper hygiene, diet, exercise, rest, and mental attitude. They were fundamentally different in their outlook on health and disease than their provaccinist opponents, seeing the sick body not as a fortress invaded by hostile organisms, which could then be destroyed by serums or chemicals, but rather seeing disease as a manifestation of systemic imbalance or distress. They thus argued for therapeutics that sought to restore the balance by nurturing the body's innate powers to resist disease. This holistic view may have harkened back to midcentury therapeutic nihilism, but it also had an explanatory power that bacteriology lacked when it came to afflictions not caused by microbes. Advances in medical science had not yet led to "medicines that will act as sure cures," as one physician complained in 1892.[60] And little changed outside of the introduction of diphtheria antitoxin in the ensuing decade. At a time when germ theory promised far more than it delivered in the way of effective therapeutics and medical researchers had not yet elucidated all of the complexities of the human immune system, the antivaccination critique made a certain kind of sense from a lay as well as a medical perspective.

By the end of the nineteenth century, organized medicine celebrated Jenner as an exemplar of scientific medicine and vaccination "as the greatest sanitary fact which the world has ever known."[61] Physicians writing medical history created the myth of a simple country doctor's experiments, admired his persistence against the initial dismissal of his findings, and proclaimed the unalloyed beneficence of vaccination.[62] One physician observed of Jenner: "To him is due that extreme and rare credit of having devised the incalculably valuable scheme of close and patient observation without which great discoveries in the realm of science are a hopeless dream."[63] As an icon of scientific medicine and new public health, vaccination was sacrosanct and criticism of vaccination was heretical. One physician, for instance, admitted that though many of his colleagues "in their own consciences disapprove of the practice, they dare not give expression to their honest judgment, for fear of being ostracized by their fellows and by the public."[64] Vaccination became an obligatory part of medical practice, with medical journals reminding doctors "of their duty to see to it that every child in the families under their care shall be vaccinated at the proper age."[65]

Antivaccinationists fared badly in both the medical and popular press. The *New York Times* referred to antivaccinationists as "grotesque creatures" who "advertise their own lack of the reasoning faculty."[66] In 1902, one practitioner accused antivaccinationists of "ignorance, dishonesty and insanity," implying that they were lunatics and criminals who sought "to disturb, obstruct and overwhelm the normal order of prevention and safety."[67] To engage in serious debate, to admit that the science behind vaccination had some problems, was to admit that the entire enterprise of scientific medicine, germ theory, and laboratory science likewise might prove problematic. And scientific medicine had not yet fulfilled its potential to discover cures as well as causes for disease. Organized medicine simply could not afford to accord antivaccination any respect—its own position was too fragile.

The elite community of AMA medical reformers shunned physicians who publicly expressed qualms about vaccination. Just a few regular practitioners in Massachusetts openly opposed vaccination, with many of the most prominent antivaccination physicians adhering to homeopathy, a medical sect that had a testy relationship with the AMA during the nineteenth century but was moving toward "eventual integration . . . with the orthodox medical world" by the early twentieth century.[68] Although antivaccinationist homeopaths often had highly respected practices, especially in Boston, they still represented a minority in their own sect. Organized homeopathy through the medium of its medical societies officially proclaimed its allegiance to vaccination in order to distance itself from the odium attached to antivaccination.[69] By the early twentieth century the vast majority had accepted vaccination as part of the greater drive to assimilate with regular medicine.[70] Dr. Horace Packard, for instance, appeared before a state legislative committee in 1902 to represent the Homeopathic Medical Society, declaring that "it grieved him very much" that many people assumed homeopaths opposed vaccination when in fact "they did believe in it and practice it." Only "a mere handful" of homeopaths opposed vaccination.[71] Homeopathic practitioners who spoke out against vaccination thus fell afoul of their own professional societies.

By 1902, antivaccinationists in Massachusetts had developed a network of sympathetic physicians active in the exemption certificate trade, and they had organized to lobby for the abolition of compulsory vaccination. At least fifteen Boston physicians publicly took a stand against vaccination in 1901 and 1902.[72] A number of lay and medical activists worked in and around Boston, many of them connected in some way through homeopathic practice or antivivisection interests. Established practices, academic appointments, and influential friends made it easier for some physicians to buck their peers on the issue of vaccination. An eminent homeopath like Conrad Wesselhoeft, for instance, could criticize vaccination without fear of censure. Educated at a German university and an 1856 Harvard Medical School graduate, he could count among his patients the novelist Louisa May Alcott. In addition to his successful private practice, Wesselhoeft held a professorship at Boston University School of Medicine, served as president of the American Institute of Homeopathy, and was on the staff of Massachusetts Homeopathic Hospital. He had a national reputation for his contributions to medical scholarship.[73] Their adversaries may have liked to characterize those who opposed vaccination as cranks, quacks, and lunatics, but that description was more of a rhetorical device than one based on reality.

Significantly, two leading Boston antivaccinationist physicians were not only homeopaths but also women, a group that the AMA campaign for medical education reform would ultimately marginalize. Women physicians had made great gains by the turn of the century, especially in Boston, where they represented 18.2 percent of that city's physicians in 1900, with homeopaths accounting for slightly more than half of the female practitioners even though as a whole homeopaths accounted for only about 8 percent of the medical profession.[74] This statistic was not a coincidence. According to Anne Taylor Kirschmann, "homeopathy had developed a reputation for having a more progressive viewpoint of women in the profession than regular medicine." Female homeopathic practitioners in Boston and elsewhere took active roles in their professional organizations and "often developed lucrative private practices."[75] By the turn of the century, they could look back proudly on the professional stature they had achieved. Even so, it took a lot of courage to stand up to other practitioners' disdain when they raised concerns about vaccination.

Caroline Eliza Hastings

One of several Boston homeopaths defying the official homeopathic stance on vaccination was Caroline Eliza Hastings, a respected veteran of the Boston medical, political, and social reform scene. Born in Barre, Massachusetts, and sixty-one years old in 1902, Hastings could claim a certain social status as a descendant from "ancient families" who could trace their residency in New England back to the early colonial period. Although she began her training as an apprentice to an eclectic physician, Dr. Aaron Bassett, her mother's illness and death forced her to interrupt her studies to take care of her family. She resumed her medical education a few years later at the New England Female Medical College, graduating in 1868. When the Female Medical College merged with Boston University School of Medicine in 1873, Hastings embraced homeopathy and was retained on the faculty until 1881 as a demonstrator and lecturer noted for her "clear, orderly, and illuminating presentation of the dry details" of anatomy and embryology.[76] One of the first women inducted into the Massachusetts Homeopathic Medical Society in 1874, she joined also the International Hahnemannian Society.[77] In 1897, she organized and served as first president of the Twentieth Century Medical Club, a pioneering women's medical society in Boston. Known as "a fine parliamentarian herself," Hastings "believed that women needed training in such technicalities in order that they might have confidence when presenting their views in public."[78]

Hastings took on a public role in feminist and social reform circles, lecturing in the 1870s with Abba Goold Woolson on dress reform and physiology, emphasizing the damage corsets and long skirts wrought on women's health.[79] An 1873 encyclopedia of homeopathic physicians described her as "a lady of great independence and decision of character, possessing every natural qualification, as well as the acquired, to win a high position in the medical ranks, worthily maintaining her position among her compeers, and winning her way upward with the passage of years."[80] Hastings never married, but lived for many years with her friend, the homeopathic physician Julia Morton Plummer.[81]

A large part of her medical practice incorporated public service in Boston. From 1887 to 1894, Hastings served on the Boston School Committee, but her most engrossing work involved the New England Female Moral Reform Society's lying-in hospital for unmarried pregnant women, considered "one of the leading private institutions in Boston."[82] Founded in 1836 by evangelical Protestant women, the society had chapters all over New England and had long focused on rescuing women from prostitution, but Hastings changed its mission when she took on a leadership role in 1869.[83] Serving as its president for many years, she redirected its efforts to that of providing a "door of hope" for unwed first-time mothers at the Talitha Cumi Home.[84] The thirty-seven-bed home provided discreet, high-quality maternal care in "an up-to-date hospital . . . with beautiful grounds" in a "secluded setting."[85] Although it took some charity cases, most of the clientele were paying customers referred by physicians, ministers, or relatives. Hastings worked for a time as the attending physician, attaining a reputation for expertise as an obstetrician and gynecologist. She urged conservatism in surgical interventions, arguing for caution in gynecological surgery to the consternation of some of her colleagues in one 1900 paper.[86] Her practice also seemed to reflect this attitude—the Talitha Cumi Home had a very low rate of instrumental deliveries with no puerperal fever cases.[87]

By the turn of the century, Hastings had attained a highly visible position as a respected senior leader not only among Boston's women physicians but also in public sector work for schools and charities. Her work at the Talitha Cumi Home made her known in Boston's religious, medical, and social circles, and in return she probably knew a lot about the private histories of many respectable Boston families. She had had a long career of public speaking and organizing by the time she took up the antivaccination cause in 1902. Her opinions carried serious weight in Boston society.

Testimony before the Joint Committee on Public Health sorely tested Hastings's composure and confidence in 1902. Her assertions about bacterial contamination of vaccine lymph so infuriated the Boston heath department chairman Samuel Durgin that he attempted to humiliate her publicly by smearing her integrity both in the press and medical community. Refusing to cave in, Hastings defended herself with spirit and grace. The two sparred verbally, trading pointed questions and barbs throughout the hearings, much to the delight of local newspapers seeking sensational stories to boost their sales.[88] Hastings's reasoned assessment of the issues even convinced one mainstream Boston editor to support the abolition of compulsory vaccination.[89]

Sara Newcomb Merrick

In 1903, the Boston homeopath Sara Newcomb Merrick took over the office of secretary-treasurer of MACVS. She served in this capacity for several years, even making her medical office the organization's headquarters.[90] Publicizing the plight of antivaccinationists who had run afoul of the law, she appealed for donations to support their court costs and lawyers' fees in notices and articles about their appeals.[91]

Like Caroline Hastings, she had a distinguished lineage that featured Mayflower ancestors and some prominent characters in the Revolutionary War. Born Sara Julia Newcomb on Prince Edward Island, Canada, in 1844, she was orphaned at seven and moved to the United States in 1860 to live with an older brother. Another brother, the celebrated astronomer Simon Newcomb, was considered "the most influential American scientist of the late nineteenth century," and spent his career at the Naval Observatory in Washington, DC. He was widely admired by literate Americans in the late nineteenth century and could count Senator Charles Sumner and President James Garfield as personal friends. Awarded the Copley Medal by the Royal Society of London, the most prestigious scientific honor of the pre-Nobel era, he authored many articles about economics and science read in popular nineteenth-century periodicals. His daughter and Sara's niece, the physician Anita Newcomb McGee, was famed for her army service in the Spanish-American War as Acting Assistant Surgeon and her work for the Red Cross in Japan.[92]

Before she surfaced as a leader among the Boston antivaccinationists, Merrick had a successful career as an educator and businesswoman in Texas. After graduating from Girls High and Normal School in Boston in 1867, Sara Newcomb embarked on a long teaching career. First, she moved to Manassas, Virginia, which is close enough to Washington, DC, to have allowed fairly frequent contact with her brother Simon.[93] There she taught both regular school and organized scripture lessons on Sundays. In 1872, she moved to San Antonio, Texas—an adventurous choice for a young woman at that time. There she taught in the Freedmen's Bureau School for Colored Children and then served as the principal of the Third Ward Colored School for eighteen years. She married Morgan Wolfe Merrick, a surveyor and Confederate Civil War veteran in 1876. After losing her first baby shortly after his birth, she had a daughter, Julia, in 1878.[94] Merrick also wrote on education for the *Texas School Journal* and was highly thought of as an educator, according to one source, who claimed "it is through her work that San Antonio has long borne the reputation of having the best primary schools in the State."[95] After suffering terribly from writer's cramp, Merrick invented and patented a pen holder in 1887.[96] She also invested successfully in real estate in San Antonio. Considered "a good businesswoman," she became president of that city's Business Woman's Association and retired from teaching around 1890. She also participated in the San Antonio chapter of the Daughters of the American Revolution and took an active part in that city's social life at least until 1892.[97]

In the mid-1890s, she began a new career—medicine—leaving her husband behind in San Antonio. Why Merrick left her husband is a mystery.[98] Returning to Boston, she attended the homeopathic Boston University School of Medicine, graduating in 1897 at fifty-three years of age.[99] From its inception in 1873, this

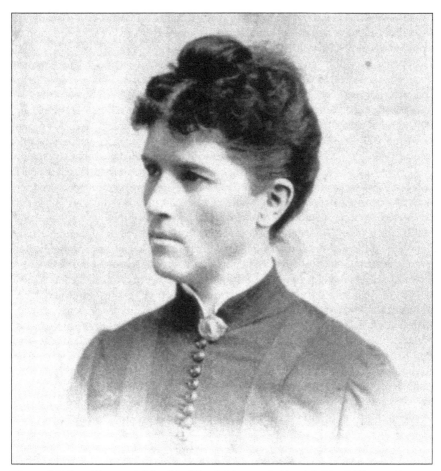

Figure 5.3. Sara Newcomb Merrick. "Sarah Newcomb Merrick," in *A Woman of the Century: Fourteen Hundred-Seventy Biographical Sketches Accompanied by Portraits of Leading Amercan Women in All Walks of Life*, ed. Frances E. Willard and Mary A. Livermore (New York: Charles Wells Moulton, 1893), 500.

school was no diploma mill. By the 1890s, it had already instituted a number of academic innovations: it was one of the first medical schools to require either an undergraduate degree or passage of an entrance exam for admission, and it had a rigorous four-year graded curriculum that included significant laboratory and clinical work. The Massachusetts state legislature regularly granted it significant financial support.[100] The physicians it graduated would have been considered among the best trained in the nation, ranking with Harvard and Johns Hopkins graduates. Merrick worked as physician and pharmacist for one of its outpatient clinics, the Roxbury Homeopathic Dispensary, which provided free or discounted medical care to the poor.[101] Practitioners coveted such positions because they indicated institutional approval and recognition of their academic work and provided a regular (albeit it small) salary while giving them the opportunity to develop a private practice.

Merrick probably got involved with antivaccination through her interest in antivivisection. In 1901, she supported an antivivisection bill, writing a letter "regarding certain cruel experiments she had seen and had herself performed on un-anaesthetized animals" as a medical student—the same bill that Hastings and Bell testified on at the State House.[102] Throughout her career, Merrick emphasized the role of nutrition, exercise, cleanliness, and rest in preserving health. She argued that a positive outlook coupled with hygienic living could prevent and even cure disease, advertising a "prospectus of lessons in HEALTH CULTURE and DIET for six cents in stamps" in *The Liberator*.[103] She apparently lectured frequently on a variety of topics in women's clubs around Boston. One 1905 talk counseled hygienic living to prevent tuberculosis.[104] Another in 1912 took on childrearing practices, where she argued against corporal punishment, warning members of the Fathers and Mothers Club that such an approach only inculcated a habit of striking back that could manifest in later life as criminality.[105] She also lectured on marriage, proposing that the federal government establish a special bureau to help young men and women find appropriate mates—a position that indicates she favored state intervention in personal lives at times.[106] The antivaccination editor Lora Little noted that the physician suffered for her outspokenness, "thereby incurring all the odium attaching to those in advance of their fellows in a matter which has stirred up so much bitterness as Anti-Vaccination."[107] The "odium" attached to Merrick may have led her family to distance itself at least publicly from her. Her brother, Simon Newcomb, never once mentioned her in his 1903 memoir, *Reminiscences of an Astronomer*, although she authored a loving tribute to him and their father for *McClure's Magazine* in 1910.[108]

Charles E. Page

Another Boston practitioner of the regular school of medicine, Charles E. Page, wrote fervently against vaccination.[109] He debated vaccination with Harvard president Charles Eliot, defended Immanuel Pfeiffer, and criticized germ theory before the American Social Science Association.[110] He corresponded with Joseph M. Greene, who published his letters in *The Animals' Defender*.[111] Page promoted the idea that better sanitation more effectively prevented smallpox than vaccination and publicized the Cleveland chief health officer Martin Friedrich's abandonment of vaccination in favor of disinfection and a cleanup effort. Contending that Boston also could eliminate smallpox if its health department took steps "to thoroughly cleanse the slum districts and all tenement houses, backyards, and fumigate the dens throughout the city," he championed sanitation over vaccination in the press for many years.[112] As late as 1916, he continued to argue that "vaccination was sprung on the poor devil laity about the time that marked improvements in personal and general sanitation began," and the medical profession, taking "coincidence for evidence," attributed the decline in smallpox to vaccination rather than to sanitation.[113]

Charles Fessenden Nichols

Charles Fessenden Nichols, a distinguished Boston homeopathic physician and popular author, also published several books criticizing vaccination. Nichols had solid social connections, coming from a New England family that could trace its ancestry to 1667. Born in 1846 at Salem, Massachusetts, Nichols's parents educated him in both public and private schools.[114] He married twice: first to Grace Belle Houston in 1884, and then to Anna Jenetta Van Arenberg in 1898. He had two children: a daughter, Cherry Elizabeth, and a son, Fessenden Arenberg.

Nichols possessed impressive academic credentials, undertaking studies at institutions of the highest caliber. He worked as curator of coins in the Peabody Academy of Science from 1860 to 1864 until he left to study in Europe. Educated in Germany for two years, he then attended Harvard Medical School, graduating in 1870. He also studied homeopathy with William P. Wesselhoeft, "one of Boston's earliest and most distinguished homeopaths," in the years between his admission to Harvard Medical School and his return from Germany.[115] Nichols interned at Massachusetts General Hospital and worked as the house physician at Carney Hospital.

After his graduation from Harvard, Nichols traveled to Hawaii in 1870 at the invitation of Chancellor and Chief Justice of Hawaii Elisha Hunt Allen, who introduced him to the Hawaiian royal family. There he practiced for over two years, "successful enough to number among his patients members of the royal family and chiefs as well as foreign residents." Nichols took a special interest in leprosy during his time in Hawaii, "testing the merits of homeopathic treatment" in that disease.[116]

When Nichols returned to Boston, he worked first as Wesselhoeft's assistant and then later his partner for fifteen years. In 1874 Nichols became the editor of the *New England Medical Gazette*, a leading homeopathic journal. From 1891 to 1892, he served on the editorial staff of *Science*, where he commented on the controversy over Robert Koch's tuberculin treatment in "widely read" articles.[117] Nichols also published many articles in popular magazines, including *Harper's*, *Popular Science Monthly*, and *Review of Reviews*.

Nichols's 1895 article in the *Review of Reviews* about the potential healing properties of the dry climate of the American Southwest for tuberculosis victims inspired the formation of the American Invalid Aid Society, which financed rest cures for consumptives in that region. As a vice president of the organization, Nichols served alongside Dr. Edward Everett Hale as president and Julia Ward Howe as the other vice president. He was friendly with notable reformers Helen Hunt Jackson, Wendell Phillips, and John Boyle O'Reilly.[118]

Nichols thus stood out as an eminent, respected physician with a national reputation who associated with some of the best-known social reform and literary figures of his time. His articles in popular magazines made his name familiar to a wide audience. He wrote and published prolifically on medicine and home-opathy.[119] He also published several monographs against vaccination: *A Blunder in Poison* (1902), inspired apparently by the Boston health department vaccina-tion order; *The Outrage Vaccination* (1908); and *Syphilis and Vaccination* (1911).[120] In 1903, he appeared with MACVS members Immanuel Pfeiffer, Charles Asbury Simpson, James W. Pickering, and Aurin F. Hill to testify extensively about "his personal knowledge of vaccination and its results" at State House hearings.[121] He probably knew Pfeiffer anyway since he kept his medical office in the same building, the Hotel Pelham, at the time.[122]

A Blunder in Poison

Although Nichols wrote *A Blunder in Poison* to marshal the antivaccination argu-ment for "the Thinking World," events in Boston clearly shaped his writing.[123] Sprinkled throughout *Blunder* are references to the Boston Board of Health, Immanuel Pfeiffer, and vaccination resistance in Boston and Cambridge. He even quoted extensively from an editorial against compulsory vaccination in the *Boston Courier* in order to discuss some of the constitutional ramifications of the debate.[124] Citing Alfred Russel Wallace as "a leader of present thought," Nichols asserted that vaccination would "rank as the greatest and most pernicious failure of the nineteenth century."[125]

Nichols documented his case against vaccination with objective facts and sci-entific analysis, relying for instance on a recent report of the Surgeon General of the United States Army that showed high rates of smallpox even among recruits who had been vaccinated several times.[126] He cited various medical authori-ties, arguing that "we reach evidence of very serious aliments or destructive dis-eases . . . directly due to vaccination," and "every practicing physician is aware of cases of life-long disease from vaccination, and of deaths in proportion." Nichols believed that physicians feared the censure of their colleagues if they publicized cases of infection after vaccination in medical journals. Although newspapers and antivaccination journals had reported many instances of bad outcomes from vaccination, the medical profession as a whole resisted open and frank disclosure of such problems because it regarded vaccination as sacrosanct. To attack vaccination was to attack the foundations of scientific medicine.[127]

Nichols had personally experienced this dilemma. He had once routinely vaccinated in the course of his medical practice, but then started to see patients for vaccine-related infections, treating "a due proportion of patients in acute or fatal sickness as a prompt sequence of vaccination." Eventually he decided "at last to stop vaccinating, in which I had persevered through a certain sort of respect for established authority."[128] Nichols rejected vaccination not because he had any previous prejudice against it—indeed his proclivity had been to support the practice—but because he had encountered too many patients who experienced bad outcomes after vaccination.

Cleveland's experience with bad vaccine in the summer of 1901 especially struck Nichols as providing very clear evidence of the stupidity of compulsory vaccination. In Cleveland, the health officer Martin Friedrich found so many people with severe infections after vaccination that he halted it altogether and substituted a strict program of case tracing, isolation, and disinfection in its stead. Like many other antivaccinationists, Nichols hailed Friedrich for his "foresight and administrative ability" and declared that "Cleveland's experience promises to repeat that of Leicester."[129] Nichols lauded "Dr. Friedrich's elasticity . . . in strong contrast with the conduct of Massachusetts health boards, where, with death-rates actually doubling, after a year of rigid vaccination in Boston, resistants are pinioned by police officers and vaccinated."[130] Stricter isolation protocols and better sanitation offered an alternative approach to smallpox control, but Boston's Durgin obstinately refused to consider these measures where Cleveland's Friedrich acted honestly and openly to address the issue. To Nichols and other antivaccinationists, Friedrich's decision to halt vaccination seemed more in line with other types of municipal reform that sought to expose corruption by opening the administrative process to public scrutiny.

Nichols believed that "respect for established authority" had been carried too far in Massachusetts. Compulsory vaccination laws originally "obtained solely through promises of protection, life-long and complete, with warrant of the absolute harmlessness of the operation" had led to terrible results. When states enforced vaccination laws indiscriminately they needlessly forced many people to risk their health and even life. He noticed that "while a reputable physician may defend his patient from jury duty, he is practically unable to protect him from vaccination." Even those with an "acute illness . . . about to undergo serious operations, or weak in convalescence, alike are frequently forced into compliance."[131] Nichols believed that physicians and their patients, not the law, should decide when or whether to vaccinate. He did not object to the state's right to protect public health, but questioned its usurpation of physicians' medical judgment when it demanded vaccination regardless of individual circumstances.

Events in Boston and Cambridge clearly served as a touchstone for Nichols, and he celebrated "thirteen resisting citizens at Boston and Cambridge" who "brought the subject of personal right to appeal in the higher courts, holding for the time law at bay."[132] A few daring and stubborn individuals refused vaccination in the face of legal sanctions. Embracing the tenets of classic civil disobedience they accepted their tickets and then went to court to fight them. When they lost, they appealed. Nichols wrote his book in large part to bolster their cases with a handy compendium of evidence against vaccination for the "great silent following" of sympathizers who feared to speak out.[133]

Rueben Swinburne Clymer

Immanuel Pfeiffer introduced a young Pennsylvania physician, Rueben Swinburne Clymer, to the Massachusetts antivaccination scene in 1902.[134] They had corresponded previously about vaccination and tetanus in 1901, with Clymer holding that "vaccine is a poison, no matter how it is prepared."[135] The twenty-four-year-old Clymer, who signed himself as "Physician and Surgeon to St. Luke's Hospital" in Philadelphia, impressed Pfeiffer, who hired him "to take charge of the Boston end of the doctor's business" in early February 1902.[136] Although Clymer had yet to actually receive his medical school diploma, his abhorrence of compulsory vaccination got him the job. To prevent smallpox, he advised dosing with a mixture of sulphur, cream of tartar, sugar, and water twice a day, drinking lemonade, and taking cascara sagrada, a laxative. To ward off ill effects from vaccination, he recommended washing the site with alcohol, soap, and dressing it with "pure vaseline and the best powdered sulphur."[137]

Initially trained as an eclectic, Clymer became intrigued with a new therapeutic approach, osteopathy, which rejected drug therapy in favor spinal and joint manipulation to achieve internal balance that then allowed the body to heal itself.[138] After filling in for Pfeiffer for a few months, Clymer moved on to work as the superintendent of the Health League Sanitarium in New York City in order to study osteopathy with its founder, Dr. August F. Reinhold.[139] Born and raised near Allentown, Pennsylvania, Clymer returned there to open a practice in late 1903. Although Clymer at first obtained a license to practice medicine in Pennsylvania, the Lehigh County Medical Society challenged it in court, and Clymer lost his case.[140] One acquaintance later claimed that Clymer got into trouble "as a result of his untiring labors in endeavoring to enlighten the oppressed people on the fruits of vaccination."[141] This legal battle might have forced Clymer out of Pennsylvania for a time to practice in Oklahoma, where he wrote a book based partly on his Boston experiences, *Vaccination Brought Home to You.*[142]

In *Vaccination Brought Home to You,* Clymer used well-known antivaccinationist sources, but he also quoted extensively from public health officials and vaccine maker's publications to document the dangers of vaccination. Like Nichols he highlighted the Cleveland experience to demonstrate how bad results had driven a supporter of vaccination to utterly reject it.[143] Although Clymer spent only a little time in Boston, events there clearly shaped his argument, for he referred several times to the 1901–2 Boston vaccination controversy. In a section titled "Some Fruits of Vaccination," he described the plight of Annie Shore and Jennie Leavitt, the Boston infants first noted by Pfeiffer in *Our Home Rights.*[144] He described Boston's citizens as "rising like slaves" to submit to compulsory vaccination from physicians who bragged, "with virulent virus we tattoo the skin," but "the might of law shall prevent any fuss."[145] Although all of the antivaccination writers brought up the issue of appropriate limits to state health authority, Clymer was the most strident in his emphasis on personal rights: "When people of America learn their constitutional rights, and demand them . . . then will such dark age brutalism and Russian coercion stop."[146] To Clymer, individual rights and personal autonomy trumped public health concerns. Unlike Pfeiffer, whose politics leaned to socialism, he would remain fiercely devoted to a libertarian vision of America for the rest of his life.

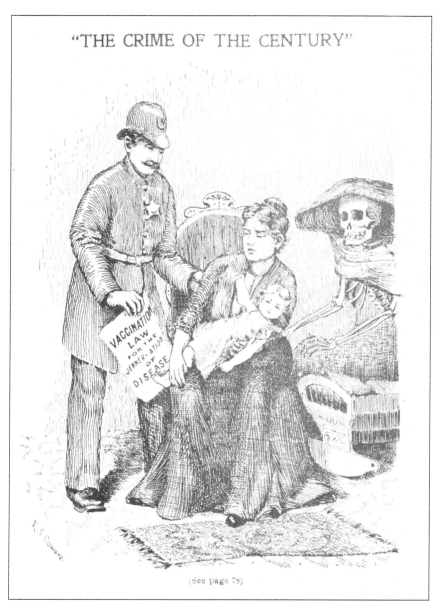

"THE CRIME OF THE CENTURY"

(See page 78)

Figure 5.4. Frontispiece from Rueben Swinburne Clymer's *Vaccination Brought Home to You* (Terre Haute, IN: Press of G. H. Hebb, 1904).

By 1902, a loose network of antivaccinationists had coalesced to create a community of activists formally organized as the Massachusetts Anti-compulsory Vaccination Society. Only a few of the physicians involved, like Pfeiffer or Clymer, had questionable credentials. The others possessed reputable social connections, rigorous medical educations, and solid practices that made it difficult to easily dismiss them. Except for Clymer, whose involvement in MACVS was peripheral at best, they tended more toward progressivism and populism in their political outlook than libertarianism. Some of the most outspoken and prolific writers among the antivaccinationists in Boston were homeopaths bucking the trend for support of vaccination among their medical society colleagues. Perhaps their professional seniority, impeccable social standing, and strong academic credentials bolstered their courage, making them unafraid to challenge the status quo. These physicians contested the validity of vaccination on scientific grounds, proclaiming that they had just as much right to question its legitimacy as any other medical expert, much to the consternation of public health officials like Samuel Holmes Durgin. Their determined advocacy, academic background, and influence over wealthy families made them a force to be reckoned with in Boston health politics. Yet, as we shall see in the next chapter, it was a regular physician with a mysterious medical background, Immanuel Pfeiffer, who stood out as the most notorious champion of antivaccination in Boston.

Chapter Six

Immanuel Pfeiffer versus the Boston Board of Health

At the 1902 annual meeting of the Massachusetts Association of Boards of Health, the biologist William T. Sedgwick argued that health officers ought to take antivaccinationists seriously by responding respectfully to their criticisms rather than automatically categorizing their opposition as lunacy. Dr. Samuel Holmes Durgin, chairman of the Boston Board of Health, reacted sardonically to his colleague's entreaty. Alluding to his many difficulties with the antivaccinationists, Durgin declared: "I think he has betrayed a more tender and considerate feeling than has been produced within me in the last few months. . . . I have no sympathy with the men and women who are publishing rash and unfounded charges against vaccination."[1] In the last months of 1901, Boston's antivaccinationists had publicized illnesses and deaths after vaccination and criticized his management of the epidemic, leading vaccination rates to drop off.[2] As the smallpox epidemic steadily worsened, Durgin had to issue a controversial general vaccination order in a desperate attempt to control the growing epidemic.

Samuel Durgin may have lacked "tender or considerate" feelings for Boston's antivaccinationists, but one more than any other proved especially irritating. From the beginning of the epidemic, Dr. Immanuel Pfeiffer, the "special champion of the opposition to vaccination," stood out as Boston's leading antivaccinationist.[3] Throughout the fall of 1901, Pfeiffer conducted a one-man crusade against vaccination, Samuel Durgin, and the Boston Board of Health in the pages of his magazine, *Our Home Rights*, and in every public forum he could find. Focusing his wrath on Durgin, Pfeiffer criticized his management of the isolation hospital and questioned his motives in sending vaccination squads only to poorer sections of the city.

Durgin, the consummate public health professional, resented Pfeiffer's allegations. In many ways, Pfeiffer and Durgin each represented two important strains of reform that had emerged in the late nineteenth century, populism and progressivism. Durgin epitomized the progressive ideal of scientific expertise in government service where trained professionals supposedly brought high standards of scientific objectivity and impartiality to previously partisan appointments. Pfeiffer personified the democratic, populist impulse of the time. He fought against state regulation of medical practice and supported government attempts to break up or regulate corporate trusts and monopolies. He espoused causes like the single tax, a "uniform tax on all land whether developed or not" to free up land for building "more homes and factories, thereby lowering rents, increasing profits and wages, and alleviating unemployment and urban congestion."[4] With his "stalwart figure and imposing carriage," Pfeiffer flamboyantly advocated for pacifism, socialism, women's rights, and freedom of speech. Compulsory vaccination drew his particular ire, and he raged against its implementation in late 1901.

Pfeiffer's duel with Durgin captivated the Boston press in the early months of 1902 when he accepted Durgin's dare to wager his life on his antivaccination beliefs by exposing himself to smallpox without first undergoing vaccination. Durgin then allowed Pfeiffer his freedom after this exposure, although he quietly set police to track the physician. When the health department chairman admitted that Pfeiffer had slipped through his surveillance, the whole city panicked. Durgin had made a massive error by assuming that he could easily snatch Pfeiffer before he became infectious.

Both men understood the power of the press and they used it adroitly to publicize their positions, hoping to sway public opinion in their favor. Each man promoted a different vision of the proper role of government authority in health issues. Durgin regarded himself as Boston's supreme guardian of public health, a medical expert entrusted with ultimate power to protect the health of the community. Confident in his authority and expertise, he brooked no interference with his management of the epidemic. Pfeiffer saw himself as a crusader for civil and medical liberty, advocating complete personal autonomy over his body and medical decisions. Pfeiffer embodied the extreme of antivaccination resistance and distinguished his position from that of those who merely objected to the compulsory component of vaccination: "I believe vaccination to be detrimental to the human family, and I will do all I can to educate the masses up to this standard, and do all in my power to wipe from the statutes the obnoxious vaccination laws."[5] He willingly risked his life to serve his cause, while Durgin deliberately gambled with public safety to make of Pfeiffer a supreme object lesson for all who still avoided vaccination.

Immanuel Pfeiffer: Medical Populist

Born in Denmark, Jens Paulus Immanuel Pfeiffer claimed to have studied medicine in Europe before immigrating to the United States in the late 1860s.[6] At the beginning of 1902 he was nearly sixty-one years old, married and the father of seven children.[7] He owned a sixty-acre dairy farm, Orchard Farm, in Bedford, Massachusetts, a house described as "one of the largest and most pretentious in appearance in the town," and also kept an office in Boston.[8] At first, Pfeiffer promoted himself as a "natural physician," but an obituary later characterized him as a "specialist in nervous and chronic diseases." In 1901, he "held that proper diet, cleanliness, and hygienic conditions were the only reasonable, efficacious means of warding off disease, whether classed as contagious or not."[9]

Pfeiffer apparently struggled to establish his medical practice, moving around a lot before he landed in Boston. In 1890, he practiced in New Bedford, Massachusetts, and then a few years later in Jackson, Michigan. In 1896, he opened a health bread bakery in Chicago in conjunction with his medical practice, according to a Chicago paper that exposed his cures as fleeting at best. Chicago must not have worked out, because by 1899 he had relocated to western Massachusetts in Pittsfield and North Adams, Berkshire County. Finally he opened an office in Boston in late 1900 or early 1901.[10]

Although Pfeiffer had official status as a registered physician, he was "a vigorous opponent of the law requiring the registration of physicians," perhaps because his own academic and professional history would not bear close scrutiny.[11] Pfeiffer claimed that he received his medical education at a European university as a regular physician, but he never specified where or when this happened. With increasing pressure to certify medical competency through credentials and exams in the late nineteenth century, older physicians who may have received their training as apprenticeships or never completed their studies were allowed to continue their practices only by special dispensation—a rule that could change at the whim of the legislature. Pfeiffer, with his mysterious academic history, had been allowed to register under this rule, but he was not happy about it, and he may have feared the possibility that he might have to take an exam at some point if the rules changed. In March 1901, he petitioned the state legislature to abolish the examination requirement for a license to practice medicine in Massachusetts.[12] The "Pfeiffer bill" never made it out of committee, much to the satisfaction of the local medical press, which called it "a very sly endeavor to practically cripple the present Board of Registration entirely."[13] Undeterred, Pfeiffer established the Medical Rights League of Massachusetts, a legally chartered corporation to legitimize his battle against "the corrupt-monopoly Registration Board," and he unsuccessfully sought repeal again in 1903.[14]

Pfeiffer also achieved "considerable notoriety" for undertaking two long fasts, one for twenty-one days in 1900 and another for thirty days in the summer of 1901, which gave him much publicity.[15] Declaring that he would "cheerfully recommend everybody to fast, at least once a year, for a few days" in order "to throw off impurities," Pfeiffer also believed that fasting conferred great psychological benefits: "If you have a desire to create will power and practise [*sic*] concentration, there is no better plan than to fast, not to speak of the development of self-esteem." He cheerfully acknowledged that he worked outside the medical mainstream by emphasizing the psychology of illness, or as he put it, "suggestion, that grand system which of late has played so important a part in the treatment of the sick."[16] When a reporter likened this approach to that of Christian Science, Pfeiffer agreed: "I believe in a great many of the doctrines embraced by Christian Science. A person who cures himself by the so-called 'faith cure' really cures himself by suggestion—by hypnotism, just as I and my assistant cure our patients."[17] He even gave demonstrations and lectures "to prove the truth of his gospel by the illustrative phenomena of hypnotism." In recognition of these efforts and his fasts, the American Psychic Society supposedly made Pfeiffer its president.[18]

Pfeiffer sought a wide audience for his medical and political views. In April 1901, he started his own journal, *Our Home Rights,* for which he claimed ten thousand subscribers.[19] Intended as a forum for the discussion of all sorts of reform movements "from an independent and progressive standpoint," Pfeiffer's magazine contained articles on a wide range of subjects including, but not limited to, "Socialism, Vegetarianism, Anti-war, Pure Foods, Women's Dept., Therapeutic Suggestion, Single Tax, Medical Freedom, Spiritualism, Capital and Labor, Women's Rights, [and] Anti-Vaccination."[20] Pfeiffer's eclecticism attracted criticism from *American Medicine*'s George Gould, who labeled his endeavor as "anti-medicine": "It is this maniacal hatred of everything medical that inspires and unites the Falstaffian crowd of warriors. Antivaccination, antivivisection, anti-everything-medical is everywhere in these pages full of folly and fury." Pfeiffer certainly detested organized medicine and its agenda of reform for medical education and licensing, at least as the American Medical Association envisioned it. He questioned the utility of serum therapies and "magic bullet" cures, instead promoting a regimen of diet, hygiene, rest, and exercise as the only sure way to prevent disease, even infectious disease. He railed against compulsory vaccination laws as well as legislation that regulated medical practice. His blatant self-promotion seemed shameless to a medical press bent on re-creating physicians as disinterested objective scientists. Even though many aspiring physicians sought to increase their standing in the profession by founding, editing, or contributing to a medical journal, Pfeiffer's magazine sought a popular as opposed to a professional audience. Other medical editors and elite practitioners automatically dismissed him. Gould certainly refused to accord *Our Home Rights* any serious regard, calling it "one of the best examples of American humor we have seen, and that means, of course, that the fun is not intentional."[21]

Leading physicians at that time were particularly sensitive to the profession's lack of social status compared with the other learned professions. In 1902, John Allen Wyeth deplored this situation in a presidential address before the American Medical Association: "It is a painful fact to acknowledge that of the three so-called learned professions, the ministry, law, and medicine, ours is accorded the inferior position." Although many physicians achieved great respect and affection for their individual accomplishments, he argued that as a whole, physicians "are incapable of wielding by organization and discipline the powerful influence of a united profession aiming at high and honorable purpose." Only reform of medical education and reorganization of the profession would help physicians overcome "this evident weakness of the profession."[22] Wyeth insisted that the AMA must work to obtain legislation that raised educational and licensing standards—precisely the sort of laws that Pfeiffer opposed.[23]

The AMA also frowned on physicians who indulged in advertising and mail order medicine. In 1905, for instance, when the reporter Samuel Hopkins

Adams published his investigations of patent medicines and medical quacks in *Collier's Weekly*, the AMA quickly published the articles in book form under the title *The Great American Fraud*. There, Adams outlined the parameters of quackery: "Any physician who advertises a positive cure for any disease, who issues nostrum testimonials, who sells his services to a secret remedy, or who diagnoses and treats by mail patients he has never seen, is a quack."[24] According to AMA standards of professional conduct, Pfeiffer skirted the edge of medical decency when he obtained notoriety by publicizing his fasts, but he really transgressed when he offered to provide medical advice by mail without personally examining his patients.[25] By 1903, he also proffered "Nine Type-Written Lessons," for ten dollars—lessons that promised to teach the "Pfeiffer Principle," with which "you can defy disease."[26] Pfeiffer's mail-order business eventually got him into trouble with the United States Postmaster, with whom he had a running battle on the issue of the postal laws regulating third- and fourth-class mail.[27] Pfeiffer violated other AMA standards as well. He issued unfitness certificates to all who applied for them. This practice infuriated Durgin, who retaliated by petitioning the state legislature to amend the current law to provide that the certifying physician must personally verify the child's condition. Pfeiffer may have also dabbled in the patent medicine business. In 1901, he ran ads for the Howard Health Company in *Our Home Rights*. Located conveniently across the street from Pfeiffer's office, this company offered a remedy against both smallpox and the aftereffects of vaccination.[28] Featuring such a product in his magazine surely added to Durgin's distaste for him along with all the other purveyors of "nostrums and propositions" who took advantage of "a time like this, the height of a smallpox scare when people are willing to try almost anything offered for the protection of their health."[29]

Pfeiffer thus ran afoul of practically the whole program for medical reform—as the American Medical Association envisioned it—in his mail-order practice, opposition to medical regulation, and endorsement of a patent medicine business. Even worse, as an antivaccinationist, he was anathema. The AMA had endorsed compulsory vaccination since the 1860s. Now more than ever the AMA leadership pushed for legislation mandating vaccination. Declaring "such ignorance or indifference to the immunizing power of vaccination is a matter of surprise in an advanced stage of civilization," AMA President John Allen Wyeth exhorted his colleagues to campaign vigorously for compulsory vaccination: "It falls upon us as physicians to labor unceasingly to impress upon the communities in which we reside the necessity and safety of this immunizing process." To Wyeth and other leading physicians in the AMA, physicians like Pfeiffer were little better than charlatans, part of "the horde of uneducated and misguided persons who . . . take charge of and treat human beings suffering from disease without submitting themselves to the state examination legally required of us."[30] Nearly every local and state Massachusetts medical society, whether regular or homeopathic, publicly supported vaccination.[31] At this time, many physicians practicing at the elite level sought to unify the medical profession under the aegis of science and steer it away from partisan bickering and competition by reforming medical education, licensing, and organization. They sought to enhance the power and prestige of the profession as a whole, and consequently sneered at practitioners like Pfeiffer, whom they felt lacked both scruples and dignity. Thus one Boston newspaper, citing health department sources, noted that Pfeiffer was "considered a crank by many people," albeit one who "had a brain of unusual power and activity."[32]

Pfeiffer probably did not worry much that the state and local medical societies might regard him as an outlaw, or that his self promotion and flamboyance galled health officials. Like most physicians at that time, he did not belong to the AMA, and consequently he did not believe that the organization should have any power over his ability to practice medicine. The AMA Committee on Reorganization, for instance, reported in 1901 that "not more than 33,000 physicians in this country belonged to medical societies," out of an estimated 100,000 to 120,000 regular physicians in practice. That meant that more than two-thirds of American physicians did not belong to the AMA or even their local medical societies, a situation that the committee declared "a revelation that accounts for the wretched condition that our profession is in as a body politic and as a social factor in many ways."[33] Disapproval from the local medical society probably did not much affect his practice, since his patients would not have necessarily discerned any great difference between his credentials and those of any other practitioner.

The War with Durgin

Not the least fazed by his exclusion from the ranks of the medical elite, Pfeiffer regarded himself instead as leading the vanguard of medical reform. When Durgin insinuated that antivaccinationists lacked good citizenship, Pfeiffer derided it as a slur "unbecoming a scientific gentleman," citing findings of the British Vaccination Commission critical of vaccination and the fact that other states had repealed or modified their vaccination laws to argue that Massachusetts should do likewise, taking "its place among the enlightened states."[34] Durgin openly expressed his exasperation with antivaccinationists: "I have no patience with those who say vaccination is useless and harmful. Their arguments are too foolish to be considered. . . . I wish the smallpox would get into their ranks instead of among innocent people."[35] Pfeiffer responded loftily: "We leave it for any fair-minded person to form their own opinion of a physician, chairman of the board of health (?) who wishes other people to get the smallpox."[36] Pfeiffer usually appended a question mark to any health department reference to imply that its policies did little to promote health as he saw it. This exchange marked just the opening salvo in a war of words between the two men.

Pfeiffer also pestered other public health experts. When the Ladies' Physiological Institute invited the Boston City Hospital physician and smallpox expert John H. McCollom to lecture on smallpox in December 1901, Pfeiffer frequently interrupted him to challenge his assertions about vaccination's safety and effectiveness. Eventually the discussion degenerated into an exchange of insults with McCollom refusing "to enter into further discussion, for I am firmly convinced that you know nothing."[37] Although the Institute had not officially invited Pfeiffer to speak, the press covered his debate with McCollom in detail, granting his views wide exposure in the city. Even though some regarded him as a rude interloper, Pfeiffer had managed to present his views before an audience of politically active middle-class women with a long-standing interest in matters of health reform.[38]

By the end of 1901, Pfeiffer was the most flamboyant and aggressive antivaccinationist in Boston. He admonished his readers to "wake up" and fight the compulsory vaccination laws in the pages of *Our Home Rights*, enclosing a copy of the repeal bill for their perusal: "it will take more than one car load of Drs. Durgin and Shea to keep the old, tyrannical, stupid, degrading law in force. It must go,—by the Eternal—as Andrew Jackson said."[39] He railed against "Dr. Durgin and the whole pack of vaccinators, including the law makers, who were hoodwinked into passing the compulsory vaccination law" in the first place."[40] Pfeiffer had declared war on compulsory vaccination, and with the health department's vaccination order, repeal became ever more pressing to the antivaccination community.

Pfeiffer Visits the Isolation Hospital

Throughout the fall of 1901, Pfeiffer and Durgin took turns baiting each other in the press. In January 1902, their conflict took a new twist after Durgin dared antivaccinationists to test their theories by exposing themselves to smallpox. "Now is the best time that people of the anti-vaccination belief could have to exhibit themselves. People who are silly enough to permit an exposure to smallpox without vaccination will now have a grand opportunity, not only to test their belief, but to give an object lesson to the people at large. . . . If there are among the adult and leading members of the anti-vaccinationists, those who would like an opportunity to show the people their sincerity in what they profess I will make arrangements by which that belief may be tested and the effect of such exhibition of faith, by exposure to smallpox without vaccination. I do not believe there is a man or woman among them who will volunteer to take an exposure to smallpox with those who are vaccinated."[41] Durgin probably did not truly believe that anyone would prove foolhardy enough to accept his invitation, but his taunt backfired. Not one to shy away from a challenge, Pfeiffer called on Durgin sometime in January 1902 to take him up on his offer, declaring that he wanted to visit the hospital "for the purpose of scientifically looking into the disease in all its various forms, and with close observation be able to get such facts which will enable a physician to diagnose smallpox cases with as much certainty as possible." Pfeiffer obviously took care to phrase his request in terms that Durgin could not easily deny—after all Durgin had frequently and loudly complained about physicians' inability to correctly diagnose smallpox throughout the fall of 1901. Pfeiffer also alluded to his own "considerable experience, gathered in Europe," as a riposte to Durgin's aspersions upon antivaccinationists' scientific acumen.[42] On 20 January, Durgin answered that he would honor his "offhand" pledge to Pfeiffer, "not knowing you to have been recently vaccinated." Cautioning Pfeiffer, "this will constitute an exception to our rules," he added that he would not allow "any other person in similar condition to expose themselves at present."[43] Pfeiffer boasted, "if I ever was vaccinated, it was over sixty years ago," and believed that since he had "been frequently exposed to the disease for many years" he could not catch smallpox.[44] Durgin did not press him to get vaccinated, even though the general vaccination order issued 26 December 1901 gave him such authority.

Pfeiffer visited the isolation hospital on Gallop's Island on Thursday, 21 January 1902. Taking no particular precautions except to don a "duck robe," he toured the premises and examined patients.[45] He took "an Elevated car which was crowded" home, and later that night "attended a public meeting at Tremont Temple," brandishing and waving "a handkerchief which I used freely while in contact with the smallpox cases . . . in the faces of my friends at the church."[46] Although Durgin did not publicize the visit, Pfeiffer sent a letter describing his experience to several Boston newspapers and gave an interview to the *Boston Post*.[47] He later claimed that he publicized his visit for two reasons: first, "to draw the public's attention to the smallpox hospital" to stimulate a public investigation, and second, to show that smallpox is less contagious than the health department purported it to be, that "only 5 per cent will get the disease by coming in contact with it."[48] Pfeiffer boasted, "I freely handled the most desperate cases of smallpox and inhaled the breath of the worst case, (it was very bad,) and was about going away from the hospital without even washing my hands; but Dr. Corson, the physician in charge, kindly offered me water, soap and towel." He pointed out that the physicians had allowed him to leave "without any precaution for the safety of the people," rather than make any special arrangement to isolate him from the public. Although he praised the hospital physicians, he condemned Durgin as "either a fool or a knave" who "was himself criminally liable by permitting me to do as I did."[49]

Not surprisingly, the press sought an explanation for this remarkable event from Durgin. In an interview with the *Boston Globe*, he explained that he had allowed Pfeiffer's visit as a professional courtesy, as "a concession to him, . . . and as he had announced himself as a physician and opposed to vaccination I allowed him to go without requiring him to undergo what he was opposed to." Playing the innocent victim of Pfeiffer's machinations, he declared, "had I thought he had so little regard for the people at large, he would not have received permission to visit the hospital," condemning the physician for mingling with people after leaving the hospital. "To me it seems very much as if instead of wishing to find out anything about the disease he desired only a chance to gain notoriety, and that by a means that will, it seems to me, be looked upon by the public as contemptible, if not worse. If he exposed unsuspecting friends and strangers to contagion, as he says, he must be a scoundrel. There is no way that I know of offhand to deal with such a person legally, but I am sure the citizens will not fail to characterize his action as it deserves."[50] To an audience of fellow health officers, Durgin questioned Pfeiffer's mental stability: "it must be either an insane man or a scoundrel who would do anything like that in any community."[51]

The Hunt for Pfeiffer

Soon after his visit, Pfeiffer attended hearings on compulsory vaccination before the Joint Committee on Public Health at the State Legislature. On 29 January he testified before the committee, seemingly quite well in the eyes of onlookers who described him as a youthful-looking "man of vigorous, robust constitution, in excellent health, nearly 6 feet in height, and weighing not far from 200 lbs."[52] Then he disappeared from public view, "his absence so conspicuous" that Durgin pointed it out to the committee on Monday, 3 February, noting that Pfeiffer had vanished just thirteen days after his visit to Gallop's Island—right at the time when Durgin had expected the "full development of the incubation."[53]

As news of Pfeiffer's absence spread, reporters questioned Durgin about the propriety of his decision to allow Pfeiffer's visit. Durgin again played the innocent victim, but argued that he had not failed in his duty to protect the public: "Knowing Dr. Pfeiffer to be a registered physician I had no objection to granting his request, whether his visit was to be that of an honest physician with honest purpose, or that of an unprotected representative of the antivaccinationists, with, however, the purpose on my part of keeping him under observation for the protection of the public."[54] Durgin was not completely reckless: he had quietly detailed a policeman to watch Pfeiffer upon his return from Gallop's Island. He calculated that if Pfeiffer had indeed contracted smallpox, he would not pose a threat until the incubation period had passed—around twelve to fourteen days after exposure—and later declared "emphatically that until the eruption which accompanies the disease made its appearance, there was not the slightest danger of anyone becoming infected by contact with him."[55] Still, Durgin's loose surveillance seemed a risky proposition, given the tendency for this type of smallpox (variola minor) to manifest so mildly that many victims continued to go about their daily routine. Some might question the sincerity of his professed regard for public safety when he could have held Pfeiffer in quarantine rather than allow him his freedom after the hospital visit.

A few newspaper editors worried over that precise point, wondering why Durgin had not taken greater care in the matter. The *Boston Post* declared Pfeiffer's visit "a most injudicious relaxation of the rules of the health authorities."[56] Another editor insisted that "the best thing for the public" would have been "a strict police quarantine with police assistance."[57] Such criticism forced Durgin to soften his initial condemnation of Pfeiffer in order to save his own reputation as a conscientious health officer. When asked on 10 February about his role in Pfeiffer's visit, Durgin defended his decision, claiming that every precaution had been followed: "Dr. Pfeiffer left the island with an exterior condition as free from carrying contagion as any other visiting physician. He did nothing that was not perfectly proper for a physician to do."[58] Durgin even went so far as to assert that Pfeiffer "washed his hands, face, and beard and hair in disinfecting liquid" before he left the hospital, a fact that Pfeiffer later disputed as "untrue," claiming no one ever asked him to do so.[59] Far from panicking that his agents had blundered in allowing a smallpox victim to wander at large, Durgin, previously rather terse about Pfeiffer's visit to Gallop's Island, now spoke openly to spin the story his way, declaring "the board of health has simply done its duty in the matter, just as it would have done in the case of any other case in which there should be suspicion and apprehension."[60]

Nevertheless, Pfeiffer was no ordinary case. Durgin had made quite an exception for him, one difficult to reconcile with his purported mission to protect the public's health. Pfeiffer later observed: "Now is it not plain that if I am to be blamed, that Dr. Durgin ought to come in for the bigger share, as without his permission I could not have either gone to the hospitals on the island, nor left."[61] Yet the small matter of his complicity in Pfeiffer's visit and his failure to contain him afterward apparently did not trouble Durgin's scruples. He later defended his decision: "I believe that the greatest good to the largest number would result by allowing Dr. Pfeiffer such a visit."[62] Durgin had expected Pfeiffer to come down with smallpox from the very beginning—thus providing a supreme object lesson to those who still balked at vaccination.

Pfeiffer's disappearance received considerable coverage from all the Boston newspapers. Reporters scrambled to obtain news of Pfeiffer and they besieged his office for information. There, they encountered his new assistant, Dr. Reuben Swinburne Clymer, just arrived from Pennsylvania, who confirmed that he had met with Pfeiffer in Philadelphia over the weekend and that Pfeiffer had hired him "to take charge of the Boston end of the doctor's business."[63] Although Pfeiffer's clerk, Mrs. S. I. Boardman, then told them that he had since traveled to New York, "and everybody there ridiculed the idea that the doctor had smallpox," speculation that he had not really left the city was rife.[64] Witnesses claimed to have seen him at various places and times throughout the week.[65]

Police detectives attempting to trace his movements first went Mrs. Boardman's home in Charlestown. They believed that as a nurse and "a great friend," she would be the first person Pfeiffer would seek if he were indeed ill.[66] She denied seeing him and "refused to confirm or deny" any theories about Pfeiffer. The janitor of her apartment house, however, told a different story. While standing at the back door of the building, he encountered Pfeiffer and Mrs. Boardman late Thursday afternoon. The janitor declared he had spoken with the doctor and that although he "is usually a man of great physical energy, he appeared somewhat weak as he walked down the stairs and up the street"—a statement that must have sent chills up Boston's collective spine. Two other witnesses saw a man and a woman enter a cab from the same back entrance that afternoon, which sent detectives flying about the city to locate the hack in question.[67]

Boston health authorities finally caught up with Pfeiffer by maintaining a watch on Mrs. Boardman. Early Saturday morning, Pfeiffer's son called on her and then left. At one o'clock that afternoon, she took a hack bound for Bedford, an 18-mile trek from Boston. Boston police detailed Officer Reilly to take the train to Bedford. There he hunted up the town selectmen in lieu of a board of health because like many other small towns, it lacked an independent board. The selectmen appointed a local physician, Dr. Edward B. Hamblin, as their agent, and together they called on Pfeiffer at his farm.[68] Hamblin confirmed that Pfeiffer had "a thoroughly developed case of smallpox" and he notified both the State Board of Health and the Boston Board of Health.[69] By this time, Mrs. Boardman had also arrived. She and the Pfeiffer family were placed immediately in quarantine. Each agency sent out physicians to examine Pfeiffer that night—a decision indicative of the importance health authorities accorded Pfeiffer as a celebrated smallpox case.

When Pfeiffer finally turned up with smallpox, "the victim of his own folly and professional vanity," the press exploded with articles and editorials about his illness.[70] Every major local paper and a number of medical journals covered the story, as well as the *New York Times*, which declared the announcement of Pfeiffer's illness had caused "a sensation" in Boston.[71] The *Boston Globe* asserted "He May Not Recover," citing health officials who declared that "he may not live more than 48 hours or three days at most."[72] The *Boston Herald* declared "Anti-Vaccinationist May Not Live" in a front-page headline.[73] The *Boston Post* also ran a front-page story complete with a portrait of Pfeiffer that announced "Pfeiffer Dying of Smallpox—Noted Anti-Vaccinationist Who Risked Exposure Is Dying."[74] Thomas B. Shea, the Boston health department physician on the scene, sadly declared, "Dr. Pfeiffer certainly got it as hard as it could come to him," and practically wrote him off.[75]

When interviewed about Pfeiffer's whereabouts throughout the week, the family presented conflicting stories, with Pfeiffer's wife maintaining he had come home Thursday evening and his son declaring that he had returned from New York on Friday.[76] Although it seemed a small discrepancy, the timing was important because Pfeiffer's two unvaccinated daughters attended school on Friday.[77] The eldest, Hannah, had taken a streetcar with fifteen other pupils to her high school, while the younger girl, Alice, had attended the local grammar school. Although they posed no real threat to their schoolmates, since they would not have been infectious until after the incubation period had passed, the Bedford school superintendent ordered all students vaccinated or to remain at home. That Sunday, the *Post* reported, "fathers and mothers gave up church in order to get their children vaccinated."[78]

In an atmosphere of heightened anxiety about smallpox and with some degree of uncertainty about the exact nature of its transmission, Bedford residents reacted with understandable irritation. Many were quite upset because the Pfeiffer family, not quarantined until Sunday, "conducted quite a milk farm," its customers coming and going all day on both Friday and Saturday, even though the doctor lay sick in bed with no public contact.[79] One newspaper reported

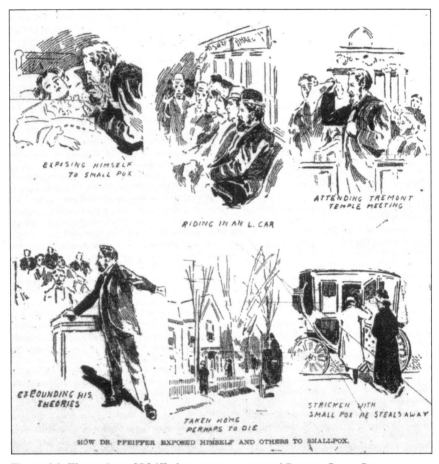

Figure 6.1. Illustration of Pfeiffer's movements around Boston. *Boston Post*,
10 February 1902, 1.

that "sympathy for him is entirely lacking in the neighborhood, and the epithets
applied to him are neither mild nor elegant, one of the least suggestive being
that he is 'an old chump.'"[80] Another declared, "Bedford is up in arms."[81] Until
Pfeiffer's case, "quite a number of people" in the community opposed vaccination to the point that "the place has been divided in regard to this question."[82]
News of Pfeiffer's illness, however, impelled many to "rush to doctor's offices"
seeking vaccinations.[83] Boston residents were likewise perturbed. Even the
Boston Post, which had reported favorably on Pfeiffer in the past, deplored the
many contacts he must have made as he traveled about Boston in its streetcars,
and asked, "when he was walking among the people . . . did he bring danger to
others as well as himself?"[84]

Pfeiffer's Side of the Story

Newspapers reported that many of Pfeiffer's neighbors, "intensely indignant" at his failure to report his case to the Boston health authorities, had condemned his selfish flight.[85] Pfeiffer saw his situation differently—he fled because he feared the pesthouse at Gallop's Island, which he knew quite well since he had inspected it and found it wanting. Recalling his situation a few months later he explained that he knew Durgin's ultimate objective—to carry him off ignominiously to the isolation hospital—a fate he desired to avoid at all cost. "Had I been a bank cashier, who had absconded with the bank funds I could not have been pursued with more persistency and hatred by a flock of paid hirelings, who held before them their instruction: 'Bring Dr. Pfeiffer, alive or dead, to the pest house and you shall get your reward.' The detectives had the hearty co-operation of the police and an army of reporters, who were eagerly seeking sensational news." If he had not concealed his whereabouts, the Boston Board of Health would have certainly taken him into custody and placed him in the smallpox hospital. Pfeiffer later defended his flight as an act of self-preservation: "Is there any one who believes I would have got away from the island alive, or at least marked for life?" Like many of his contemporaries, he preferred to be ill at home, attended by private nurses and his family rather than take his chances in the city isolation hospital. "Some have gone so far as to condemn me because I went home. Is this not a good place to go to when you are sick? I remember the time when we treated all small-pox cases in the patients' homes, and who will deny they had better treatment than given in our modern pesthouses, controlled by unscrupulous politicians, and certainly we had fewer deaths."[86] The Bedford selectmen quarantined the Pfeiffer family, since like many other small Massachusetts communities, they lacked a pesthouse. Pfeiffer knew this and judged that he would be far more comfortable at home than in the clutches of his enemies.

Nevertheless, Pfeiffer did not escape health department ministrations. The State Board of Health sent medical officers Frank L. Morse and Dr. Wright to examine him, while the Boston health department sent the smallpox expert Thomas Shea. According to Pfeiffer, the three "semi-wild" physicians came "rushing into the house, crazed with the thought, 'Found at last,'—asking questions in all directions." Ignoring attempts to bar their entry into the sickroom, they pushed in and proceeded to examine the sick man, using a lamp to illuminate the room even though Pfeiffer's son tried several times to remove it because the light hurt his father's eyes. "The three doctors rushed to my bed and commenced to handle me in all kinds of ways. . . . They tore my shirt-sleeve open in trying to find any recent vaccination mark, and one of them expressed surprise in not finding any recent mark of vaccination, as he certainly thought I had lied . . . and the kind finishing touch was applied by Dr. Shea in telling my wife that there was no prospect for my recovery, and that I would only live about three days." The health department physicians apparently displayed little in the way of kindness to the sick man or his family. Desperate to pin down

Pfeiffer's movements for the last week, they took the house by storm, interrogating Pfeiffer's daughters and wife separately to ascertain whether there were any contradictions in their accounts of Pfeiffer's whereabouts. One doctor cornered twelve-year-old Alice in the kitchen to ask, "'Was your father's face broke out on his arrival?' 'When did he get home?'" Pfeiffer indignantly called this tactic "a sneaking way of trying to get a child to contradict her seniors," affronted at the health officers' invasion not only of his home but also of his parental rights.[87]

Pfeiffer charged that the health department physicians provided no medical care, even though they believed him to be in a "critical and dying condition": "The great experts (?) were so delighted—they reminded me of Indians having a war dance after a successful battle—and so anxious to find out particulars of when I arrived, etc., etc., that not one of them gave one word of advice to my nurse, who was present." Offering neither treatment nor assistance to Pfeiffer, "no effort was made to get me an experienced physician" until the next morning. Pfeiffer later learned that Shea had expressed grim satisfaction at his plight by remarking to a railroad conductor: "'Yes, Dr. Pfeiffer has not only got the small-pox, but he has it bad, and it is a damn good thing he has.'"[88]

Although every person in the house submitted to vaccination, Bedford quarantined the family and their visitor at great expense ($1,000) and even considered suing Boston for the costs of guarding them, declaring "the disease was imported because of the inexcusable negligence of the health authorities of Boston."[89] The family's quarantine cost them dearly—it lasted five weeks and extended even to the livestock, although no one else in the household fell ill and the Bedford authorities understood that vaccinations provide immunity in about eight or nine days. Although Immanuel Pfeiffer, Jr. was vaccinated and applied "several times" for release in order to maintain his veterinary practice, the town authorities denied him. Yet, as Pfeiffer noted, they allowed Pfeiffer's physician, E. J. Alley, also vaccinated, to come and go at will. Pfeiffer later complained that his son "complied with the compulsory vaccination law, and ought to have had his liberty. It looks as if the pro-vaccinationists after all don't believe vaccination protects." The Pfeiffer family was not allowed to sell their milk or eggs, and they were forced to dump "about $100 worth of milk."[90] Immanuel Pfeiffer, Jr. later sent the town of Bedford a bill for the lost milk that also included "the loss of his professional services."[91] Pfeiffer felt that public health authorities had treated him harshly because of his political stance: "had I not taken a lively part in the anti-vaccination movement there would not have been anything said in the papers about me, and the Board of Health (?) of Boston would not have done a thing."[92]

Pfeiffer was mistaken if he believed that the Boston health department would have done nothing to track and isolate him if he had been an ordinary smallpox case—such actions were standard tactics in epidemic control. But he was no innocent victim, and thus became an object lesson of supreme value in the propaganda war. His case was extraordinary, and this notoriety tempted health authorities to take advantage of his plight to make a public point about the value of vaccination. Dr. Morse of the State Board of Health attempted to photograph the sick man as his illness reached its apex, but had to back off when Pfeiffer's attending physician objected. A picture of Pfeiffer's swollen face covered with pustules would indeed be worth thousands of words, and he well knew it when he complained that "perhaps engraving my face would have given the most satisfaction" to the health department officials.[93]

Although Pfeiffer thought the health officers seemed insensitive, their primary duty did not lie with the victim, but rather with the public at large. Their first priority was disease containment, and they had to trace his contacts even if their interrogation seemed overly intrusive to Pfeiffer's family. Although their failure to offer treatment or advice seems cruel on the face of it, they did not come into his home as caregivers, but rather as detectives determined to limit the damage Pfeiffer might have done as he moved about the Boston area. They also thought he would have been better off in the isolation hospital where he could have received expert nursing care. Indeed Pfeiffer reported that Dr. Shea told his son that they had no desire to make the sick doctor any more miserable. "Your father thought we wanted to get him down to the island to kill him or do him harm; far from it, we would have been very kind to him." Nevertheless, Pfeiffer was not impressed when he heard of Shea's sentiment: "Yes, 14 detectives hunted me day and night for a week, for the purpose of giving the pro-vaccinationists a chance to be kind to me."[94]

Pfeiffer eventually recovered, his case less severe than first reported, and he declared that "the disease of smallpox, dreadful as it is said to be, never caused me pain for one minute." He maintained that he bore up well under the onslaught of smallpox: "I never lost control of my mind for one minute." He even "laughed and told jokes and played games most of the time." Pfeiffer blamed overtiredness for his susceptibility: "I had good reason to believe I was immune, and I honestly believe now that had I not been immensely overworked as many of my friends know I was, harm would not have come to me."[95] The anti-vaccinationist physician Charles E. Page agreed that Pfeiffer caught smallpox because he was "excessively fat, soft, and physically untrained; living a sedentary, indoor life; overworked and generally run down, he might well have come down with the disease if he had remained away from Gallups Island."[96]

Pfeiffer asserted that his experience showed the difficulty of communicating smallpox because he had contact with so many "clerks, stenographers, and others in my office" as well as his family, yet none came down with smallpox. Pfeiffer further alleged that the only people sick in Bedford were the recently vaccinated, including a man who usually worked on his farm, but had been "sick for two weeks, unable to do his work" because of his vaccination. Defiant to the end, Pfeiffer denied that his neighbors were angry with him, arguing instead that they were upset about the outcomes of the vaccinations they had hastily procured in the panic after his arrival. "Here in Bedford is a large number of people who curse the day they permitted themselves to be vaccinated, and there are many who declare they will use a shot gun next time an attempt should be made to vaccinate them. Although it is now several weeks since the people here got vaccinated, still there are many who suffer yet greatly from the effect."[97]

Immanuel Pfeiffer did not regard his illness as a humiliating debacle. Instead he saw it as an ordeal imposed on him by overreaching public health officials intent on punishing him for standing up to them. From his perspective, he was a hero, not a laughingstock.

Aftermath

Just a day after news of Pfeiffer's condition broke out throughout Boston, the health department undertook yet another vaccination sweep, this time in the North, South, and West ends. Perhaps not so coincidentally, the 125 physicians employed to give the vaccinations "met with but little objection," finding "that the case of Dr. Pfeiffer had helped their cause amazingly."[98] Every major Boston newspaper continued to cover the story of his illness as it progressed, providing an ongoing account of his travails to edify the Boston public.[99] The *Boston Medical and Surgical Journal* declared that "as an object lesson the case has proved of the very greatest value," and several months later observed that "vaccination received a new impetus as soon as the circumstances of his illness became generally known through the daily papers."[100]

The medical press crowed over Pfeiffer's misfortune, characterizing him as a fool who deserved his fate. In New York City, the *Medical News* jubilantly proclaimed: "This is a case in a hundred years for the cause of prevention of smallpox.[101] The *Journal of the American Medical Association* concurred in the edifying effect of "a Boston anti-vaccinationist crank" (obviously Pfeiffer) for the cause of vaccination: "If a few more of the blatant anti-vaccinationists would only furnish an object lesson like the eastern physicians mentioned it could perhaps be said they did not suffer or die in vain."[102] For the *Boston Medical and Surgical Journal*, Pfeiffer merely demonstrated "the utter want of common sense by which the experimenter becomes victim of his own folly."[103] Although Philadelphia's *American Medicine* criticized Durgin for allowing Pfeiffer's exposure as one of "two bad methods of fighting the antivaccination craze," it regarded Pfeiffer and other antivaccinationists as "criminals and insane."[104] When Pfeiffer announced a few months later that he remained committed to his antivaccinationist beliefs, the same journal commented that "a belief not founded upon reason and evidence is affected neither by reason nor evidence."[105] *American Medicine* continued to lambaste Pfeiffer regularly over the course of the next few months.[106]

Other commentators were not entirely convinced that Pfeiffer had provided an object lesson in vaccination. Although the *Boston Post* had observed that Pfeiffer's case would discredit the antivaccinationists, it also wondered if perhaps Pfeiffer's overly provocative attempts to expose himself by deliberately inhaling a victim's breath had somehow rendered him more susceptible than a more ordinary exposure. "Can anyone say that vaccination alone would have warded off the disease? Dr. Pfeiffer is the victim of rashness in testing his theory. It has failed in his personal case. He was not immune, and he was unvaccinated since infancy. But can we draw the general inference from this negative evidence

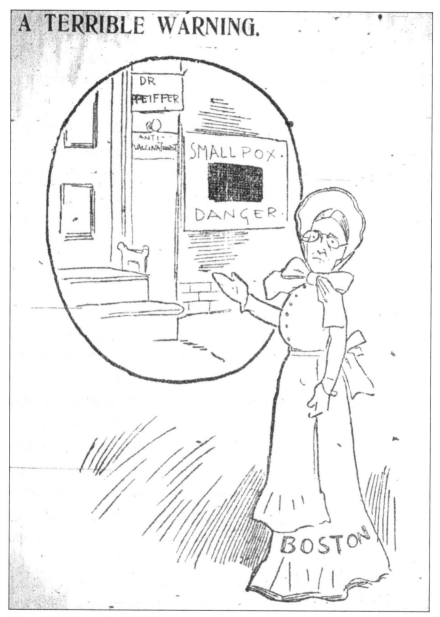

Figure 6.2. Illustration depicting Boston as a prim old lady deploring the danger Pfeiffer represents. Cartoon in the *Boston Evening Record*, 10 February 1902.

in a single case, that the practice of vaccination is everywhere preventive? The question must be decided on broader grounds, by the experience of communities rather than of individuals—more especially when the individual conducts himself so recklessly as did Dr. Pfeiffer."[107]

Pfeiffer's case may have resulted from very unusual circumstances, circumstances unlikely to occur for most people, and it proved nothing about the need to vaccinate an entire community when cases of smallpox crop up. The antivaccinationist physician Charles Fessenden Nichols asserted that the case of Immanuel Pfieffer had "no bearing upon the large problem," explaining that "thoughtful opponents of vaccination have reached their conclusions by massing large results."[108] Others faulted Durgin's carelessness rather than lack of vaccination for the continuing epidemic. State Senator Chester B. Williams, who sat on the Joint Committee on Public Health, asserted that Durgin was remiss in his duty as a public health officer. "If there is an epidemic of smallpox in Boston at this time, it is directly traceable to the office of Dr. Durgin, and it comes from permitting physicians to go from smallpox cases direct to the public. . . . If Dr. Durgin thought Dr. Pfeiffer had smallpox, as it seems he did so think by his action in tracing him around the city, I think he ought to have quarantined him instead of allowing him to expose himself so generally to other people."

Representative Walter E. Nichols, another state legislator on the Public Health Committee, admitted "that Dr. Pfeiffer needlessly exposed himself," but criticized Durgin for allowing Pfeiffer "to come up to the city and expose himself to other people without thorough fumigation." Refusing to heed the so-called object lesson, Representative Nichols could not "see how the case of the antivaccinationists is affected by this illness of Dr. Pfeiffer. . . . It is not their contention that smallpox is not contagious and neither is it their contention that persons cannot catch it. What they do contend is that a person if exposed to smallpox, is as likely to catch the disease if vaccinated as he would be if unvaccinated. I think the case of Dr. Pfeiffer bears out this very claim. Dr. Pfeiffer was vaccinated in his childhood or youth, I understand, and he has taken the disease."[109] Although Durgin repeatedly emphasized the need for revaccination to protect against the present smallpox epidemic, many people like Nichols may not have completely understood his message. Thus it is possible that some read Pfeiffer as an instance of vaccination's failure to protect rather than as an example of the fate wrought by failure to get vaccinated. Still others saw him in heroic terms. Another legislator sympathetic to the antivaccinationist cause, Representative John F. Foster, later admired Pfeiffer for demonstrating "the courage of his convictions,"hand compared him to "John Brown of Harper's Ferry and Carrie Nation of Kansas" as examples of other Americans who took controversial actions to effect social justice and progress.[110] Thus for some observers, albeit a minority, Pfeiffer stood out as an object lesson in courage rather than folly.

The *Boston and Medical Surgical Journal* boasted that Pfeiffer's case convinced "a great mass of the wavering who will take the lesson to heart."[111] In the estimation of his peers, Durgin had succeeded brilliantly in making Pfeiffer into an object lesson for vaccination. Yet had his gamble had paid off in the eyes of the public? Although health department physicians in Boston noticed a more cooperative spirit in their vaccination sweeps shortly after the discovery of Pfeiffer's illness, Cambridge residents remained less inclined to open their doors when vaccinators called several weeks later. Pfeiffer's lesson may have been less salutary for the cause of vaccination than it first appeared after people learned that he had survived smallpox relatively unscathed.

In the end, however, Samuel Durgin got exactly what he had asked for when he had publicly dared antivaccinationists to step forward and expose themselves to smallpox. Immanuel Pfeiffer became an object lesson for the people, one that apparently convinced many to accept their vaccinations without protest just as the Boston health department conducted one of its sweeps. Even with the power to compel vaccination, the Boston health department still ran into resistance over vaccination as it started door-to-door visits in various sections of the city. Newspaper coverage of Pfeiffer's case provided crucial publicity for the value of vaccination just when Durgin needed it the most. Pfeiffer conveniently acquired smallpox just as the health department began another vaccination sweep and the Joint Committee on Public Health concluded its hearings on a bill to abolish the compulsory vaccination law. Sensational accounts in every major paper of the search for Pfeiffer and his illness served to remind Bostonians that smallpox lurked everywhere. The *Boston Post*, for instance, lamented that Pfeiffer "came and went like any other resident of the city, coming in contact with hundreds of people." In a story designed to maximize general anxiety, the paper dwelt in lavish detail upon Pfeiffer's movements about the city. "Stopped at a street crossing by a passing car or vehicle, he rubbed elbows with other passersby. Riding in a crowded Elevated train, as the car swung around one of the sharp curves in the subway he was thrown against the man or woman who was clinging to the next strap. Meeting a friend or acquaintance, he took his hand and shook it heartily, laughingly reiterating his opinion that there was no use in vaccination. When the anti-vaccination hearings were held at the State House, he attended the first two sessions, there coming in contact with many people, some vaccinated, others believers and followers of his own theories."[112] The moral of this story is clear: only the recently vaccinated were safe—all others flirted with death. Samuel Durgin could not have gotten better publicity for the value of vaccination if he had written it himself. A *Boston Herald* editor deftly summed up the situation when he observed: "Chairman Durgin comes up smiling."[113]

Chapter Seven

The 1902 Campaign to Amend the Compulsory Vaccination Laws

Early in 1902, Massachusetts antivaccinationists almost achieved one of their dearest objectives, a change in the state vaccination law to allow adults the same medical exemption privilege as that accorded to schoolchildren. Boston Board of Health Chairman Samuel H. Durgin had petitioned for a bill to strengthen the existing vaccination law by requiring that physicians personally examine the children for whom they provided exemption certificates. When the bill came to the senate floor for debate in 1902, legislators sympathetic to antivaccination successfully proposed an amendment to include adults as candidates for medical exemptions, and the amended bill passed by a narrow margin. Nevertheless, provaccination senators managed to reopen the bill for consideration the next day. In another very close vote, this time the senate voted *not* to allow adults the exemption.

These votes present a unique opportunity to gauge the extent of sympathy for antivaccination in Massachusetts. Antivaccination bills to abolish or weaken the vaccination law simply never came up for floor votes—the legislature's Joint Public Health Committee always voted them down, serving as a very effective gatekeeper to preserve compulsory vaccination. Thus state legislators never got a chance to debate these abolition bills or vote on them, giving a false impression that they all overwhelmingly supported compulsory vaccination. But Durgin's bill passed easily through the committee, providing a rare opportunity for legislators sympathetic to antivaccination to debate and amend the existing law. The closeness of the back-and-forth votes on the amendments shows that antivaccinationists had gained substantial public sympathy for their position.

Looking at this contest closely can tell us a lot about where support for change was strongest in the state and helps explain how the Massachusetts vaccination statutes—among the strictest in the nation—would eventually soften to allow various exemptions to its requirements. Public interest in changing the vaccination law ran high in 1902. Hearings on petitions for vaccination bills were packed to overflowing with supporters from towns and villages all over the state. They demonstrated enthusiastically for witnesses who disparaged vaccination and booed those who supported it. Even though these bills never made it out of committee, such attendance shows that there was significant popular support for changing the state compulsory vaccination law. The press reported on these hearings in detail, and this coverage reached people who might have had some doubts about vaccination but were unlikely to attend a lecture or read a pamphlet. The mere fact that newspapers devoted so much space to these hearings indicates that these editors agreed that compulsory vaccination was a controversial issue that deserved their attention. If such coverage boosted circulation, so much the better.

The Massachusetts Boards of Health and Antivaccination

At the beginning of 1902, the smallpox epidemic that had begun eight months earlier still plagued the cities, towns, and villages of Massachusetts. As new cases continued to crop up despite health officials' efforts to isolate, quarantine, and vaccinate, confidence faltered that they would soon contain the disease. By 30 January 1902, when the annual meeting of the Massachusetts Association of Boards of Health convened in Boston, smallpox and vaccination unsurprisingly dominated the discussions. Composed of officers from local health boards as well as health officials from other states, the Association had become by 1902 the premiere professional public health organization in the United States. It counted among its members leading public health figures such as Samuel Holmes Durgin (who, as its vice president, served as de facto leader of the organization), Charles V. Chapin, Hibbert W. Hill, William T. Sedgwick, Theobald Smith, and C.-E. A. Winslow.

That January evening, anywhere from seventy-five to one hundred health officials gathered to dine together at the Parker House Hotel and consider the latest public health issues.[1] After dinner, the Boston health department physician Thomas B. Shea gave a talk about vaccination in which he deplored how Boston's antivaccinationists had subverted the health department's vaccination efforts: "Yesterday morning I was at the State House, and listened to our friends, the 'antis,' making another assault upon our vaccination law. I must confess that they during the past five or six years have been up and doing."[2] First passed in 1855, the Massachusetts vaccination law required parents or guardians to vaccinate children before they were two years old and forbade public schools to admit any unvaccinated pupils.[3] It required vaccination for inmates in prisons, jails, asylums, and other public institutions, as well as employees of large manufacturing concerns. Called by one historian "the most advanced stand ever taken by States," it also granted local boards of health the power to order the vaccination and revaccination of all inhabitants during smallpox epidemics, with a fine of five dollars levied for refusal.[4]

Although this law was one of the strictest in the United States, some Massachusetts public health experts believed that it had significant shortcomings. State Board of Health Secretary Samuel Abbott called the law "defective, and wrong in principle" because it only required universal vaccination after an epidemic had already taken hold.[5] He noted that in "several instances the

presence of one antivaccinationist upon a local board of health has so influenced the action of the board as to result in serious harm to the community, by
delaying public vaccination." Even worse, the law allowed a piecemeal response
when smallpox epidemics were "not confined to the boundary lines of cities or
towns": "The neglect of one town or one state may prove also a serious menace to the people of another town or state. Again, the non-voting part of the
community, the women and, especially the unprotected children, may become
victims of the neglect of the voting portion." Even worse, Massachusetts antivaccinationists weakened this law in 1894 when they convinced the state legislature to amend it to allow registered physicians to certify some children as unfit
candidates for vaccination.[6] Originally intended as a humane measure to allow
sickly children to put off vaccination temporarily yet still attend public school in
the meantime, the amendment had become a convenient dodge for those who
objected to vaccination on principle. Some physicians who believed that vaccination endangered all children colluded with antivaccinationist parents to certify
even healthy ones as unfit for it. Parents who wanted to avoid vaccinating their
children yet still send them to public school could do so easily with the help of
an obliging physician.

Nevertheless, antivaccinationists wanted more. During this latest smallpox
outbreak, after the Boston Board of Health had ordered compulsory vaccination—an order applicable to all adults—they began a campaign to abolish the
state's general compulsory vaccination law. A state representative revived a bill
to abolish the law just a few weeks before the meeting of the Association, and
the Joint Committee on Public Health had already started hearings on it. Thus,
at the Association meeting, Shea warned his colleagues that the antivaccinationists had managed to gain quite an advantage over public health officials.
Their literature had proved very effective in spreading their arguments to the
larger public. Now their campaign had moved into the State House and public
health authorities had no formal plan to counter their attack, not even witnesses
pledged to testify for vaccination at the current hearings.

William T. Sedgwick, a Massachusetts Institute of Technology professor
and biologist who worked closely with the State Board of Health, also gave
a talk that night at the Association meeting. He noticed how adeptly antivaccinationists reached out to the general reader, whereas physicians and health
officials tended to confine their rhetoric to the pages of professional medical
journals and reports in a mistaken attempt to keep the debate on a scientific
level, feeling that such matters were beyond the scope of lay consideration.
Health officials resorted to blanket condemnations of antivaccinationists, and
Sedgwick feared that they would lose the battle for the hearts and minds of the
general public, a bad strategy "in America, especially where we have popular
government." He felt that health officials needed to take antivaccinationists
seriously and "to listen to the arguments of honest objectors and endeavor,
if possible, to meet the arguments and convince their advocates." After all,
he argued, the whole public health edifice rested on the will of the voting
public that he hoped "will pay attention to arguments if they are put forward

in a dispassionate, honest, and straightforward way." Health officials had to recognize that antivaccinationists made some valid points concerning personal liberty and vaccine quality, and they must address those objections in order to gain the confidence of the general public: "Compulsory vaccination is a very serious infringement of personal liberty. The whole idea of our government and our living is that, in general, a man's house is his castle, and that his body and his religion and his politics are his own." Sedgwick noted that although infringements to personal liberty existed as matter of course in American law and everyday life, compulsory vaccination posed a unique problem because it meant the injection of disease into an unwilling, healthy subject: "it is a serious thing to take a man . . . and thrust a disease germ into him against his will; for the cow-pox is a disease, of course, and . . . this is a serious infringement of personal liberty." Until health officials were willing to come up with reasonable arguments that such an intrusion was justified, they could expect even more resistance. They had to find a way to convince people to accept the "mild disease" of vaccinia as a community good, "to prevent . . . distributing the fatal disease to others." Although Sedgwick believed that the argument ultimately revolved around the simple issue of individual sacrifice for the common good, health authorities seemed to have difficulty in communicating it adequately to the public at large. Even when vaccination sometimes resulted in infection, as its opponents charged it too often did, Sedgwick maintained that such outcomes were nothing compared with the toll smallpox took on its victims before vaccination: "An occasional bad arm, or even an occasional lost leg, if you prefer, doesn't compare for a moment with the fear and pain and anguish and sorrow that came only too often in the old days. Our opponents suffer from a lack of perspective, from a failure to look at things in a large way, and see where the most beneficent results, after all, have come in." The supporters of vaccination needed to enlarge the perspective of the public to remind people just how loathsome and horrible smallpox unchecked by vaccination could be.[7]

Antivaccinationists found support in books with mass appeal like Alfred Russel Wallace's *The Wonderful Century,* but Sedgwick found no one of similar stature writing to defend vaccination for a general audience.[8] Instead, the medical establishment fostered an attitude of exclusivity in its literature that tended to put the latest medical findings beyond the intellectual reach of the average reader. He charged that little "readable" literature promoting vaccination was available to lay people, yet a plethora of antivaccination literature seemed to inundate Boston. Medical journals were too difficult and "your ordinary citizen, who goes up to represent his town or his city at the State House, does not get time to go through them, he is not familiar with the statistics and medical terms." Health officials needed to reach out to "honest, well-meaning people, who really have a grievance . . . by bringing forward the facts. We need very much, it seems to me, a simple, straightforward account of the whole matter, which shall be readable, and which can be put into the hands of those who are honestly seeking information."[9] Sedgwick believed that health officials who dismissed antivaccinationists merely as a bunch of lunatics or hysterics had made a serious mistake. They needed to muster statistics and facts to address the contentions of the antivaccinationists rather than just to call them names.

Although Sedgwick had "no very deep fear" that the antivaccinationists could overturn the compulsory vaccination law, he warned his audience that they could not "afford to pooh-pooh the whole thing, pay no attention to it, and simply laugh at it, because, if we do, we shall some day wake up to the fact that these people, by their incessant arguing and mistaken statements, have persuaded the legislature to follow their wishes."[10] Others at the meeting agreed that they must do something to counter the antivaccinationists. Samuel Durgin admonished the health officials to organize: "if this is not a body of men who have convictions upon this point, I should not know where to look for them." Durgin urged them to protest against any attempt to change the existing vaccination laws, scolding his colleagues: "Now, shall we sit by and permit our statute laws, which mean protection to our citizens, to be emasculated in that way? It is just what will be done if you and I don't show a spirit of resistance. Will you go, or will you submit to these inroads upon wholesome laws?"[11]

Inspired by Durgin's remarks, the Boston physician Edwin L. Pilsbury motioned that the Association present a formal resolution supporting compulsory vaccination to the Public Health Committee.[12] The Association adopted the resolution with great enthusiasm. Twenty-eight members volunteered to form a committee pledged to attend the hearing, and they elected Durgin, over his protests, as their spokesman.[13]

Public fervor over vaccination led one newspaper to observe that "no question coming before the Legislature of late years has so stirred up public sentiment at the State House."[14] Massachusetts antivaccinationists provided some steep competition for the Association's health officials. Streaming into Boston's State House, they overwhelmed the 1902 legislative vaccination hearings as they boisterously applauded statements they liked or jeered those they hated. Interest in proceedings was so strong that the largest committee room in the State House could barely accommodate all who wished to attend.[15] One newspaper noted that "more than half the auditors were women, and among them were some of the most ardent anti-vaccinationists."[16]

Out of all the health officials in the state, Durgin especially drew antivaccinationists' ire. He seemed to relish the attention, however, as both sides worked assiduously to manipulate public perceptions of vaccination to gain their objectives. He wanted to toughen exemptions to the existing law and obtain an appropriation to build a state vaccine facility. Antivaccinationists wanted to either abolish compulsion or amend the statute to allow adults a medical exemption from vaccination. They had organized the Massachusetts Anti-compulsory Vaccination Society (MACVS) primarily to petition for changes in the compulsory vaccination laws and to organize testimony before the state legislature's hearings on vaccination.

In Massachusetts, individual citizens could present a petition for legislation to a member of the House of Representatives or the Senate, who presented the bill for a "first reading." Then the bill was assigned a committee for a review, which would hold hearings for public input and vote to recommend or reject the bill. If the bill passed through committee, the legislature would then submit the bill to two more votes, called a "second" and "third reading." In order for a bill to become a law, it had to pass on its third reading. Bills concerning public health that originated from either the House or Senate went before the Joint Committee on Public Health, which then decided whether or not to pass them on for a second reading on the floor.[17]

The first 1902 abolition bill, introduced by Representative John F. Foster of Somerville, originated from a bill held over from the last session.[18] It asserted that state officials could neither "compel any man or woman to be vaccinated against his or her consent" nor "order any child vaccinated against the will of the child's parent or guardian."[19] Accompanied by petitions signed by citizens in several towns, Foster's bill had fairly substantial popular support and it became the focal point of well-attended legislative hearings. Feelings about vaccination ran deep on both sides of the issue: in Provincetown, 110 residents signed a petition to abolish compulsory vaccination, whereas 33 signed a remonstrance to support it.[20] In Rockland, 111 citizens also signed abolition petitions.[21] Significant numbers of women signed the abolition petitions, though none signed the pro-vaccination remonstrance.

Other bills to amend the vaccination law flooded into the legislature during 1902. Representative Foster not only revived the 1901 abolition bill but he also introduced several bills to grant adults the same medical exemption as children.[22] If antivaccinationists could not obtain a repeal of the compulsory vaccination law, they sought to soften it by amending the existing law to include adults. Other legislators also endorsed bills to amend the compulsory vaccination law. Representative Fred C. Gilpatric, a Republican from Boston, called for legislation to restrict the authority of public health officials to penalize objectors to compulsory vaccination and repeal the five-dollar fine.[23] The attorney James W. Pickering, who later represented several antivaccinationist objectors in court, appeared to testify for this bill, declaring that the law as written lacked "an adequate remedy for persons injured by the acts of public officials," and this bill would restrict the power of boards of health that had "acted with autocratic power and forcibly assaulted persons to vaccinate them."[24] Immanuel Pfeiffer also petitioned for abolition of compulsory vaccination by outlawing the injection of "any poisonous substance without first obtaining the consent of such person."[25]

The first public hearings to take testimony on vaccination began in late January.[26] Despite the plans laid at the Massachusetts Association of Boards of Health meeting for its members to descend on the hearings en masse, antivaccinationists had already packed the room by the time they arrived. The *Evening Transcript* noted that "they [antivaccinationists] were out in such force that they captured all the seats before their opponents arrived, and the result was a room crowded to suffocation with a large contingent standing."[27] Each day of the hearings, antivaccinationists overwhelmed the 240-seat room, occupying every single chair so that "the sergeant-at-arms was at his wit's end to provide accommodations for the doctors who came up to the State House to enter their protest against any change in the law."[28] Massachusetts antivaccinationists took these hearings seriously as a battle in a grim war they waged against state authority and tensions ran high. They made their presence known, "hissing such statements as they disapproved and applauding those they liked."[29] The *Evening Transcript* commented on the partisan nature of the audience at the hearings. "There never has been so much interest manifested in this question as has been shown this year, and the determined and aggressive spirit shown by the opponents of compulsory vaccination was emphasized by the way in which the remarks of the speakers have been received at the two hearings given. Many of the spectators came from distant parts of the State, and they resolutely continued in their places until the last word was spoken, whether it was for or against the cause they espoused."[30] Antivaccinationists clearly seemed determined to use these hearings as a public platform from which to air their views. The two committee members sympathetic to their cause, Senator Chester B. Williams and Representative Walter E. Nichols, dominated the proceedings with questions designed to embarrass health officials and expose their callousness about vaccination injuries.

Representative Nichols, a druggist, identified strongly with the antivaccination movement. When he explained to a reporter why he opposed vaccination, he used the pronoun "we" to describe his position: "What we do contend is that death and disease is caused by vaccination, and if it is thrown in our face that an occasional death from vaccination is not to be regretted if the whole public is benefited by vaccination, we throw it back by saying if there is an occasional death from smallpox what of it, if the whole public is benefited by refraining from vaccination?"[31] Even though Nichols was a druggist, he opposed vaccination—an interesting position given that he probably stood to lose business if his principles stood in the way of vaccine sales.

On the other hand, Senator Williams actually supported vaccination and only rejected compelling it on the unwilling. In a newspaper interview he noted that when antivaccinationists "claim to be as well informed on it as are the advocates of vaccination," he could not support "forcing other people to be vaccinated." Given the differences of opinion between medical experts on vaccination, he felt the matter was best left up to individuals to decide in consultation with their physicians: "The medical profession itself does not agree on the matter. I can't agree with both sides, and I do not wish to contest the opinion of experts that vaccination is a good thing. For my own part, I prefer to leave myself in the hands of my family physician, and to allow other people the same privilege." Senator Williams thus took the stand that the state had no business interfering in the private relationship between patient and physician. The real source of his hostility, however, lay less in his opposition to compulsory vaccination and more in his dissatisfaction with Samuel Durgin's management of Boston's smallpox epidemic. Williams blamed Durgin for the continued spread of smallpox, charging that he allowed health department physicians who treated smallpox patients to mingle with the public without taking precautions necessary to prevent exposure: "If there is an epidemic of smallpox in Boston at this time, it is directly traceable to the office of Dr. Durgin."[32]

Nevertheless, the nine colleagues who supported the existing compulsory law outnumbered Senator Williams and Representative Nichols. Eleven legislators—three senators and eight representatives—sat on the Joint Committee on Public Health.[33] This committee had a history of antipathy for proposals to fund state production of vaccine lymph, supposedly because some of its members were druggists who opposed the idea. It did not, however, have a problem supporting compulsory vaccination, and had yet to pass any repeal bill on to the legislature for a second reading.

As leading antivaccinationists from all over Massachusetts showed up to testify, Representative Nichols and Senator Williams provided them with an excellent venue in which to express their views to a sympathetic audience.[34] A number of physicians from varying medical sects appeared before the committee. Immanuel Pfeiffer charged that "boards of health were made up of politicians who could not make a living in any other place" and that Boston's free vaccination stations were "unfit for cattle."[35] Charles E. Page read a letter from Dr. Martin Friedrich describing his problems with vaccination in Cleveland, Ohio.[36] James D. Judge, who had treated smallpox victims at a boys' school during the 1872 epidemic, observed that the vaccinated had the worst cases, and "said he believed vaccination was all rot and a humbug, and it was a shame that in this enlightened age men should be submitted to a poison of the system."[37] The Boston homeopath William B. Sanders pointed out that "the medical schools were divided on the question of vaccination" and he contended that "medical science, next to theology, was the greatest fraud in the world."[38] Sanders had quite a reputation: his testimony in 1894 supposedly persuaded state legislators to add the controversial exemption amendment to the vaccination statutes, and like Pfeiffer, he was one of the most prolific purveyors of the certificates in the state.[39]

The most damning evidence, however, came from the homeopath Caroline E. Hastings. Declaring that "an investigation by the United States government" of vaccine had found massive amounts of contaminated lymph from all producers, she went right to the heart of the most potent anxiety about vaccination—that it could wreak havoc through blood poisoning or other infections. Hastings claimed that she had approached Boston Board of Health Chairman Durgin for his opinion about various vaccine lymph producers and he had recommended the National Vaccine Company to her. Yet, according to her testimony, a recent federal report found that this company's lymph contained up to 1,380 colonies of bacteria per point. Other companies had even worse contaminations that ranged as high as 89,000 colonies per point. Hastings concluded: "I believe it is impossible to procure pure vaccine. I don't believe the State can make any better vaccine matter than can these companies, and that the proposed manufactory to be established by the State Board of Health will produce no better result."[40] Hastings believed that these reports indicted all vaccine producers.

Contamination would continue to plague vaccine lymph no matter who produced it and state control would not solve the problem.

This testimony outraged Samuel Durgin—he had lobbied the Massachusetts legislature unsuccessfully for years to authorize a state-run vaccine facility. Early in December 1901, Durgin proclaimed that he would try yet again, even though a similar effort "a few years ago" had "met with strong opposition and failed."[41] Thus when Durgin took his turn before the committee on the second day of the hearings, he not only stood up to defend the existing law but he also attempted to lay out a foundation for his petition for state control of vaccine production. After insisting that vaccination with pure lymph could cause no harm whatsoever, Durgin acknowledged that "he had no doubt" people had been vaccinated with impure lymph. Only state control of production could ensure its purity.[42]

Resenting Hastings's testimony, Durgin rebutted by attacking her sincerity: "There is hypocrisy here . . . and I wish to refer to a specific case of it. I refer to Dr. Caroline Hastings."[43] Before he could go on, Hastings interrupted "with much show of feeling and her customary emphatic utterance," demanding an opportunity to respond to his slur.[44] After the committee cleared him to continue, Durgin explained that she was misrepresenting herself as an antivaccinationist in order to get back at him for his refusal to help her land a lucrative vaccination contract. "She came to me and wanted my influence in getting her the job of vaccinating all the people of a large manufacturing concern."[45] According to one newspaper, the company was the New England Telephone and Telegraph Company, and Durgin declared, "I want to ask Dr. Hastings if she did not say to me: 'If the work has to be done, I might as well do my part of it!'"[46] Hastings replied simply: "That is false."[47]

Durgin's attack on Hastings backfired. It must have seemed ludicrous, given her status in Boston society as a pioneering social and moral reformer. Newspapers published detailed accounts of her testimony. The *Boston Courier* even responded with a sympathetic editorial, while another noted her civility and gentility in the face of this public humiliation. In the *Courier*, Hastings explained that she criticized vaccination only because few in the medical profession seemed willing to subject it to a real scientific study. If a strictly objective scientific analysis demonstrated its safety and efficacy, then vaccination should be required to protect the community. If, however, it could not, then health officers should respect and even expect dissent about the procedure. "If it can be proved beyond a question . . . that the introduction of a certain poison into the human body protects that body from the invasion of a dreadful disease, and that it does not carry with it other forms of disease no less to be dreaded, then it may be the duty of the guardians of public health to compel everyone to receive this poison and the duty of everyone to receive it without protest; but if a careful study of cause and effect and an honest admission of all the facts in the case demonstrate that there is actual failure to secure the desired protection and also the actual introduction of other forms of disease equally to be dreaded, then we may well hesitate to blindly follow tradition, and, indeed, may find that duty compels us to arraign even a time-honored tradition before the tribunal of later and greater knowledge." Hastings argued that in the light of recent medical history, the medical profession should mistrust its high regard for vaccination: "Once venesection had as ardent defenders as does vaccination at the present, but who defends or advocates it now?"[48] In noting that physicians had once regarded bloodletting as a therapeutic *sine qua non*, but now discredited it as a useless and even harmful treatment, Hastings berated physicians for according vaccination similar iconic status. What if scientific study showed that vaccination also did more harm than good? Would physicians discard it or "blindly follow tradition"?

Hastings's remarks went to the heart of the issue. Impure vaccine had caused a number of infections in the Midwest and on the Eastern seaboard during the summer and fall of 1901. Additionally, vaccine of poor quality had rendered many vaccinations useless. In medical journals and symposiums, physicians discussed these problems at length. Newspapers and antivaccination literature publicized tales of death and injury resulting from bad vaccine. If public health officials expected to restore public confidence, then they had to acknowledge these problems and remedy them. Bland assurances and stubborn insistence on its safety and efficacy were not sufficient—they had to convince the public that they had subjected vaccination to scientific scrutiny and it had passed the test.

Durgin countered by presenting the Cambridge city bacteriologist Eugene A. Darling as a witness, hoping perhaps to take advantage of the growing popular willingness to grant scientifically trained experts great credibility. Durgin may have hoped that Hastings would seem quaint in comparison, a relic of the mid-nineteenth-century medical tradition pitted against a scientific expert. Yet Darling's testimony proved equally unsettling. Although he dismissed the idea that modern vaccination with glycerinated lymph could transmit scarlet fever, tuberculosis, or syphilis, he acknowledged that given conditions of poor after-care, infections like tetanus or blood poisoning could follow vaccination. He cautioned the committee not to take statements about the presence of bacteria on vaccine points too seriously, however, pointing out that "the great majority of bacteria are harmless and are simply air organisms; that ordinary milk, 24 hours old, contained more bacteria than the ordinary uncleansed vaccine virus."[49] However valid Darling's point, an audience fixated on the idea of the inexorable connection between germs and disease simply did not get it. Bacterial contamination, whether or not it posed a real threat, provoked disgust.

Newspaper reports focused on the bare fact of vaccine contamination without explaining about relative levels of harm posed by various microorganisms. Both the *Globe* and the *Evening Transcript* featured detailed reports of Hastings's revelations, but gave Darling short shrift. The *Boston Globe* called Darling "the most interesting witness of the morning," but the *Evening Transcript* failed to even mention his testimony, even though both papers covered the hearing until it closed.[50] Hastings so impressed the *Courier* that it published a long editorial sympathetic to the antivaccinationists' case, which concluded that the Board of Health should devote its efforts to sanitation rather than vaccination. "In the light of modern science, indeed, vaccination as a specific against smallpox is coming to take its place alongside that other superstition of medical practice a century ago, bloodletting for the cure of fever. The true method of prevention is sanitation. An epidemic of small pox may spread to the invasion of cleanly communities, but it does not have its origin or its aliment there. Let our boards of health be required by law to clean out our slums, to ventilate and purify our tenement houses, to enforce rigid sanitary regulations in crowded and filthy habitations, and the source of evil will be reached in an effective manner."[51] By indicting the health department for its failure to cleanse the city, the *Courier* editor alluded to the contention that adequate sanitation could prevent smallpox epidemics. For many Bostonians who associated smallpox with filth such a conclusion seemed only sensible. Hastings's testimony had touched a nerve, serving to underscore that feeling.

The Committee on Public Health also took testimony from opponents (called remonstrants) of the repeal bills. In a highly charged atmosphere, William T. Sedgwick, Samuel H. Durgin, John H. McCollom, and William T. Shea, among others, stood up to defend vaccination and the medical profession. They presented the Massachusetts Association of Boards of Health petition in support of the current law as they had pledged. Then they each gave testimony in favor of vaccination. For instance, McCollom, a Boston City Hospital physician with a record of over twenty years of service in the health department, cautioned that "one vaccination may last a lifetime, but it is better to vaccinate frequently."[52] Sedgwick took the stand to refute charges that "the medical profession in a large way was commercial and grasping and ignorant." He stoutly declared: "No profession in the world has done so much for philanthropy and humanity as the medical profession."[53] Yet he undermined these sentiments by sternly affirming that vaccination must continue even when impure vaccine had caused infections because the greater good must prevail.[54]

Senator Williams and Representative Nichols clearly directed their interrogations to please the antivaccinationists in the audience. In one exchange with Durgin, Williams asked if the committee members could inspect the isolation hospital. Durgin replied they certainly could, if they complied with his rules— they must first submit to vaccination. To which the senator replied: "Dr. Durgin, no one shall ever vaccinate me."[55] Antivaccinationists "broke into vociferous applause" at this riposte, "which required the chairman to rap for order."[56]

Understanding the theatrical nature of the hearings, Samuel Durgin convinced medical experts representing nearly every medical organization or institution in the city to appear in support for compulsory vaccination.[57] Durgin also mustered support from other important sectors of society. At least six representatives from large business establishments appeared to lodge their protest against abolishing compulsory vaccination.[58] The archbishop of the diocese of Boston sent word supporting vaccination, as did the bishop of Springfield. The Cunard, Furness, Leyland, and Dominion shipping lines also joined the protest against repeal.

As vice president of the Massachusetts Association of Boards of Health and as longtime chairman of the Boston Board of Health, Durgin personally knew many leaders in medicine, education, and business. No stranger to the art of conducting meetings, Durgin attempted to direct his witnesses' testimony by interrogating witnesses himself and passing notes to them to influence their answers. Passions ran high during the proceedings, and MACVS leader William Bassett frequently challenged Durgin for these breaches of protocol. When Durgin tried to read letters from influential individuals to the committee, Senator Williams and Representative Nichols "manifested such objection" at Durgin's "playing to the galleries" that the letters were merely placed in evidence instead.[59] Durgin managed to get what he wanted by giving one of the letters, that of Harvard president Charles W. Eliot, to the press, which they obligingly published that day. By that evening every reader of the *Globe* and other papers knew that Eliot objected to repeal as a "barbarous and merciless proposal."[60]

Unimpressed by Durgin's orchestration of knowledge and power, Nichols and Williams subjected these provaccination witnesses to hostile interrogations, compelling them to admit to worrying about vaccine contamination. When the president of the Massachusetts Medical Society, Dr. Francis Draper, appeared "to enter a protest against the proposed legislation," Nichols launched into an attack, asking him "whether he would care to be vaccinated with virus whose source was not known." Draper replied that "he would want to know where the virus came from." Dr. Horace Packard of the Homeopathic Medical Society also acknowledged that problems with quality and purity in vaccine lymph had led to accidents, that vaccine production "was done in almost a promiscuous way, and under no legal restraint . . . and in the rush of commercial competition there was liable to be carelessness in its preparation." But such remarks could be construed to bolster Durgin's agenda for state vaccine production. Nichols may have hoped to highlight concerns about purity and quality that had made many Bostonians hesitate over vaccination, but the remonstrants' testimony also indicated the need for state control—one of Durgin's long-cherished ambitions.[61]

In the end, despite all the impassioned testimony against vaccination, none of the bills that sought to abolish or amend the vaccination law made it out of committee. By April 1902, they had all been withdrawn. Again and again Senator Williams and Representative Nichols provided the only dissenting votes when the Committee on Public Health reported against the various antivaccination bills.[62]

Samuel Durgin's Bills

Boston's Board of Health Chairman Durgin also petitioned for changes in the vaccination laws. Now he sought once again to gain approval for state funding by inserting vaccine lymph in the annual request for money to make antitoxin.[63] He also wanted to tighten the exemption clause of the existing law to ensure that physicians actually examined the children they certified as unfit for vaccination.[64] In this way, Durgin hoped to halt the traffic in unfitness certificates that had plagued Boston's public schools. Durgin apparently wrote the legislation himself and was the sole signatory on the petitions.[65]

Auditors again crowded into the hearing rooms, "with many ladies in attendance."[66] Testimony focused on Durgin's bill to require physicians personally to examine children before they certified them as unfit subjects for vaccination. Joined by several public school medical inspectors, schoolmasters, and the Boston superintendent of schools, Durgin argued that antivaccinationists and their physicians had "taken advantage" of the exemption clause as currently written to declare "no child is a fit subject for vaccination." The result, according to the medical inspector Edward M. Greene, was that at the six schools under his purview, "many robust looking children came to school with certificates stating that they are unfit subjects for vaccination." Suspiciously, he found that "all these certificates came from only three doctors, and from these doctors have come no certificates of vaccination." Another medical inspector of five Boston schools, Dr. William F. Temple, noted that of thirty children presenting certificates of unfitness, he could find "not one whom he considered an improper subject for vaccination." Still another medical inspector, William H. Grainger, declared that "at least twenty per cent of the children in the public schools of Boston were unvaccinated."[67]

Two schoolmasters testified to the effects of parents' resistance to vaccination at their schools. Master Young of the Prince School found a proliferation of unfitness certificates among his pupils, "which greatly embarrassed him in the administration of his school." Even more disturbing, Master Mead of the Chapman School in East Boston found that "twenty percent [of his pupils] did not show marks of successful vaccination" despite having certificates that attested to their vaccination.[68] Thus one out of every five students supposedly protected from smallpox at the Chapman school was not at all immune—a fact that helped explain why this school had several smallpox cases. Mead's testimony implied that some physicians had either knowingly provided false vaccination certificates to help parents evade the vaccination requirement or they were so incompetent that they had utterly failed to follow through by checking to see if the vaccination had taken, yet signed the certificate anyway. Either way, it seemed that a significant proportion of Boston's physicians and parents opposed vaccination, even to the point of blatant subversion of the law.

In closing that day, Samuel Durgin displayed an advertisement from the notorious antivaccinationist physician Immanuel Pfeiffer, "in which Dr. Pfeiffer offered to grant 'unfit' certificates to any children."[69] Durgin argued that the only way to combat such open disregard for the law's intent would be to require public health officials to countersign all unfitness certificates. On the next day, he even brought some unfitness certificates that he knew "had been issued indiscriminately." A "lively tilt between opposing factions" then ensued, as Durgin's nemesis, Caroline Hastings, asked how he had managed to obtain the certificates. When he replied that "teachers and others" had given them to him, an audience member demanded to know, "by what right Dr. Durgin questioned the honesty of any registered physician who issued a certificate?" When the committee chairman invited Durgin to respond, "irate antivaccinationists" in the audience shouted: "only a scoundrel would!" At that point "it looked very stormy for a moment," until Hastings rose and declared: "No one has better reason to feel bitter toward Dr. Durgin than I, but I utterly disown any such expressions as those of the last speaker."[70]

Antivaccinationists rebutted with testimony to support the idea that the state had no business mandating vaccination—it should remain a personal decision made in private consultation with the family physician. Dr. Cates, a Wakefield homeopath, described a case in which a young girl had died from blood poisoning subsequent to vaccination. Although he had been "strong for vaccination" previously, this girl's death changed his mind and he had since stopped vaccinating, which "called forth applause" from the assembled onlookers.[71] Several spoke to the problem of the state invading the sanctity of the physician-patient relationship. A member of the Massachusetts Anti-compulsory Vaccination Society, Walter C. Wright of Medford, declared for "freedom of private judgment on vaccination."[72] The Boston "allopathic physician" George C. Hale "held that the family physician alone should decide whether a child is a fit subject for vaccination." Hale defended some of the physicians who had signed unfitness certificates as standing "eminent in the profession" and he declared it "unkind . . . to intimate that they have acted improperly." Hale noted cases of blood poisoning after vaccination in Paterson, New Jersey, and Chicago, Illinois. And his own child had been "sick with the sore for fourteen weeks" after vaccination. Hale also declared that until the state could ensure with certainty both the purity and efficacy of vaccine lymph, "compulsory vaccination should be a crime."[73] Another Boston physician, Dr. Wheeler, "a Harvard graduate," argued that Durgin's bill represented an attempt "to take away the power of judgment of the minority of doctors," whom "the majority of physicians represented by Dr. Durgin, want to outlaw."[74] Francis J. Garrison declared that it would "put a despotic power in the hands of the board of health."[75] Representative John F. Foster, sponsor of a failed abolition bill, closed the session by noting that several towns in Massachusetts had voted in officials sworn not to enforce the vaccination law, and "the State should not pass laws which could not be enforced by public sentiment."[76] Thus most of the remonstrants expressed anxiety about state interference with their professional judgment just as much as they pointed out the potential for harmful effects from vaccination.

The Vote on Durgin's Bill

Antivaccinationists' qualms about Durgin's bill failed to move the Joint Committee on Public Health: it was the only vaccination legislation on which the committee reported favorably, although Senator Williams and Representative Nichols dissented. Once the bill (House no. 1113) made it to the floor of the Senate, however, Senator Williams offered an amendment to allow adults the same right as children to claim medical exemptions from vaccination, contending that "honest people . . . are convinced that vaccination is unsafe, and when you find 300 to 400 persons coming to a hearing it is good evidence they are in earnest." Impressed by antivaccinationists' sincerity and numbers, he believed that extending the law to cover adults would give individuals a chance to choose for themselves which medical theories to follow: "We are not here to make good business for any particular profession or clique."[77] He intended only to level the playing field, not necessarily support either side.

Although the chairman of the Public Health Committee, Senator J. Frank Porter, "vigorously opposed the amendment, urging that it was catering to those whose desire was to overthrow entirely all vaccination laws," the Massachusetts State Senate passed the bill with Williams's amendment by two votes.[78] The Republican Party overwhelmingly dominated the Massachusetts legislature, holding thirty-two out of forty seats (thirty-three, counting the lone Republican Independent senator). Six of the seven Democratic senators represented Boston districts. Thus community sentiments rather than partisan politics underscored this vote: two Democrats, one Republican Independent, and fourteen Republicans voted for the amendment, while four Democrats and eleven Republicans voted against it. Forty-three percent of the Massachusetts State Senate supported softening the law in order to accommodate personal health circumstances, and only 38 percent of the senate stood against the Williams amendment when it first came to a vote. Six senators, or 15 percent of the total senators, declined to participate in this vote by abstaining.[79] Senator Williams's rationale for proposing the amendment had convinced his colleagues that extending the medical exemption to adults compassionately adjusted the law to accommodate personal health needs.

Some papers proclaimed the outcome of this vote as a triumph for the antivaccinationists.[80] Sadly for the antivaccinationists, their triumph did not last. Fearing that the recent past traffic in certificates of unfitness for children would soon be duplicated among adults as ruse to escape vaccination, Senator Porter proposed a new amendment the next day to restrict the exemption once again only to children. After a bit of wrangling with the abstainers, Porter managed to scrape together a majority and it passed by four votes.[81]

Analysis of the Two Votes

Most votes in the Senate were not actually counted. Instead the president of the Senate asked for a voice vote on the bill before the body. The president usually declared the vote, based on his sense of majority from a voice vote. If a member objected, then individual votes were tabulated.[82] The votes on these two amendments are unusual because the 1902 *Journal of the Senate* provides a list of how each senator voted—an exception to its usual practice of simply noting that bills were read a second time and ordered to a third reading without giving any details of the vote.[83]

A breakdown of both votes reveals where antivaccination sentiment was strongest in Massachusetts. Senators who represented coastal communities steadfastly supported allowing the adult medical exemption through both votes. Their districts included about one-half of Boston, most of Cambridge, a swath of Middlesex, and the eastern coastal counties of Essex, Plymouth, and the Cape. But senators from western and central townships either opposed the amendment, abstained from the vote, or dropped their support later. The two senators representing Berkshire districts on the western border, for instance, both abstained from the initial vote. Four of the five senators who represented Worcester districts in the center of the state voted against it, with the fifth senator abstaining from both votes on the measure. The nine senators who represented Suffolk (Boston) split evenly on the issue, with four voting for the Williams's amendment and four against with one abstention. Three of the seven senators representing Middlesex (Cambridge and towns to the north and west) supported the amendment. Although four senators representing other districts in the western part of the state and towns to the southwest of Boston voted for the amendment initially, they ultimately backed off and abstained when Senator Porter counterattacked. Thus the vote roughly reflects an east-west split, with Boston, Cambridge, and their suburbs divided as well.

Although the Williams amendment lost some support on the second vote, a hard core of thirteen senators, 33 percent of the Senate, stood fast by it through both votes. That one-third of the Massachusetts State Senate held firm in support of amending the law to allow adult exemptions shows a high degree of sympathy for the civil liberties of antivaccinationists. Only two senators switched sides, and they deliberately paired their votes to cancel each other. All the rest either stuck with their original position or bailed out by abstaining, which led to 20 percent abstaining from voting on the Porter amendment to limit the exemption once again to children.

The fact that one-fifth of the senators decided to dodge the issue altogether on the vote to restore the old language of the law demonstrates that compulsory vaccination may have touched a political nerve. Cornelius R. Day, for instance, abstained from both votes. As a member of the Public Health Committee listening to all the testimony, he might have just wanted to avoid raising the ire of either side among his constituents. Charles S. Sullivan, who represented three Boston wards and one Cambridge ward, also abstained from both votes, perhaps because he considered vaccination a political quagmire. Most Massachusetts towns did not have many smallpox cases compared with Boston, and some communities were notable for their antivaccination activists.[84] Senators from such towns might have worried more about the political repercussions of compelling vaccination on unwilling constituents than smallpox itself. They took the path of least resistance—neutrality.

Some senators who stood by adult exemption represented communities where antivaccination was strong. Chester Williams, who proposed it, lived in Wayland, home to Mrs. Jessica L. C. Henderson, who testified that she would go to jail before she vaccinated her children. She eventually became president of MACVS.[85] The four Boston senators who supported him through both votes also represented wards noted for opposition to vaccination—East Boston, Roxbury, West Roxbury and Dorchester. The senator who lived in and represented Cambridge wards where antivaccination dominated stuck by adult exemption as well. And the senator for Lowell, home to large textile mills that routinely enforced the vaccination laws on unwilling employees, voted for the exemption both times.[86]

Disquiet over vaccination in Plymouth County and Cape Cod swayed their three senators to consistently support Williams. A 1901 abolition bill had originated with Issac M. Small, who represented Barnstable County and lived in North Truro on Cape Cod. Provincetown, another Cape Cod community, manifested pronounced hostility to vaccination by electing antivaccinationists to its board of health in 1901.[87] Rockland, located in Plymouth County, was a notable antivaccination stronghold in which Hulda B. Loud, the owner and editor of the *Rockland Independent*, periodically whipped up public antipathy for vaccination. Senator Elisha T. Harvell supported the Williams amendment, and he lived in Rockland. Perhaps he and the other Plymouth County senators favored adult exemption because they feared they might face a rocky election if they voted otherwise.[88]

Senator Chester Williams's rationale for changing the Massachusetts vaccination statute hinged more on a respect for personal liberty than any antivaccination sentiment. In the end twelve of his fellow legislators stuck with him, their reasons for changing the compulsory vaccination law lodged somewhere between concern for civil liberties and anxiety about vaccination. As Senator Williams explained to the press, antivaccinationists' testimony and numbers had persuaded him that they reasonably feared injury from vaccination and deserved protection of their individual rights. "All they ask for is exemption from what they consider an infringement on their rights. It is certainly no greed or hope for gain that prompts their requests. They are not cranks, because they are too numerous. On the other hand, the advocates of compulsory vaccination were the members of the profession which does the vaccinating and the representatives of the business interests that the Boston board of health has so effectively at its call."[89] The antivaccinationist campaign to organize testimony and flood the audience with its supporters paid off: it had convinced him that antivaccinationists were reasonable, sincere people who merited not only intellectual respect for their position but also legal recognition of their right to choose. Durgin's mustering of leaders in business and the medical profession to testify before the Joint Committee on Public Health did not impress Williams. The too conveniently close relationship between business interests and government entities like the Boston Board of Health seemed suspicious and only gave the antivaccinationists greater credibility as far as he was concerned. Possibly other legislators felt the same way and thus voted to support Williams.

Nevertheless, the medical establishment and public health authorities managed to convince the state Senate to shore up the existing vaccination law. Taken as a bare fact this vote at first glance seems to demonstrate that the Massachusetts legislature strongly supported compulsory vaccination. The fact that nearly one-half of the legislature initially supported modification of the law disappears from historical view.[90] Yet a closer look at the intricacies of the legislative process reveals a sharp, nearly even division over vaccination in Massachusetts. Our system of majority rule often obscures the existence of significant differences over legislation. In this case, compulsory vaccination prevailed in Massachusetts, but just by a narrow margin. The will of the people was anything but unified on the matter.

Chapter Eight

Criminal Prosecution of Antivaccinationists

In official reports, Boston's chief health officer Samuel H. Durgin represented his vaccination efforts in neutral terms, claiming that he began by merely recommending vaccination in 1901. Only when it became clear that people had failed to heed his advice did he resort to a compulsory vaccination order in which people were "visited and vaccinated if willing to be vaccinated." Refusals were respected, given an opportunity to change their minds, and only summoned to court if they persisted in their obstinacy.[1] Yet this benign characterization is belied by the fact that force and coercion played a prominent role in Durgin's approach to vaccination. He routinely sent police to accompany his health department vaccinators, and he exercised his authority to its fullest extent to get people vaccinated. When his exhortations and free vaccination stations failed, he resorted to various legal sanctions to compel vaccination. Local health departments could quarantine, if they desired, any establishment in which they found smallpox cases, and Durgin used this threat to nudge local businesses into vaccinating their employees. When business owners made vaccination a condition for continued employment, nearly every worker complied. Before he issued the general vaccination order, Durgin sent out squads of health department physicians, accompanied by policemen specifically tasked to restrain resistors, to conduct a vaccination campaign in various lodging house districts. Confronted with physicians backed up by policemen, most people chose to oblige the doctors. Those who did not were pinioned by police and summarily vaccinated. Only later, during official vaccination sweeps, were refusals accorded due process of law.[2]

Durgin regarded antivaccinationists not only as fools but also as criminals deserving punishment, grumbling: "It is dangerous to allow such teachings to continue, and some day in the near future I will bring some of those fellows into court."[3] The Massachusetts vaccination law penalized vaccination refusal with a five-dollar fine—a seemingly mild penalty. Yet as the homeopath Conrad Wesselhoeft pointed out: "The rich man can pay his fine and thus save his family from assault, while the poor man who cannot pay the fine, must go to jail and languish there till it pleases the Board of Health to allow him to be discharged."[4] Although many health officials argued that persuasion yielded the best results, some, like Samuel Durgin, were determined to cow the opposition and routinely pushed the vaccination law to its limits. Others, like Cambridge's E. Edwin Spencer, hesitated in applying the full weight of the law to refusals. This chapter explores the ways in which health officials used their legal authority to limit opposition to vaccination.

Compulsory Vaccination in Massachusetts, 1901–2

Only a few Massachusetts towns and villages besides Boston and Cambridge issued community-wide vaccination orders. Samuel Abbott of the Massachusetts State Board of Health complained in 1902 that some local boards hesitated because they were "composed (at least partially) of men who opposed vaccination": "In several instances the presence of one antivaccinationist upon a local board of health has so influenced the action of the board as to result in serious harm to the community, by delaying public vaccination, until the common sense of the community compelled them to act."[5] Elected officials ran many boards and they may have found the prospect of forcing vaccination on the voting public a bit daunting. Even professional public health officers had to deal with mayors and council members sensitive to the political implications of foisting any compulsory health measure on their constituents. Thus health departments preferred voluntary vaccination and their responses to the threat of smallpox varied.

At the end of 1901, Henry P. Walcott, chairman of the State Board of Health, declared that "general neglect of vaccination throughout the State" coupled with "greatly increased facilities for transportation from one town to another" had led to the speedy dissemination of smallpox on the railroads throughout Massachusetts. Cases appeared in every town located on "one of the principal lines" or "upon one of the branches" of the state's rail system.[6] In a circular issued to local health boards in 1899 and 1900, the State Board of Health "earnestly recommended that a general vaccination of all unprotected persons be made, and that the local authorities of cities and towns be requested to carry out this recommendation."[7]

Yet few towns went to the expense and trouble of declaring vaccination compulsory, despite state health department urgings. Medford, a city of 18,244, had five cases of smallpox in 1901. Although it vaccinated 1,982 individuals "at the expense of the city," it did not issue a general vaccination order.[8] Brookline, with just three cases in a population numbering 19,935, declared that over half its people had sought vaccination in "the past four months." Although worried that "there are still several thousand not recently vaccinated, and some, chiefly domestic servants from the provinces, who have never been vaccinated at all," it did not make vaccination compulsory for the entire population in either 1901 or 1902.[9] Somerville had just four smallpox cases among its 63,727 residents in 1901. It merely "authorized" three physicians "to perform free vaccinations to such as might apply to them" and also put out a public appeal for vaccination in the press and asked for "co-operation of other city departments . . . in getting their employees vaccinated."[10]

Newton had four cases among its 34,934 inhabitants in 1901 and simply offered free vaccination at its board of health office and supplied free vaccine "to physicians for non-paying patients" and "large employers of labor."[11] In 1902 with eighteen cases of smallpox, it still opted for the voluntary route, reporting, "in case vaccination was refused the exposed person was quarantined for two weeks."[12] Two smaller communities close to Boston apparently decided not to undertake any extraordinary effort to vaccinate their citizens. Hyde Park, a town of 13,547, had eight cases of smallpox and Quincy, with 24,593, had six cases.[13] Neither community apparently did anything noteworthy to encourage or order vaccination.[14] Yet Watertown, with no cases of smallpox, instituted free vaccination, "of which 900 persons took advantage."[15]

Still, several communities did issue general vaccination orders. As its smallpox cases mounted to sixty-eight in 1902, Somerville finally resorted to compulsory vaccination, although forty-one residents "openly refused" it.[16] Southbridge's forty cases in 1902 forced a general vaccination, however only as a last-ditch resort when "professional incompatibilities" subverted its quarantine efforts.[17] North Adams, in the far northwestern part of the state, also ordered compulsory vaccination in 1901.[18] Compulsory vaccination, then, remained the exception rather than the rule in Massachusetts towns and villages.

The provision of free vaccinations clearly troubled some boards of health. The Worcester health department decided to provide free vaccinations "without asking any questions" about applicants' financial status, but it had to defend its stand: "Consequently, a great many people appear with children who, perhaps, can well afford to pay for vaccination to the regular physicians, but we have felt that the sanitary good that is derived from the thorough vaccination that we know we do more than offsets the cost and trouble of vaccinating those children." As a result of this liberal practice, Worcester vaccinated "in the course of a year" about "2,500 to 3,000 children." Worcester health authorities also abjured quarantine, preferring instead simply to vaccinate "everybody who has been exposed in any way to the patient," boasting, "we have had no difficulty in stamping out the disease."[19]

Like Worcester, many other Massachusetts localities with very small numbers of smallpox cases limited their costs by offering rather than demanding vaccination. Boston's experience with smallpox, however, was on an entirely different scale. Although Boston initially tried to follow a similar protocol, by late December 1901, smallpox cases had mounted into the hundreds, with no end in sight. Compulsion seemed the only answer. Cambridge, too, faced with mounting smallpox cases, announced compulsory vaccination in February 1902. Thus resistance centered in these two cities despite the existence of antivaccinationist sentiment throughout Massachusetts.

Coerced and Forced Vaccination

People who worked in factories, hotels, stores, and on railroads had the choice to be vaccinated or lose their jobs. Anyone housed in public institutions had no choice at all. State law mandated vaccination in jails, prisons, reform schools, asylums, and orphanages. It also required that "incorporated manufacturing companies" had to vaccinate their workers whenever a local board of health required it.[20] The state health department frequently sent vaccination circulars to various employers and institutional leaders, reminding them to make vaccination a condition of continued employment, enrollment, or membership. Coercion fell heaviest on those who could least resist it—the institutionalized poor, insane, orphans, prisoners, and working-class people who could not afford to lose a job over vaccination. Many people submitted to vaccination not because they personally desired it but because their circumstances made refusal all but impossible.

Business after business required vaccination—some because they feared an outbreak would cause "considerable inconvenience and imperil their business" and others because the local board of health had ordered it.[21] In 1902, for instance, the Melrose board of health ordered vaccination for "2,000 persons employed in Fells rubber shop."[22] Anxious that rumors of smallpox cases among their employees might drive away holiday shoppers to stores in other towns, Boston department store owners prevailed on Durgin to issue official notices declaring their clerks smallpox free.[23] In Cambridge, the Manhattan Market advertised, "we have caused every person connected with our establishment to be vaccinated."[24]

Nearly every large firm ordered its employees vaccinated. One Boston physician noted that "nearly all employers are requiring that only vaccinated persons shall work for them."[25] According to the *Boston Post*, "practically all the large retail firms have issued notices to their employees to be vaccinated at the firm's expense."[26] In Cambridge, "almost every firm in this city employing a dozen or more persons" vaccinated their workers, with "more than a thousand" vaccinated at the National Biscuit Company alone.[27] The C. E. Osgood Furniture Company hired a physician to vaccinate its workers "at the request of the firm" in December 1901.[28] Earlier in September 1901, the Boston Elevated Railway Company had ordered its employees "who cannot show satisfactory scars" to obtain vaccinations.[29] In November, a Boston factory vaccinated five hundred workers, and Postmaster George A. Hibbard requested that all postal employees in the greater Boston district submit to vaccination.[30] At the end of November, with cases spreading to all the outlying districts and across the Charles River to Cambridge, Boston Mayor Thomas N. Hart officially required all city employees to obtain vaccinations.[31] Rear Admiral Mortimer L. Johnson, Commandant of the Charlestown Navy Yard, likewise ordered all "on duty and at work in connection with this station" to be vaccinated.[32] In December, the general manager of the Boston and Maine Railroad mandated vaccination for all of its twenty-five thousand employees.[33] Frank C. Bostock, "the animal king," proprietor of the Animal Arena, ordered all of his employees vaccinated also in early December.[34]

Employees had little choice but to comply for fear of losing their jobs. Although business owners avoided openly admitting that they made vaccination a condition for continued employment, one Boston physician testified that "one member of a large firm . . . told me yesterday that he had told his employees that if they did not submit to vaccination he would not have them in his employment."[35] One man working for the Boston Elevated Railway Company described how the employees marched along "in single file with sleeve rolled up" for their vaccinations. "Some of the men, when they come near the young dignitary [the vaccinating physician], faint and fall out of line, while others begin to vomit. If any declare that they will not submit to the disgraceful treatment, they are told, or given to understand, that they can settle up with the Co., which I think is an act of intimidation. The men, as a rule, take the poison rather than give up their positions."[36] The proprietor of Clark's Hotel in Boston stipulated in November 1902 that all employees "must be vaccinated or leave."[37] The Waltham Watch Company issued a similar edict in March 1902. One of their employees, Miss G. Williams, complied though "she did not desire it," but "being the only support of a widowed mother, she took the risk."[38] In testimony before the Joint Committee on Public Health of the State Legislature, John Shepard, of Shepard & Norwell Company, affirmed that he had stipulated "that all who were to remain in their employ must be vaccinated."[39]

Some sought compensation for injuries resulting from coerced vaccinations. One employee, G. D. Gillard of Medford, brought a lawsuit against his employer, U.S. Shoe Company of Boston, "for $20,000 damages for enforced vaccination" that had resulted in injury. The suit went against him because he had "stood in line with other employes [*sic*] and did not seem to be unwilling to be vaccinated" at the time, although it was understood that refusal meant immediate discharge.[40]

Although no law mandated forced vaccination, health officials occasionally resorted to outright force when faced with resistance from those thought to threaten public health by virtue of their race, ethnicity, or predicament. Deemed to pose a special hygienic menace, African Americans, Asians, the homeless, and non-Anglo-Saxon immigrants often received quite different treatment from white native-born Americans. In Philadelphia, health authorities forcibly vaccinated an African American congregation of three hundred persons during a Sunday evening prayer meeting in late 1903. Forty physicians accompanied by forty policemen held the congregants hostage until they all submitted to vaccination.[41] In early 1902, in St. Louis, Missouri, the discovery of a smallpox case among the passengers on a train brought local health officers to vaccinate everyone in the affected car. When several Italians resisted, the train crew and other passengers held them down for vaccination.[42] Grain traders in the Minneapolis Chamber of Commerce received similar treatment when "policemen guarded the doors" to prevent their flight from health department vaccinators.[43] In Philadelphia, health department physicians accompanied by policemen surprised a gang of Italian, Polish, and African American men laboring on the city water system. When one Italian ran off and hid in a drain pipe, "the two physicians grabbed him by both heels and dragged him out of the pipe. Then they vaccinated him."[44]

These incidents provoked little public outrage. Antivaccinationists complained of injustice, but the mainstream press took a more a lighthearted perspective.[45] The *Philadelphia Evening Bulletin*, for instance, called the surprise visit to the pipe layers an "expedition" that generated several "amusing experiences," one of which included extracting the above-mentioned laborer hiding in the sewer pipe to vaccinate him.[46] The *Boston Globe* captioned its story about the Italian passengers' forced vaccination as "Held Up the Train," a play on bandits who "held up" trains in the late-nineteenth-century American West.[47] In 1901, one newspaper described the forced vaccinations of American Tobacco Company female factory workers as "a lively time," as if the women had participated in some amusing outing when policemen locked them in and dragged them "screaming, struggling, and kicking" to the vaccinators.[48]

In Cambridge, Yee Kee, "the popular proprietor of the American Chinese hand laundry," tried to explain to health department physicians that he not only had smallpox once before but had also been vaccinated twice. The physicians ignored him, losing "no time . . . in arguing with a heathen and a foreigner. John [Yee Kee] was unceremoniously tipped over on his back, his arm was bared and before he could say three words, the job was done." Ironically, the Cambridge health department vaccinated Yee Kee the same week that it finally got around to swearing out a criminal complaint against five other residents who had refused vaccination months earlier. One of them, the Rev. Henning Jacobson, had also immigrated to the United States, albeit from Sweden. Jacobson, a Lutheran minister, received not only due process of law but also preferential treatment from the Cambridge health department. Jacobson's Christianity and Nordic ethnicity evidently led it to assume that he would not infect anyone, even though as a minister he might visit a parishioner sick with smallpox, contract the disease, and then spread it. But health officials would not grant Yee Kee the same degree of trust even though he owned a successful business. His Chinese ethnicity marked him as dangerous, so alien that the mere fact of his existence in Cambridge posed a threat to public health, even though the editor noted "a case of smallpox has yet to be reported from a Cambridge laundry shop conducted by a Chinaman."[49] Although Yee Kee's medical history revealed that he posed less of a public health threat than Jacobson, who had not been vaccinated since childhood, he was forcibly vaccinated whereas Jacobson was not. Both men were immigrants, but Yee Kee was "a heathen and a foreigner," thus forever an alien and far more dangerous in the eyes of public health officials than Jacobson.

Health department authorities also treated the predicament of homelessness as an a priori threat to public health. Called tramps, hoboes, or "Weary Willies," homeless men aroused a great deal of fear in Boston. Newspaper articles paid particular attention to cases of smallpox found among them. A series of three front-page stories in the *Boston Evening Record* focused especially on tramps. One story about a physician's chance encounter with a sick homeless man, Richard

Roche, emblazoned the word "tramp" in huge bold capitalized font: "TRAMP, Stopped By Doctor Had Smallpox."[50] The next day, headlines cried, "ANOTHER Tramp Found Ill With Smallpox," and then a few days later exclaimed, "ONE MORE Tramp with Smallpox in Court Sq."[51] A fourth story explained how "habitues of the old court house are much worked up over the fact that as yet no steps have been taken to clear the corridors of tramps, who have no other ostensible means of warmth and shelter." A physician diagnosed a case of smallpox in one of the men resting there, and court house employees rebelled at the prospect of close proximity to potentially infected individuals: "no one in the building is quite reconciled to the idea of having a case of smallpox at close range every little while."[52] They called for the city to keep the tramps out, but raised no similar objection to the considerable traffic of other persons who constantly went in and out of the building—people who also might carry smallpox, as did Councilman George A. Flynn "who visited City Hall while indisposed" with ambulatory smallpox.[53] They assumed the homeless posed a special threat by virtue of their plight rather than their actual medical condition.

Newspapers depicted the homeless as singularly dangerous and dirty, congratulating Samuel Durgin for his "vigilance" in sending "virus squads" out nightly to inspect "all the large lodging houses of the cheaper class."[54] One *Boston Post* reporter casually documented forcible vaccinations of homeless men as humorous episodes in which "hoboes in virtuous indignation refused to bare their arms to the needles of doctors" and "were very much averse to rising from their warm couches and submitting to the vaccination process." The ensuing "lively argument" resulted in policemen throwing "the struggling 'pads' upon a bed and while the disgusted looking bluecoats held the victim the doctors did their prettiest."[55] Another reporter at the *Globe* related the work of two virus squads in the North End and South End one cold November night in 1901 as an amusing anecdote in which the health department physicians and police laid out a "plan of campaign" against wily tramps. "The policemen knew the natural aversion which frequenters of cheap lodging houses have for water or anything else that is cleanly, and they guessed they would object to the attentions which the board of health desired to show them." One policeman blocked off the sole exit, while the others assisted the physicians by physically restraining resisters. "A good many of the men kicked and clawed and also fought with teeth and heads against what some of them declared was an assault upon their rights as otherwise free and independent American citizens, but none of the men that the doctors and policemen tackled escaped inoculation. Every imaginable threat from civil suits to cold-blooded murder when they got an opportunity to commit it, was made by the writhing, cursing, struggling tramps who were operated upon, and a lot of them had to be held down in their cots, one big policeman sitting on their legs, and another on their heads, while the third held the arms, bared for the doctors." In one instance a policemen clubbed a man who attempted to defend himself. After vaccinating him the physician sewed up his head, "and then they let him go back to bed, cursing the entire medical profession and uttering bloodthirsty threats against all policemen."[56]

This attempt to depict casual brutality as an amusing anecdote appalled at least one reader. Joseph M. Greene of *The Animals' Defender* called the virus squads' work a "cowardly outrage" and chastised the *Globe* for its insensitivity in writing "as if the whole affair were a humorous one" that "spoke of these victims as 'tramps' and 'hoboes,' as if, therefore, they had forfeited all personal rights." Calling Durgin "our little medical czar," Greene fumed at the hypocrisy evident in the health department vaccination campaign: "Dr. Durgin well knows that he *would not dare to commit such an outrage on anyone of wealth, power or influence in this city.*" Greene surmised that "the only reason he dared through his hirelings to attack these unfortunates was because they were poor, friendless and powerless."[57] When the Board of Health later asserted that it did not use force to vaccinate, Greene responded: "When a squad of police accompany vaccinating doctors to lodging houses, what is the natural inference?" He declared that "proprietors of lodging houses" had told him "that force has been used; that inmates have been held and vaccinated; that those objecting have been compelled to get up, dress, and leave with the officers, as an intimidating device to influence others."[58] Despite Greene's protest, Boston health authorities continued forcible vaccinations of homeless men into 1902.[59]

The health department also regarded drunks as fair game for forced vaccination. Two policemen escorting some inebriated men to jail were exposed to a smallpox case. At first health officers demanded that everyone must be vaccinated: "There was every indication of a promising row, for the policemen said they had all been vaccinated six weeks ago and they wouldn't stand for it, but the doctors still insisted, and the policemen intimated that there were not enough men around the pest house to make them stand for another jab of vaccine virus, so the matter was not pressed." Although detained for hours and then fumigated, no one forced vaccination on the officers, but foisted it on two unwilling intoxicated prisoners. The *Globe* sympathetically acknowledged that the experience had insulted the officers' dignity, and "no words yet invented are equal to doing anything like justice to those feelings."[60] The policemen's outrage at the proposed violation of their personal bodily integrity was perfectly understandable, but the reporter treated the forced vaccination of the intoxicated prisoners with approbation: drunks posed a threat to society and therefore did not deserve any special respect or tenderness for their feelings.

Compulsory Vaccination

Although itching for a fight with the local antivaccinationists, Durgin waited until the day after the holiday shopping season had ended to order general compulsory vaccination for Boston on 26 December 1901. Now the health department could bring the full weight of the law into middle-class homes, whereas previously it had restricted its "virus squads" to poorer lodging houses and flophouses patronized by the homeless poor.

On 2 January 1902, the Boston Board of Health began sending vaccinators out to canvas door-to-door, but it did not use the vaccination order to ensure that every Boston resident got vaccinated. Instead, it implemented the order only in selected districts, making "vaccination sweeps" of neighborhoods in which cases of smallpox kept cropping up almost daily—the working-class districts of "East Boston, South Boston, Charlestown, the North End and West End, and a portion of Roxbury and Dorchester." Beacon Hill, the Back Bay, and Bay Village—the enclaves of Boston's elite citizens—escaped the ministrations of the Board of Health physicians. In these sweeps, physicians accompanied by policemen went door-to-door, offering free vaccination and recording the names of those who refused. After allowing a "short time in which to change their minds," the health department issued a court summons for any remaining recalcitrants.[61]

Lodging houses, crowded with a transient population, especially worried Durgin, and he concentrated his vaccination efforts on their inhabitants. One newspaper explained this strategy as an efficient allocation of resources: "The physicians from the health department are visiting as many of the so-called cheap lodging houses throughout the city as possible, and compelling all inmates to submit to vaccination, as it is considered that in these places there is the greatest danger of the spread of this disease."[62] As immigrants flooded into Boston in the late nineteenth century, the middle classes fled to suburban neighborhoods connected to its central core by streetcars and subways. Boston's inner sections became densely populated as landlords converted old single-family homes into duplexes, triplexes, lodging and rooming houses, and tenements.[63] Durgin thus initially concentrated his public vaccination efforts on multifamily housing in densely settled districts. Other sections of Boston may have harbored many who supported antivaccination either openly or covertly, but he chose to leave them alone.

Durgin branded these congested sections dangerous to the public health, decrying the "conversion of old single dwellings into tenement houses" as "one of the greatest evils and . . . a source of much annoyance." Throughout 1901 he had directed his department to conduct "a most thorough and systematic inspection of the tenement houses," believing their inadequate light, ventilation, and crowding to pose a public health problem in general.[64] Intimately acquainted with these districts, Durgin readily sent his "virus squads" to buildings that the health department assumed were filled with characters who practiced questionable hygiene. The vaccinators visited lower Roxbury, "the land of the lower middle class," but not West Roxbury, which "belonged to families of the central segment of the middle class." In Lower Roxbury "three deckers, cramped two-families, and brick row houses" predominated, whereas single-family homes characterized the highlands of West Roxbury.[65] Health department physicians also visited parts of South Boston, where settlement house workers had observed housing so wretched that they lamented, "in these haunts of disease human life is sacrificed to the fetish of property."[66]

On 26 January the health department expanded its operation, sending 125 physicians to East Boston with "no warning of the impending invasion" in order "to surprise the people in their home on a Sunday, when it was expected the entire family would be at home at more leisure than on a week day."[67] In 1902, the island community of East Boston still remained relatively isolated from the rest of Boston, accessible only by ferry or boat.[68] Its physical separation from Boston, according to one early twentieth-century analyst, favored the development of a strong sense of community remarkable among Boston's districts: "In no other portion of the city will one find anything like so well knit and humanized a population and one so fitted to participate in local affairs. Not only is it easier to stay in East Boston than to cross the channel, but there is a decided local tradition which favors this provincialism." Known as "a great working-class section in the very best sense of the term," East Boston's native-born craftsmen gradually gave way to Irish, Italian, and Jewish immigrants who moved into the district after 1895. Still, the community continued to flourish: "Most of the people owned their own homes, attended near-by churches, and met at various gatherings in the homes of their friends and neighbors: there was real neighborship up and down the streets. . . . Local shops were prosperous, and furnished social centers of a certain degree of significance."[69] East Boston's cohesion and community granted its residents a sense of possession and security that those living in other districts lacked.

East Boston offered the first real resistance to Durgin's vaccination order. Neighbors of long standing who knew one another intimately and gossiped together felt more comfortable defying intruding health officials. Homeowners felt more justified in refusing entry into their premises than those living in rooms rented from week to week. Secure in their homes, friends, churches, and lodges, East Bostonians regarded outsiders like the Boston health department physicians with suspicion. More unvaccinated children attended school in East Boston than those in other districts. For example, nearly 20 percent of the pupils at the Chapman School in East Boston went unvaccinated, as compared with a 6.2 percent rate for the city overall.[70]

"Invasion" thus proved an apt description, as many East Bostonians objected to admitting unexpected strangers, even if they claimed to be physicians on city business, into their homes: "The people were taken by surprise, and many of them did not like the idea of being vaccinated in that way, while others refused outright to be vaccinated or to permit the doctors to examine or vaccinate any member of the family. No amount of persuasion would avail in these cases, and some of the doctors were roundly abused for their trouble." To the health department's chagrin, the doctors vaccinated far fewer people than they had expected, convincing less than five thousand to do it, when the Board of Health "had expected that at least three times that number would be vaccinated during the day."[71] The surprise visit backfired, as many people met the door with demands to see the physicians' credentials and doubts about the legality of their claims.

When a health department physician, accompanied by a policeman, called on the Mugford family, the father, John Mugford, declined vaccination. Declaring that he had "studied the question too long to allow any poison to be put into my system," Mugford also refused to vaccinate his two youngest children.[72] Canadian immigrants of English descent, the forty-two-year-old Mugford and his wife, Bessie, had lived in Massachusetts for over twenty years. They had five children: Eva (5), Walter (8), Bertha (12), Lillian (13), and Roy (18). They owned at least two businesses: John owned a grocery store in Somerville and Bessie ran a milk and cheese shop on the same street as the family's dwelling. Surrounded by neighbors who worked in various crafts and trades, the Mugfords represented quintessential East Boston—a solid working-class community of skilled English and Irish immigrants who owned or rented homes and duplexes.[73] Mugford received a summons to court for his refusal, along with ten other East Bostonians.

The next day, 115 physicians canvassed South Boston homes in search of the unvaccinated. By the turn of the century, many of South Boston's residents worked as teamsters, longshoremen, or laborers in and around its freight yards and wharves. Machine shops, foundries, the American Can Company, and the Gillette Razor factory also offered good jobs. About sixty-five thousand people lived in the district, distributed in housing that ranged from congested tenements of the lower section to pleasant single-family residences in the hilly upper section. Dominated by native-born families of Irish descent, South Boston was one of the most stable districts in Boston, with generation after generation electing to remain within its precincts, maintaining "in spite of the modern unsocial impersonal city customs a local identity and loyalty." Despite its overall reputation as a good place to live, one part of South Boston, Ward 13, offered such grim housing conditions that it had the highest rates of infant mortality, tuberculosis, and death in the entire city. This ward occupied the lower section, cramming its inhabitants into shabby tenements "no longer suitable for dwellings" that were "forlorn in appearance and invite careless, unwholesome living." The other wards, however, compared "favorably with such a suburban region as West Roxbury," in terms of their high proportion of home ownership.[74]

The health department experienced similar difficulties in South Boston: the *Globe* reported that "it was not all plain sailing for the physicians. Many people were found who did not care to be vaccinated, in fact, refused to be, on the ground that they did not believe in it; but the majority were willing."[75] The antivivisection editor Joseph Greene contended that health department vaccinators succeeded only because their "threats of arrest, fine, or imprisonment" sent women "into hysterics, some thinking that the law permits violence to be used."[76] The Board of Health estimated vaccinations at ten thousand and announced it would take legal action for refusals, so that "many of those in East Boston who refused to be vaccinated Sunday have changed their minds, and have been anxiously soliciting the local board of health physicians to vaccinate them."[77]

Durgin made good on his threat to prosecute holdouts. Ultimately, twelve people who refused vaccination in this sweep wound up in the East Boston District Court, but their resistance crumbled in the face of Judge William H. H. Emmons.[78] Of the twelve people charged, only John and Bessie Mugford pled not guilty. The rest either got vaccinated or argued that extenuating circumstances

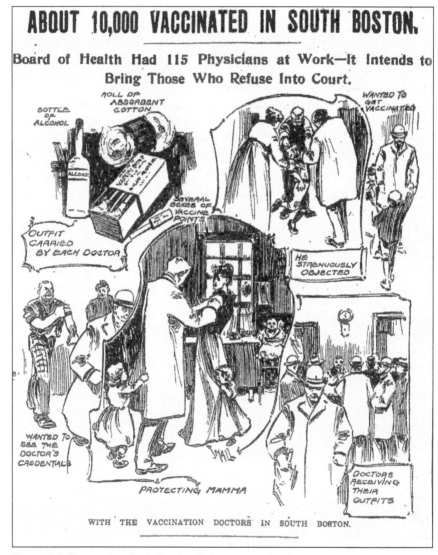

Figure 8.1. Illustration depicting South Boston vaccination sweep. *Boston Globe*, 28 January 1902, 1.

should exempt them from vaccination. Frederick B. Poole and his wife Mary answered their summons to declare that they had gotten vaccinated in the meantime. Frederick Mott, "an elderly gentleman," explained that he did not realize vaccination was compulsory. He had refused because "the last time he was vaccinated he was laid up for three months and nearly lost his arm." Despite his previous bad experience, however, he allowed a health department physician to vaccinate him right there in the courtroom. John and Kate Evans brought their family physician with them to attest that with Kate's ill health, "vaccination would be apt to injure her." Judge Emmons took this circumstance into account and ordered a continuance of three weeks to allow Kate to become well enough for vaccination. John M. Evans, her husband, managed to escape conviction for refusal on a technicality. It seemed that the health department physician had not actually asked him to get vaccinated, and he had therefore broken no law. When Duncan McKay claimed that he had refused vaccination because "he was suffering from the effects of an operation," the health department physician Wright declared the man healthy enough for vaccination. Judge Emmons continued McKay's case with the understanding that he would seek a vaccination from his family physician. Sarah Tierney did not show up—not because she intended to evade the law but because she "was too sick to appear in court" as a result of her recent vaccination.[79]

Significantly, the judge seemed more interested in mediating practical solutions than in imposing draconian measures, tempering the health department order with a degree of mercy. As the cases of Kate Evans and Duncan McKay show, he tailored his decisions to allow defendants time to seek vaccination on their own as their health permitted it. Judge Emmons also did not push the law to its absolute limit. John Evans, for instance, got off on a technicality. Since the health officers had not actually asked him to get vaccinated, he was found not guilty. Yet despite the presence of a health department physician in the courtroom, the judge did not direct him to vaccinate Evans there and then. Judge Emmons demonstrated leniency with these defendants by remitting their fines, and he dealt kindly with the Mugfords, continuing their case for a week "with the understanding that they get vaccinated." Harsh punishments were unnecessary when headlines such as "Board of Health Wins" provided priceless ammunition in the health department's vaccination campaign.[80]

Nevertheless, the Mugfords returned to court unvaccinated several weeks later. This time the judge found Mugford guilty, fined him five dollars for refusing vaccination, and then fined him fifteen dollars more for refusing to vaccinate his daughter Eva. He declared Bessie Mugford innocent for lack of evidence that the health department physician had asked her to get vaccinated. Apparently, John Mugford's refusal prevented the vaccinator from interviewing her. Mugford also escaped paying a fine for refusing to vaccinate his son Walter. Like many other East Boston children, Walter had a certificate of unfitness exempting him from vaccination. The Boston health department apparently did not ask about the older children's vaccinations, nor did it later attempt to bring them into the picture. Undismayed by this outcome, Mugford declared that he did not believe in vaccination, and determined to "take the case to the supreme court."[81]

City officials gave Mugford a lot of time to think about his decision to pursue a jury trial. They did not even swear out a formal criminal complaint against Mugford until nearly a month later, and then waited a week to file it with the superior court, taking over two months to prosecute him during a smallpox epidemic.[82] Boston city officials' procrastination indicates that they probably hoped that Mugford would give in as so many others had and make the whole problem disappear. But Mugford did not give in. Tried simultaneously on two separate charges, one for his own refusal and one for his failure to vaccinate his daughter, Eva, Mugford finally got his jury trial in superior court on 25 April 1902—the first trial of an antivaccinationist for refusing the Boston Board of Health vaccination order.[83] Judge Henry N. Sheldon presided.

From the beginning, Mugford's attorney, Frank M. Davis, laid out a defense calculated to generate rulings from the judge that he could allege as errors to appeal in a higher court.[84] First he cross-examined the prosecution witnesses to cast doubt about their certainty as to the purity of the vaccine they used.[85] Then he attempted to introduce evidence showing that vaccination sometimes resulted in various injuries, diseases, and death, but the judge refused to allow it. Davis then requested that Judge Sheldon give instructions to the jury that would allow it to find his client not guilty. Covering every possible contingency, Mugford's attorney asked instructions that would take his client's fears about vaccination into account and then for several instructions about the constitutionality of the Massachusetts vaccination law. Judge Sheldon refused the request, leaving the jury basically only one fact to decide—whether or not Mugford had refused vaccination. The jury returned a unanimous verdict of guilty.[86]

Mugford was not disappointed at this outcome—he expected to use the trial to launch an appeal that he hoped would put vaccination itself on trial. Observers understood the case's broader relevance: "The case will go, of course, to the supreme court, where we shall get a decision on the whole subject that will stand."[87] Mugford's attorney quickly filed exceptions to all of Judge Sheldon's rulings, alleging the judge erred when he did not allow evidence about vaccination, his client's concerns about vaccination, and the constitutionality of the compulsory vaccination law. Several months later, on 25 October 1902, Judge Sheldon allowed those exceptions, meaning that he agreed that these points of law deserved the review of a higher court. Then he sent the exceptions on to the Supreme Judicial Court of Massachusetts (the state supreme court) to "await the determination of the Justices."[88] Although Mugford's appeal reached the state supreme court before any other vaccination cases, it languished in judicial limbo waiting for the justices to decide whether or not to hear it.

In the meantime, the successful prosecutions of the East Bostonians hardened the health department's approach to other refusals. Whereas the East Bostonians had gotten off rather lightly, other uncooperative Boston residents now faced ruin. Resistance, for instance, nearly wrecked Charles E. Cate's life. Cate, a thirty-five-year-old laborer described as a "lumper by trade" who currently "gets his living by helping furniture movers," lived with his wife in a Boston lodging house.[89] When his wife came down with smallpox, the health department removed her to the smallpox hospital, fumigated the premises, and vaccinated everyone in the rooming house, except Cate, who "refused point blank to submit," declaring vehemently, "I'm d—d if I'll be."[90] Evicted from his lodgings, Cate wandered around Boston homeless and unvaccinated, shadowed by the policeman William Ready, specially detailed to watch "until the time has elapsed when symptoms of the disease, if he has contracted it, should be noticed."[91] Undeterred by the loss of his home, Cate continued to refuse vaccination every time the officer mentioned it. After ten days, the policeman asked him for the last time, and Cate angrily refused, declaring, "there was no law strong enough to compel him."[92] The officer arrested him. Declaring that "he was being imposed upon," Cate "flatly refused" to pay the fine and went to jail.[93]

Durgin had played an elaborate game of cat-and-mouse with Cate, but he did not have to go to such an extreme. He could have issued Cate a ticket and summons to court immediately for refusing vaccination. He could have even quarantined Cate in his rooms instead of following him about. Quarantine of individuals exposed to smallpox was a settled legal principle in Massachusetts for two centuries by 1902.[94] Indeed Cate's prompt eviction undoubtedly stemmed from the rooming house owner's fear that the health department might quarantine the premises. Unvaccinated and exposed to smallpox, the hapless Cate probably had little chance to find lodging anywhere in the immediate vicinity of his former residence—his plight pointing to the coercive threat of homelessness for those who refused to go along with the program. Cate thus wandered about and slept on the streets of Boston for ten days. Although quarantine would have cost the city his room and board, budget considerations probably did not figure here. Detailing a policeman to watch one man day after day was an expense too, but one that also provided invaluable publicity about the perils of failing to obey the vaccination directive.

Samuel Durgin warned that he would not drop the matter if Cate insisted on serving out the time rather than submit to vaccination. Durgin promised that the police intended promptly to arrest him again upon his release, and "dryly" speculated, "I don't imagine . . . that he will hold out that long. If he does, he will be the first of his kind."[95] Determined to work out his fine in jail, Cate remained obdurate when he learned of Durgin's determination. He "vowed . . . that the health board might continue arresting him and sentencing him to jail for a century, but he would not give in."[96] The Boston Board of Health turned the tables on Cate, however, by vaccinating him anyway according to the section of the state law requiring vaccination of jail inmates "whose presence in jail might be looked upon as dangerous to the health of others."[97] Cate apparently "submitted gracefully to the prison rules," noting, "I have had smallpox once when I was four years old, but your rules must be lived up to, I suppose."[98] Ironically, Cate's newfound compliance did him no good: unfortunately his vaccination did not exempt him from serving out his sentence, unless he chose to pay the fine. Several other refusal cases sent to jail also wound up in the same predicament.[99]

Durgin seemed concerned less with public safety than with teaching another public lesson. He orchestrated this incident to sensationalize the legal consequences of resisting vaccination while John Mugford awaited his second hearing. He wanted Mugford and the public to realize just what could happen when he "brought one of these fellows into court." Press coverage of the case tacitly supported Durgin's policy by not mentioning at all the danger that Cate may have posed to the community if he had fallen ill, focusing instead on the irony of his situation. The *Evening Transcript* referred to Cate as a "test case" and declared that the "Board of Health sought legal vindication of its policy and obtained it in a double sense."[100] The *Evening Record* wryly noted, "Mr. Cate of the county jail is bound to be a vaccination martyr."[101] Cate's story served as a cautionary tale for would-be vaccination resisters.

The *Record* also published a letter about Cate from the antivaccinationist physician Charles E. Page, captioned "Cate Will Know Better Next Time." The editor may have intended to poke a little fun at Cate's predicament. Page, however, was outraged "to have our citizens forcibly vaccinated in face of their protestations" and felt that it violated the "spirit of the law" that mandated only a fine or a jail sentence—not forcible vaccination—for refusal. Page noticed that the health department seemed very selective about who it went after when it decided to push vaccination enforcement to extremes. "If the law had been made compulsory to the limit; that is, that every one, rich, poor and middle class, should be vaccinated, and by force if necessary, as I, for one, could almost wish it had been, every well informed anti-vaccinationist would have armed himself for protection at any cost; though doubtless the bloody work would have ended before it begun if this stand were taken by our intelligent and self-respecting people."[102] A laborer, Cate had no clout, no money to hire an attorney, and no cadre of well-placed friends to speak for him. He thought he could evade both vaccination and the financial penalty by opting for jail time in lieu of paying his fine. Durgin proved him wrong. As Page pointed out, the administration of the vaccination law hammered the poor, whereas it just tapped the rich. In the most extreme case, a wealthier person could pay the fine and continue to pay the fine if it was levied again. The connected, informed, and relatively well-to-do could quietly avoid vaccination, whereas the poor could not. It took resources far beyond those of most individuals to obtain legal representation in order to demand a trial and fund an appeal.

This discrepancy came to the fore in the case of Mary Issacs, "a pretty table girl in a West End theatrical boarding house" who refused vaccination after her exposure to smallpox. Rounded up by Officer Ready, she insisted, "I'll go to jail before I will submit to vaccination!" Officer Ready duly wrote her a summons. By the time she got to court, however, she testified that she had gotten vaccinated in the meantime, much to the annoyance of the judge and Officer Ready. Judge Dewey agreed to release her only after she submitted to an examination of her arm. Officer Ready and Issacs "withdrew from the courtroom to an anteroom. Five minutes later both came out smiling and the judge smiled a big grin when he said that the case would be placed on file."[103]

Issacs's bravado deserted her when confronted with the reality of fines and jail time for her refusal. Waitresses were among the most vulnerable of working women, relying on their customers' tips to make ends meet.[104] Mary Issacs probably had no extra money to mount a legal defense or pay repeated fines. A jail sentence certainly would have prevented her from working—she might have lost her job as a consequence of her absence and have a difficult time finding another. Facing such a dim prospect, Issacs "saw that she was making a mistake and went to a physician and was vaccinated."[105] The economic consequences of jail and fines fell hard on working women and men. When they actually wound up in court, most capitulated because they simply could not afford defiance.

The Back Bay, West Roxbury, and Beacon Hill districts, home to Boston's social and economic elite, escaped the ministrations of health department vaccinators. Yet the vaccination order had required "that *all* the inhabitants of the city who have not been successfully vaccinated since January 1, 1897, be vaccinated or re-vaccinated forthwith."[106] Even though Durgin regarded smallpox as a threat to the entire city and its suburbs, he never once suggested that these wealthier enclaves might benefit from a house-to-house visitation of the public vaccinators. Thus relatively elevated social status insulated the upper ranks from the health department vaccination order. Even when confronted by authorities, they had many options that poorer classes lacked: they could leave town, pull their children out of public schools, hire attorneys, or pay the fines. One "large property owner" in Pittsfield, for instance, moved out of state "to save her children from the vaccination pollution."[107] In Hyde Park, one of Boston's wealthier suburbs, a parent brought a successful civil suit against the town for excluding his unvaccinated children from public school.[108] "Mortimer W. Lawrence of the Highlands" avoided vaccination only because he found legal representation and paid his fine.[109] Thus vaccination was compulsory mainly for those who lacked the ability and means to avoid it, and the Boston health department vaccination policy weighed more far heavily on the working class than wealthier segments of society.

For all of Durgin's bluster about bringing antivaccinationists into court, he kept his physicians away from the wealthier districts where many of them resided, leading the editor Joseph Greene to comment sardonically: "Boston's 'Board of Health,' after raiding all the humbler sections of the city, conveniently finds, just before reaching the hallowed precincts [*sic*] of Back Bay and other 'high-toned' districts, that the 'appropriations' for vaccination have given out!"[110] Yet these districts reputedly harbored many sympathetic to antivaccination. Charles W. Eliot, president of Harvard University, knew many wealthy Back Bay families who avoided vaccination.[111] Even though he strongly supported vaccination, he did not require it of Harvard's students; instead he merely recommended it, perhaps out of deference to parents' beliefs.[112] Possibly Durgin realized that he could ill afford the adverse publicity generated by a poor reception of health department vaccinators from the well-to-do of the Back Bay and Beacon Hill. Newspapers avid for sensational stories would have accorded any socially prominent resister expansive coverage, further fueling the fire of resistance.

Compulsory Vaccination Enforcement in Cambridge

Less severely afflicted than Boston at first, Cambridge did not issue its compulsory vaccination order until 27 February 1902. Cambridge Board of Health Chairman E. Edwin Spencer took a more comprehensive approach to vaccination than his Boston counterpart, Samuel Durgin. Instead of targeting selected districts with virus squads backed up by policemen, Spencer dispatched physicians who "went from house to house vaccinating all inhabitants whom they could find," including Harvard University students and faculty, in early March 1902.[113]

Chairman Spencer's demeanor throughout the 1901–2 smallpox epidemic conveyed little of the antagonistic bluster displayed by his Boston counterpart, Samuel Durgin. Whereas the Boston health department had teamed its vaccinators with policemen, Spencer instead adopted a low-key approach by sending his physicians out alone. The Cambridge health department physicians also took people at their word about their vaccinations. By accepting a verbal declaration instead of examining arms for signs of recent vaccination marks, Cambridge vaccinators respected residents' sensitivity about this intrusion on their person.[114] Unfortunately for Spencer, many took advantage of this trust and easily thwarted the doctors by lying about their previous vaccinations.

Spencer also trod lightly on the issue of antivaccination. Slow to pursue legal remedies for refusals, he did not initially prosecute vaccination resisters. When seven hundred "law-breakers, many of them in the wealthy districts," declined vaccination in the first sweep in March 1902, Spencer took no immediate measures to initiate formal prosecutions.[115] When they refused, he seemingly dropped the matter for months, merely warning them by letter that they could face legal sanctions at some point in the future.[116]

Spencer's laissez-faire attitude toward resistance probably stemmed from his apparent successful control of the epidemic. Smallpox cases declined markedly throughout late March, April, May, and early June.[117] Yet smallpox suddenly returned with a vengeance, reaching an unprecedented height of forty-one cases in late June. Breaking out primarily in the Cambridgeport district, the epidemic produced "nothing less than a panic."[118] Some families fled the neighborhood; schools, libraries, and churches closed, forcing Mayor H. H. McNamee to charge that "the people generally are up in arms because of this spread of smallpox in Cambridgeport."[119]

People complained to Mayor McNamee that the Board of Health "has not been doing its utmost to stem the tide of the disease." The mayor took the unusual step of attending the weekly Board of Health meeting, along with a number of irate citizens. He criticized Spencer's lax vaccination tactics, asserting, "it would be better to vaccinate all impartially so that none could possibly escape by falsifying."[120] Under this pressure the Board of Health issued another vaccination order, this time specifying that its doctors would inspect everyone for vaccination marks and prosecute refusals: "The vaccinating doctors will ask to see the vaccination mark instead of merely taking a person's word, and if the person refuses to give such evidence that he has been vaccinated, the doctors will report the matter to the board, who will feel at full liberty to prosecute."[121] Determined to keep better track of who got vaccinated, this time the health department recorded the names and vaccination status of every individual in each house it visited on a card filed at the department.[122] Yet vaccinators still encountered resistance, with a local paper reporting that "many refuse to be vaccinated, while others evade the doctors when they call at the house."[123] The health department persisted nonetheless, and a week later "many who dodged the doctors when they first went around to vaccinate came forward, humble and repentant, and eager to have the same operation performed that they formerly attempted to avoid."[124]

This latest outbreak embarrassed Cambridge health authorities and the mayor (who was up for reelection), provoking comment from cities all over the state. The *Boston Evening Transcript* condemned the Cambridge Board of Health for allowing smallpox to run rampant.[125] An editorial in a Detroit medical journal blamed the local antivaccinationists. "For years this part of Massachusetts has been a hotbed of antivaccinationists. More has been said on the subject there than in any equal area of territory anywhere in the world. Numbers of people in that part of the State, though themselves without pretense of being antivaccinationists, have shirked their duty to the public health because of the amount of talk indulged in and have put off their vaccination from year to year. A good part of the citizens are unprotected by vaccination and smallpox rages almost as in the old pre-Jenner days in England."[126] The church closings attracted commentary even from observers outside the state.[127] They "set off a debate in Cambridge," irritating not only local residents but also nearby towns who "received a considerable influx" from Cambridge churchgoers (and possible exposure to smallpox) as a result.[128]

With the entire city disrupted, Spencer scrambled to explain why his department had allowed forty-seven cases of smallpox to crop up in just eight days. He traced the outbreak to one family new to Cambridge that initially concealed the sickness, making it very difficult to contain the contagion. Once apprised of the situation though, health department physicians promptly moved to vaccinate almost everyone in the neighborhood, disinfect the premises of the sick, and remove all the victims to the hospital. He confidently declared: "it is most improbable that such an outburst will occur again, if prompt notice of all suspicious cases is given to the board of health."[129] Despite pressure from the mayor, he still refused to quarantine houses in which he found smallpox victims. He also did not file charges against individuals who had first violated the law in early March. Instead, he stalled again. Apparently he still hoped that the mere threat of prosecution would suffice in persuading the holdouts to get vaccinated.

For a few weeks, the Board of Health's strategy of vaccination, disinfection, and isolation succeeded in containing the outbreak to Cambridgeport. Then it fell apart as smallpox cases broke out all over the city in mid-July, hitting North Cambridge hard and even afflicting the Cambridge city councilman William H. Coleman. That was the last straw for the mayor, who "has been asked from all quarters what was being done to stop the spread of the disease, and has had all kinds of alarming tales poured into his ear."[130] Mayor McNamee, who had "always felt that quarantining should be the very first measure to be adopted in a smallpox case," conferred with the state board of health on the issue. Although it had at first supported Spencer's determination to avoid quarantine, it now agreed with Mayor McNamee. Backed by the state board, he took his case to the other Cambridge board members, William Rodman Peabody and Charles Harris.[131] An editorial in the *Cambridge Chronicle* supported the mayor's call for quarantine: "in this he will have the support of conservative citizens. . . . Public sentiment favors extreme measures for the protection of the people."[132]

Under pressure, Spencer still refused to back down in his rejection of quarantine, but he now signaled his intention to enforce the law by sending policemen to accompany his vaccinators.[133] The mayor's attempt to undermine Spencer's authority also prodded the health department chairman to make good on his threat to prosecute vaccination refusals. On 17 July 1902, five days after the mayor's meeting with the other Board of Health members, Spencer swore out criminal complaints against six resisters who still stood fast on their March refusals, undoubtedly to display his willingness to take "extreme measures" to protect public health.[134]

Three "prominent citizens" stood out among these individuals.[135] The Reverend Henning Jacobson was a highly educated Swedish Lutheran minister, holding a BA along with a divinity degree, and he had also undertaken advanced studies at Yale University.[136] At a time when city employment generally went only to those connected by kin or party affiliation to the mayor's office, Albert M. Pear held the position of assistant city clerk and Frank S. Cone worked for the city water department. Pear, the most politically prominent resister, had family connections that landed him a good job in the Cambridge city hall. His father, Isaac S. Pear, wielded considerable influence in the Massachusetts Republican Party, then the overwhelmingly dominant political party in the state. The elder Pear served on the Republican Party state central committee and as a registrar of voters for Cambridge.[137] Albert first won election to the post of assistant city clerk in 1895. Reelected annually, by 1902 the thirty-two-year-old Pear practically owned a lucrative sinecure that commanded a salary of $1,400 per year.[138] Both Albert Pear and his father were "widely respected" in the community.[139] Pear's income placed him well into the middle-class bracket, earning as much as some of the more highly paid food and drug inspectors who worked for the State Board of Health and far more than others in clerical positions at that time.[140]

Characterized as "one of the most strenuous antivaccinationists in the city," the thirty-two-year-old Pear declared, "I do not propose that the board of health shall dictate to me what medicine I shall put into my system."[141] For over four months, the Cambridge Board of Health accorded Pear special treatment by tolerating his open defiance of the vaccination law, even though one newspaper reported: "It cannot be said that he has made any effort to avoid a fight with the board of health on the matter, for he has never even tried to conceal the fact that he does not believe in vaccination. To say that he is strenuous on the point would be putting it mildly, for he has repeatedly talked against it in the strongest terms."[142] Pear's public stand on his refusal inspired local antivaccinationists to form their own branch of the Massachusetts Anti-compulsory Vaccination Society specifically to solicit funds for the resisters' legal fees.[143] Pear's outspokenness and political connections may have influenced Spencer initially to back off on the issue of criminal prosecution.

Pressure from the mayor finally forced Spencer to abandon his tacit policy of tolerance on the vaccination issue. Admitting that the board had chosen to defer prosecutions because it "did not consider it wise," he now declared the board "determined to hesitate no longer and to bring into court those who defy the regulations and refuse to be vaccinated." Public outcry over the renewed spread of smallpox to North Cambridge, coupled with the mayor's open frustration with the health department's rejection of quarantine, pushed Spencer to adopt a tougher stance on vaccination. Albert M. Pear, Henning Jacobson, Frank W. Cone, Ephraim Gould, Maggie Gould, and Paul Morse each received their long-delayed summons. Yet even after Spencer had decided to bring charges, he treated Pear with special restraint and delicacy, giving him one more chance to reconsider by personally talking to him about the matter days before he actually filed. Pear stood firm, and the Board of Health "decided to bring him into court, as such defiance of their authority right in city hall should not, they thought, be allowed to continue."[144]

All of the newspapers treated Pear as the star, featuring his name in the secondary headlines and including his photograph in the body of the article.[145] And Pear happily granted interviews, explaining to a *Globe* reporter that he suffered from "muscular rheumatism" and had "been under a physician's care for several years now." Pear added that his physician had provided him with a certificate "showing my condition," and he asserted, "I will not submit to vaccination without finding what my legal rights are."[146]

Yet, Pear did not bring an attorney to his hearing. Of the six resisters summoned to court on 23 July 1902, only Frank Cone brought legal counsel, James W. Pickering of the Massachusetts Anti-compulsory Vaccination Society.[147] Three of the others immediately capitulated: Maggie Gould and Paul Morse had gotten vaccinated; Ephraim Gould pled guilty "and was given a day to get the money."[148] Pickering defended Cone by arguing that the vaccination law was unconstitutional and "vaccination is dangerous to the health and life of the individual vaccinated and . . . no sure preventative to smallpox."[149] He claimed that "some doctors were in favor of vaccination, but a great many more were not in favor of it, who do not recommend it to their private patients."[150] Both Jacobson and Pear attempted to defend themselves, but the judge refused to hear them. Jacobson tried to explain how "his physical condition and his experience did not warrant him in being vaccinated," but the judge forestalled him, remarking that the statute in question made no provisions for medical exemptions from vaccination for adults. Jacobson "then tried to tell how his position reminded him of a certain minister who, etc., but the judge gently shut him off."[151] Somewhat amused by the pastor's legal naïveté, Judge McDaniels declared, "I am fond of a good story and am sorry to interrupt one, . . . but this is a court of law and when I am at leisure I shall be pleased to hear it."[152] Pear never even got to the witness stand. Once he admitted he planned to testify that his physician had advised him against vaccination, "the judge saved him the journey to the stand by saying he would not hear it."[153]

Judge McDaniels then found Cone, Jacobson, and Pear guilty, fining them each five dollars. They all appealed for jury trial in superior court, each posting $200 bonds.[154] Described as "perfectly sincere in their objection to vaccination" and "prompted neither by a spirit of bravado nor a desire to obtain notoriety," all three defendants planned "to carry the case to the supreme court, if necessary, in order to prove their point."[155] Judge McDaniels's blunt rejection of Pear's and Jacobson's attempts at self-representation taught them a lesson. Pickering would represent them at the next phase—jury trial.

Jacobson initially refused vaccination because he had experienced "great and extreme suffering, for a long period" from his own childhood vaccination and he had also "witnessed a similar result of vaccination in the case of his own son." His son, who submitted to vaccination to keep his job, "carried his arm in a sling for six months."[156] Jacobson apparently had a confrontation with health officials over vaccination years earlier as well. When his six-year-old daughter needed a vaccination in order to attend school, he refused and "took her to Dr. Abbott, of the State Board of Health . . . and asked Dr. Abbott to give a written guarantee that he would be responsible for any injury to the child resulting from vaccination."[157] Abbott refused, but granted an exemption to the little girl. This time, however, the vaccination order applied to Jacobson, who had once preached: "It happens not seldom that the state demands something when the church demands the opposite. It is an unholy act to break the law of Jesus Christ in order to be obedient to the magistrates."[158] Jacobson took a stand on principle even though contesting his guilty verdict represented a considerable hardship.[159] At that time he supported his wife and children on a salary of fourteen dollars per week.[160] Suffering "grave financial difficulties," he held services in rented rooms and "owned no parsonage."[161]

In 1902, Jacobson was forty-six years old. Born in Sweden, he moved to the United States at the age of thirteen in 1869. He was well educated, receiving his bachelor's degree from Augustana College in Rock Island, Illinois, in 1880. After marriage to Hattie Anderson in 1882 and a decade of student pastorships, he took his divinity degree from Augustana in 1892. Although Jacobson could have gone to more affluent parishes after he completed his studies, he answered the call to serve as a "home missionary" for Swedish Lutherans in Cambridge upon his ordination in 1892.[162] Though poor, his 364 parishoners were very proud of their struggle to create a solid foothold for the Augustana Church in Cambridge, and they celebrated their pastor's work with a commemorative history published in 1902.[163] They had big plans to build a beautiful church and most of their energy was directed toward raising the necessary funds to accomplish this feat. Jacobson did not mention his predicament in his church newsletter at that time, nor were his court battles a subject for reflection in any of the church's histories or his obituaries. He seemed to keep his judicial drama separate from his clerical life, perhaps because he believed it improper to ask his congregation for financial aid in such a personal quest.[164] He would not have been able to mount an appeal without the welcome help of the Massachusetts Anti-compulsory Vaccination Society.[165]

Albert Pear got the earliest trial date, 12 November 1902.[166] Newspapers covering the story referred to him as a "test case," describing his attorney as "acting for the Massachusetts Anti-Vaccination Society."[167] At trial, J. W. Pickering "offered no evidence, but agreed to the facts testified to" by the Board of Health.[168] The judge addressed the jury, explaining that the defendant had not denied the facts because he desired "to test the constitutionality of the law." The jury returned a guilty verdict "without even leaving the courtroom."[169] According to one editorial observer, the "organized antivaccinationists" were "glad of a chance to get a test case considered."[170] Pickering immediately filed his exceptions, which the Supreme Judicial Court of Massachusetts accepted for a January hearing.[171] It seemed that Pear, rather than Mugford or Jacobson, would challenge the constitutionality of compulsory vaccination.

From the beginning, Albert Pear's vaccination case took precedence over all the other 1902 vaccination cases. The legal establishment clearly accorded Pear preferential treatment. As an elected official with close family ties to the Republican Party establishment in Cambridge, Pear had status and visibility that the others lacked. His case went to trial in November 1902, whereas Henning Jacobson had to wait until late February 1903. Even though the Supreme Judicial Court of Massachusetts had accepted John Mugford's exceptions for review weeks before Pear's jury trial, it decided to consider Pear's appeal first.[172]

The state supreme court justices never gave a reason for favoring Pear over Mugford. Possibly the justices felt that Pear's case better represented the interests of the antivaccination movement because MACVS had sponsored his appeal.[173] It had set its sights on the Pear case, noting that "a Massachusetts decision would have great weight in other states."[174] Holding a respected position in his community and known for his antivaccination sentiments, Pear may have seemed the most appropriate candidate to test the constitutionality of the Massachusetts compulsory vaccination law. Thus the Supreme Judicial Court of Massachusetts scheduled his appeal for 19 January 1903, more than a month before Jacobson's jury trial.

Pear's attorney, J. W. Pickering, also represented Jacobson, and he apparently wanted to bring his other client into the appeal. Just before Pear's case came up on the supreme judicial court docket, assistant district attorney Hugh Bancroft realized that he had filed the wrong charges. Pear originally refused vaccination on 14 March 1902. In the meantime, however, the state legislature had amended the vaccination statutes, effective 19 March 1902, and Bancroft had mistakenly charged Pear under the amended law rather than the old law.[175] The court dismissed the case on this technicality. Although it gave leave to file again, and Bancroft could have quickly corrected this minor mistake, both sides agreed "the case was not in proper shape for argument."[176] Even though he could have filed immediately, Pickering took advantage of this little glitch to stall until he had finished Jacobson's jury trial.

Jacobson's case came to trial on 27 February 1903. Pickering attempted to present evidence to show that vaccination "quite often causes or results in serious and permanent injury to the health of the person vaccinated," and he tried to call Jacobson to testify about why he refused vaccination.[177] Pickering also asked the judge to instruct the jury that the Massachusetts compulsory vaccination statute "is unconstitutional and void," just as he had done at Pear's trial. The trial court judge, however, refused to give such instructions and also refused to allow this evidence and testimony, ruling it immaterial to the case. Jacobson received a guilty verdict. On 2 March 1903, Pickering filed exceptions to these rulings on behalf of Jacobson, alleging the lower court erred in excluding this evidence and refusing to give the instructions. On the same day he submitted Pear's exceptions again as well. Thus although Jacobson's jury trial took place several months after Pear's original trial, Pickering joined the two appeals together.[178]

Jacobson's exceptions challenged the propriety of excluding testimony about the risks of vaccination, an issue in which MACVS had a vested interest. MACVS noted that each case covered different issues: "in the case of Mr. Pear we made our exceptions chiefly on the unconstitutionality of the Statute, and in the case of Mr. Jacobson, . . . we sought to obtain rulings to allow *evidence* in jury trial of injuries and deaths resulting from vaccination." It decided to support both cases, "to make them test cases," emphasizing their status as "highly respected citizens."[179] Jacobson's exceptions listed fourteen points in which Pickering noted that vaccination "quite often causes or results in a serious and permanent injury," that it "occasionally causes . . . death," that it "renders a person vaccinated incapable of performing his usual duties and labors . . . sometimes incapacitating him for a period of months." He contended that vaccine lymph "quite often is impure and in a condition unfit and dangerous to be used," that it can cause "tetanus, or lockjaw, ulcers, boils, eczema, erysipelas, abscesses, various forms of blood-poisoning, . . . consumption, paralysis and syphilis." Finally Pickering brought up Jacobson's prior experience with bad effects after vaccination as a child, in which he had experienced "great and extreme suffering, for a long period," and that he recently had to watch his own son endure "a similar result."[180] With these exceptions, Pickering and the antivaccinationists believed that they could put vaccination itself on trial at the appellate court level, and they certainly hoped that the justices would agree to review the cases on those terms.

If we were to focus only on the sheer numbers of those vaccinated in 1901 and 1902, objectors like Jacobson, Pear, and Mugford appear as lonely outliers. Seen against the backdrop of routine and widely accomplished vaccination in the face of an epidemic, they certainly look like the lunatic cranks deplored in health officials' rhetoric. Yet a closer investigation of the circumstances surrounding vaccination from the perspective of the subjects of the campaign reveals that although many people got vaccinated, most did it under some form of duress. Health department claims to the contrary, they enforced vaccination unevenly in Boston, employing coercion routinely and even blunt force occasionally to selected individuals and populations. Well-to-do residents never had unpleasant confrontations with vaccinators because their neighborhoods were not canvassed, whereas the working classes had to argue with doctors on their doorsteps. Even worse, drunks and the destitute got rough treatment at the hands of the authorities. In the workplace, seemingly willing acquiescence masked the coercive nature of the situation. Most faced a stark choice—get vaccinated or lose your job. And those who openly resisted could not easily do so without financial assistance, leaving only a few stubborn individuals like Jacobson, Pear, and Mugford willing to undertake the arduous appellate process.

Chapter Nine

Jacobson v. Massachusetts

The Constitutional Context of *Jacobson*—Police Power

When Jacobson and Pear set out to appeal their convictions, they did so at a time when American constitutional law had undergone nearly three decades of challenges that had limited the scope of police power—the power of a state to make laws to promote the common good and general welfare of its citizens. The concept of "police power" is deeply rooted in American law, originating from traditions of ancient household governance and Roman law, articulated by William Blackstone in English common law, and expressed in the continental European science of police.[1] From the early days of the Republic, state legislatures did not hesitate to make and enforce all sorts of police laws, particularly those directed at promoting and preserving public health, and judges generally upheld these laws even when they deprived individuals of their liberty (quarantine) or their property (nuisance abatement).[2] Indeed, until the passage of the Fourteenth Amendment in 1868, there was no effective federal constitutional basis on which to challenge a state's right to pass such legislation.

William Novak has argued that from the colonial period up to the Civil War, American communities enacted and enforced regulations and laws covering nearly every public and private interaction "from Sunday observance to the carting of offal." Americans regarded the ideal society as a "well-regulated" one in which local authority managed both the economy and citizens' lives through a myriad of rules. They did not see government as a necessary evil that limited individual liberty; rather they saw government as a positive force obliged to protect its citizens. The arguments of political philosophers like John Stuart Mill notwithstanding, American antebellum communities never operated on a laissez-faire basis, but instead promulgated rules and regulations designed to control both markets and morals, to ensure the prosperity, health, and welfare of their citizens: "the notion of a well-regulated society secured by state police power was an essential part of the American governmental tradition."[3]

After the Civil War, Congress summarily abolished slavery in the Thirteenth Amendment (ratified 6 December 1865). The Fourteenth Amendment (ratified 9 July 1868) was intended primarily to protect the civil rights of freed slaves, but it also created a new relationship between states and the federal government by declaring: "No state shall make or enforce any law which shall abridge the privileges or immunities of citizens of the United States; nor shall any state deprive any person of life, liberty, or property, without due process of law; nor deny to any person within its jurisdiction the equal protection of the laws."[4] That is, the Fourteenth Amendment placed new restrictions on state police power. Citizens and corporations could now challenge state regulations of their conduct, property, and businesses on the basis that these laws violated their federal civil rights. After this amendment, the Supreme Court of the United States had to answer again and again how far states could go to regulate the affairs of their citizens. It had to redefine police power in terms of the amended federal constitution. It had to "'begin the nation anew'—to strike a balance of power between the national government and the states and between new public powers and new individual rights."[5] In a series of decisions after 1868, the United States Supreme Court thus worked out new limitations on state police power.

The salient case came early. In 1869, Louisiana restricted all slaughtering in New Orleans to one regulated facility in order to control pollution from animal wastes and byproducts, thus putting about one thousand butchers out of business. These businessmen challenged Louisiana's authority to take their property (their businesses) without compensation, averring that it amounted to a failure to provide due process protected by the Fourteenth Amendment. The United States Supreme Court upheld the state regulation, describing police power in a broad but vague statement: "The power is, and must be from its very nature, incapable of any very exact definition or limitation. Upon it depends the security of the social order, the life and health of the citizen, the comfort of an existence in a thickly populated community, the enjoyment of private and social life, and the beneficial use of property."[6] A more specific limitation on police power came in 1877 when Chief Justice Morrison R. Waite ruled in *Munn v. Illinois* that when "one devotes his property to a use in which the public has an interest, he . . . must submit to be controlled by the public for the common good."[7] Legal scholars regard this statement as the first important Supreme Court articulation of a boundary for state police power, one that "clearly implied that there were limits to what legislatures could do," inviting future scrutiny of police power laws for violations of the Fourteenth Amendment due process clause.[8] William Novak, for instance, argues that 1877 marked a turning point in the "postwar reconsideration of public power and private right" that ultimately wrought a revolution "in the conduct of American governance, including the 'invention' of constitutional law, the constitutionalization of police regulation, and ultimately the creation of a new American liberal state."[9] The *Munn* opinion invited, even demanded, American appellate courts to reconsider state police regulations in terms of the Fourteenth Amendment due process clause. And as the growth of railroads, large manufacturing concerns, corporations, cities, and immigration impelled states to pass more regulatory legislation, due process cases piled up "to throng the docket of the Supreme Court."[10]

In the "great police power cases of the late nineteenth century," the Supreme Court carved out a new configuration of citizens' rights versus police power, that of substantive due process.[11] Essentially legal shorthand for Fourteenth Amendment due process, substantive due process refers to the idea that if a law unjustly or unequally deprives a person of liberty or property, it denies due process of law in its substance as opposed to a procedural violation of due process. Another important development in late-nineteenth-century constitutional law was the idea of liberty of contract, in which the Court deferred to state legislatures "in cases involving public health or morals" but intervened "where other kinds of state regulations, or other industries, were concerned."[12] Although the Court tended to support state police power in cases associated with public health, it still scrutinized these state laws to determine whether they actually covered a health issue and did not violate substantive due process.[13]

By the turn of the century, legal theorists agreed that police power health regulations had to pass a test of reason. Were they truly in the public interest or did they use the public interest as a ruse to protect or punish a particular class or interest? Were they truly necessary? Were they reasonably framed so as not to bring undue hardship on persons or businesses? In 1900, for instance, San Francisco health officials imposed travel restrictions and quarantines only on its Chinese residents during an outbreak of bubonic plague. In two important cases, a federal circuit court judge ruled in favor of the Chinese plaintiffs because the health laws had not been applied equally to all citizens.[14]

It is in this constitutional context that the antivaccinationists and their attorneys sought Fourteenth Amendment protection from, as they saw it, the predations of their state on hapless individual citizens. Understanding that most police power cases tended to support public health regulations over individual civil rights, they still hoped to convince jurists that in the case of compulsory vaccination, the state had carried police power too far.

Commonwealth v. Albert M. Pear and *Commonwealth v. Henning Jacobson*

With such crucial constitutional issues at stake, the Massachusetts Anticompulsory Vaccination Society realized that it had to bring strong legal talent to the Pear and Jacobson appeals. Although James Winthrop Pickering had "given much study to this subject," it asked another attorney to serve as senior counsel for the joint appeal, sixty-four-year-old Henry Ballard.[15] Ballard, afflicted "for many years" with tuberculosis, was regarded as "one of Vermont's best-known criminal lawyers." Renowned as an "effective political speaker . . . in demand on the stump," Ballard took a prominent role in Republican Party organization in the 1870s and 1880s. He served as a Vermont state senator, as a delegate to the Republican National Convention in 1884, and as a reading clerk in the 1888 Convention. A seasoned, skillful defense attorney, he had conducted several notable cases over the course of his career, including the "longest jury trial ever held in New England." By convincing Ballard to join Pickering in the Jacobson and Pear appeals, MACVS believed it brought one of New England's finest attorneys on board, one noted for making rousing speeches before rapt audiences.[16]

Pickering and Ballard jointly prepared identical briefs for their clients, but Ballard appended a special section to Jacobson's brief. Their argument centered on the crucial issue of police power. In their view, Massachusetts carried police power "to such excess" that it overburdened "the citizen with multitudes of stringent exactions and requirements." It had "imposed almost countless conditions" on its citizens, but now it had entered a new realm, the body: "Having thus dealt with his affairs and his relations to the community, and pretty much every individual therein, the Legislature goes further and deals with his person." Ballard and Pickering asserted that Massachusetts's use of police power in this case transcended the bounds of republican government, achieving "paternalism more fully and completely than any surviving monarchy." They declared that if the court upheld compulsory vaccination, then the state would have unlimited power over people: "If the citizen has surrendered his body to the State for one purpose, he may as well surrender it for another, and surrender all the activities of his body to the service of the State which is so ready to assume so fully the regulation and management of all his private affairs."[17] The attorneys argued that with compulsory vaccination, the state had gone too far. By invading a healthy individual's body to perform a medical procedure, it asserted unwarranted control over the internal private space of the body.

Pickering and Ballard acknowledged that other appellate courts had gone to "the extreme limit in sustaining police power at the expense of the Constitution" by supporting the constitutionality of any law "*based* on the *idea* of the *promotion* and *protection* of society."[18] They argued nevertheless that the mantle of police power did not allow state legislatures to pass arbitrary or unreasonable laws that invaded civil rights guaranteed by the Constitution. They cited eminent legal scholars who declared that health and safety laws passed as an exercise of a state's police power "must not degenerate into an irrational excess," they are "not above the Constitution," and the "power is not without limitations." They warned that upholding such a law as constitutional would open "a very wide door for paternal legislation in the guise of police regulations for the benefit of public health." All sorts of medical treatments could be made compulsory, from various "hypodermic injections of the public with all the known anti-toxins" to "operative surgery."[19]

Pickering and Ballard argued that their clients had based their refusals on sincere anxieties about vaccination, anxieties supported by well-known medical facts that the law unreasonably ignored. Again and again the two attorneys hammered home the point that eminent medical authorities had criticized vaccination and linked it to a host of ailments and diseases. To bolster their credibility they focused on mainstream medical acknowledgment of widespread vaccine contamination, citing Joseph McFarland's widely read study on tetanus and vaccination.[20]

In oral argument, Pickering emphasized the need to respect personal choice in medical care, especially when the community possessed the means to prevent smallpox among those who accepted vaccination. Each person "had a right to judge for himself what medical treatment he should adopt, especially since all who believed in vaccination were . . . at liberty to become fully protected without regard to any dissenter."[21] Those who chose not to vaccinate understood the risk they took and could not pose any real threat to the vaccinated.

Henry Ballard appended a special section to Jacobson's brief that labored at length and in minute detail over each way the statute defied reason. Ballard argued that the Cambridge health department vaccination order "left no opportunity for the exercise of any discretion" because it applied to everyone regardless of his or her fitness for vaccination. It was "so sweeping in its terms—so utterly without any conditions, restrictions, or limitations, and which gave a power for its enforcement so arbitrary and despotic [that] the term *reasonable can in no sense be applied to it.*" Noting that the Massachusetts Constitution had granted to the legislature the power to make "all manner of *wholesome* and *reasonable orders, laws, statutes* and *ordinances*," he declared "all laws enacted by the General Court of Massachusetts must stand this test of reason."[22] He then devoted the rest of the attachment to showing how other state appellate courts had applied the rule of reason to support compulsory vaccination statutes that accommodated individual health circumstances. In oral argument, Ballard similarly emphasized that a reasonable law would allow discretion in its application.[23]

Pickering and Ballard focused intently on the issue of reason because police power statutes and regulations now had to pass the test of reason. The 1894 unfitness exemption for schoolchildren gave them an opportunity to challenge the reasonableness of the Cambridge health department general vaccination order. If the legislature recognized previously the injustice of refusing exemptions for children too sick for vaccination, then logic dictated it ought to extend a similar exemption to adults as well. If higher courts in other states supported exemptions then Massachusetts should too. Highlighting medical disagreement about vaccination to bolster their position, they hoped that the court would agree that the statute as written was simply too broad and thus an unreasonable application of police power.

Assistant District Attorney Hugh Bancroft authored the brief for the state. Young and relatively inexperienced, having just graduated from Harvard Law School in 1901, he had acquired celebrity as a champion rower for the Harvard crew. An academic star, he completed his four-year course of study in three years and earned a master's degree before entering law school. Well-connected to Boston's financial and legal elite through his father, William A. Bancroft, a general in the National Guard and president of the Boston Elevated Railway Company, Hugh Bancroft probably personally knew every judge on the Supreme Judicial Court.[24]

Bancroft presented identical arguments for both briefs. In a series of concise statements backed up by citations to previous leading cases, he asserted that police power, "an extensive undefined power," allowed the legislature "to pass laws for the common good," and that this power "unquestionably" includes lawmaking to protect public health.[25] Furthermore, courts had no business deciding exactly what constitutes "public good" because "the legislature determines what is for the public good, and its wide discretion cannot be controlled by courts unless its action is clearly evasive." Bancroft confidently asserted "it is not a question for the court whether vaccination is a preventive of smallpox" because "that question was for the legislature." Although Bancroft acknowledged that a court could intervene when a legislature passed "utterly arbitrary and unreasonable" laws, vaccination laws were reasonable because "vaccination is a successful and most effective known preventive of one of the most dangerous diseases." Bancroft succinctly torpedoed the contention that the statute unreasonably allowed for no exceptions by citing the smallpox epidemic as an "emergency . . . sufficient to warrant the most stringent measures" without further comment.[26]

On the question whether vaccination laws violated the "natural right to liberty," Bancroft asserted that individuals living in an "organized society" could not possess unlimited liberty. "The natural right to liberty is not an absolute right, but must yield whenever the welfare, health, or prosperity of the state demands." He tersely listed as "familiar instances" other limitations on individual liberty: quarantine, conscription, and statutes prohibiting or regulating certain trades and occupations. Bancroft also invited the court to comment broadly on the constitutionality of forcible vaccination: "If an individual submits to vaccination, against his will, because of the statute, it cannot be said that any right guaranteed to him by this article is invaded."[27]

Chief Justice Marcus Perrin Knowlton wrote the opinion handed down on 2 April 1903.[28] A seasoned jurist, the sixty-four-year-old Knowlton had served from 1881 to 1887 as a superior court judge and then on the Supreme Judicial Court since 1887. In 1902 he replaced Oliver Wendell Holmes as Chief Justice. Knowlton came from an "ancient and honorable" family that had "always had a hand in public affairs" in New England since the seventeenth century.[29] A native of Springfield, he graduated from Yale University in 1860 and was admitted to the Massachusetts state bar in 1862. Later commentators remembered him as achieving recognition early in his career "as a leading member of the bar in the western part of the State."[30] Politically active, he served both as a senator and representative in the state legislature, received honorary LLD degrees from Yale and Harvard, and had a reputation for writing great dissenting opinions over the course of his career as an appellate judge.[31]

Knowlton's respect for legislative deliberation clearly shaped his opinion on the Jacobson appeal. He deplored judicial activism and favored giving legislators credit for "intelligent consideration" of constitutional issues when they created law. In a 1901 commencement address, for instance, he noted "a tendency on the part of some courts in considering constitutional questions to give less weight to the action of the legislative department than fairly belongs to it." He thought appellate court judges should accord legislators the utmost respect: "the makers of law intend to be as regardful of their constitutional obligations as the interpreters of law." He argued that judges should presume in favor of constitutionality rather than the reverse. "A court therefore will not lightly set aside an expression of the legislative will, but will try in every reasonable way so to interpret it as to bring it within the true meaning and spirit of the constitution."[32]

Following this logic, his 1903 opinion summarily dismissed all questions as to the propriety and constitutionality of state compulsory vaccination laws in just one paragraph. "That such an object is worthy of the intelligent thought and earnest endeavor of legislators is too plain for discussion. Under the police power there is general legislative authority to make laws for the common good. . . . The rights of individuals must yield, if necessary, when the welfare of the whole community is at stake. This is true of the right to personal liberty as well as the right to property."[33] In creating such a statute, the state appropriately exercised its police power because it sought to control a pernicious disease, smallpox. In his view, the common good achieved was so evident that it hardly warranted explanation.

The bulk of Knowlton's opinion dealt specifically with Jacobson's exceptions to lower court rulings that excluded his offers of evidence to show "injurious or dangerous effects of vaccination."[34] Bancroft had argued that the lower court properly excluded these offers of proof because such "facts may be arguments against the enactment of legislation compelling vaccination, but they . . . have no place before a jury."[35] Jacobson and other antivaccinationists had failed to convince the legislature to change the law. Their beliefs and fears about vaccination provided no valid defense for refusing to comply with the requirements of the statute.

Chief Justice Knowlton, however, took a slightly different view of these points. After dismissing one point as "unnecessary and immaterial" and two others as "matters depending upon his [Jacobson's] personal opinion," Knowlton acknowledged that the other points properly asked the lower court to hear expert testimony about the safety of vaccination. Yet he concluded that if the lower court judge had allowed this testimony, he "would have been obliged to consider the evidence in connection with facts of common knowledge, which the court will always regard in passing upon the constitutionality of a statute." Among these "facts of common knowledge" was the general acceptance of vaccination. Knowlton noted that "the medical profession and the people generally have for a long time" accepted that vaccination posed a slight risk of injury, yet one "too small to be seriously weighed as against the benefits coming from the discreet and proper use of the preventive." Even if the lower court had allowed expert testimony about injurious effects from vaccination, "it could not have changed the result."[36] Knowlton inferred that the Massachusetts legislature understood these risks when it passed the law in the first place—a conclusion demonstrating his assumption that it had deliberated reasonably when passing the statute. He declared that a defense based on fear of harm from vaccination, however sincerely held, would not have saved Jacobson from a guilty verdict. Thus it did not matter that the evidence had been excluded.

Chief Justice Knowlton characterized Ballard's contentions about the statute's unreasonableness as an "elaborate argument" that failed to convince.[37] The fact that a person *might* be harmed by vaccination did not equate automatically to unreasonableness: "The theoretical possibility of an injury in an individual case as a result of its [the vaccination statute's] enforcement does not show that, as a whole, it is unreasonable. The application of a good law to an exceptional case may work hardship." Knowlton additionally noted that even if he thought that the compulsory vaccination law did nothing to promote the health of the community, it was not his place to declare the law unreasonable: "the question whether it will be for the good of the community is a legislative, and not a judicial question."[38] The legislature made laws to protect the welfare of the community, and he presumed that it acted reasonably. Thus Knowlton overruled Pear's and Jacobson's exceptions, declaring the compulsory vaccination statute constitutional and their trials free from error, provoking the antivaccination editor Joseph M. Greene to remark scathingly: "No matter how great and authoritative the evidence might have been presented to prove the 'majority' wrong, it would have made no difference, —because of the grand and glorious principle that the majority CAN'T be wrong."[39]

Yet it is important that Knowlton refused to take Bancroft up on his invitation to expand the scope of the state law to include vaccinating a person against his or her will. Even though neither Jacobson nor Pear had faced forcible vaccination, Bancroft's contention that there was nothing in the Massachusetts state constitution to prohibit it forced Knowlton to comment on the subject anyway: "If a person should deem it important that vaccination should not be performed in his case, and the authorities should think otherwise, it is not in their power to vaccinate him by force, and the worst that could happen to him under the statute would be the payment of the penalty of $5."[40] The vaccination statute made no provision for forcible vaccination. No judicial activist, Knowlton would take the law only as far as the wording of the statute allowed.

Knowlton's remark might have also served to warn health officials like Samuel Durgin to curb their zeal—Durgin's physicians had forcibly vaccinated homeless men sleeping in cheap lodging houses in 1901 and 1902, and Knowlton may have read of this practice in the *Boston Globe*. Knowlton noted too the care with which Cambridge health authorities had handled the Pear and Jacobson cases: "there is no reason to suppose that the enforcement of the requirement, in the present case, was conducted harshly."[41] Thus Knowlton emphasized the limitations of the vaccination statute as well as the relative triviality of its penalty. His concern about the harshness of treatment signaled that he would have regarded the vaccination statute as an unreasonable exercise of police power if it had permitted forcible vaccination.

Other observers noted the importance of Knowlton's qualification. One Cambridge newspaper reprinted the passage in which he declared that the compulsory vaccination statute did not give health authorities the legal power to forcibly vaccinate.[42] Some antivaccinationists celebrated this point despite their disappointment at losing the larger issues. Charles Asbury Simpson, secretary and treasurer of the Massachusetts Anti-compulsory Vaccination Society, quoted the passage in full with italics added ("*it is not in their power to vaccinate him by force*") to highlight the portions of the text most crucial to antivaccinationists: "Finally the Court gives us one ruling which we trust will stop, to some extent, the bulldozing of citizens who, from ignorance of their rights, have been compelled by threats of forcible vaccination, arrest, imprisonment with repeated fines, etc., to be vaccinated." Simpson also delighted in pointing out that Knowlton had specified "the *worst* that could happen to him under the statute would be the payment of the penalty of five dollars." Simpson felt the Chief Justice had taken notice of a point dear to antivaccinationists, asserting: "if this is the worst that could happen then *repeated fines can not be inflicted.*"[43] Many antivaccinationists had feared that health authorities could apply the fine on a daily basis, thus causing the fines to mount up to a sum impossible to pay, one intended to bankrupt resisters. Despite the loss, Simpson argued that the decision actually placed some important limits on the powers of health authorities to compel vaccination.

Simpson also articulated another important feature of antivaccination-ist sentiments about the appropriate limits of public health authority. The Massachusetts antivaccinationists campaigned against compulsory vaccination not because they believed that government had no business taking measures to protect public health. Quite the contrary, they felt that governments sometimes needed to take extreme action. "I certainly feel that I am correctly expressing the sentiments of the intelligent opponents of Compulsory Vaccination, when I say that we never argue against the interference with personal liberty in cer-tain cases, and we *accept*, and *urged* such restraint as may be found necessary in carrying out methods of sanitation which *have been* and *can be substituted* for vaccination, viz., Isolation and Disinfection." Simpson thus distinguished the "intelligent opponents of Compulsory Vaccination" from those who campaigned against it as part of a larger resistance to all governmental interference with the rights of individuals. Speaking for these "intelligent opponents," Simpson asserted that they agreed that health authorities should enforce quarantines that severely restricted individual freedom in order to protect public health. What they could not abide were "*active assaults*" perpetrated "when vaccination is inflicted upon a person against their desire" because it "*is an avowed intent to inflict a specific disease* viz., cowpox, and in many cases results in injury or death." Quarantine to prevent the spread of a communicable disease posed no harm to the health of those isolated, but compulsory vaccination statutes authorized "a personal assault upon the health and life of large numbers of citizens who are honest and respected members of the community."[44] In Simpson's view, govern-ment should trust its "honest and respected" citizens by giving them a choice to comply with quarantine orders instead of the personal invasion of vaccination.

Other antivaccinationists responded less optimistically. J. M. Greene, sarcas-tically declared that "the citizen is thus informed that, if he does not wish to obey the law, he need not,—all that he has to do is to contribute five dollars to the Government exchequer, and snap his fingers at the 'authorities.'" Greene thought little of Knowlton's distinctions, doubting he had "swept off the statute books" the law authorizing the forced vaccination of Charles Cate in the city jail along with other inmates of state institutions.[45] Immanuel Pfeiffer also dispar-aged Knowlton's opinion, asserting: "It practically says that the value of the com-pulsory vaccination law is five dollars. Cheap for those who have the money and expensive for those who do not have the money because they will be cast into prison and under the prison rules are compelled to be vaccinated."[46] Both of these antivaccinationists feared that health authorities would ignore Knowlton's fine points and continue to use coercion or force whenever they thought they could get away with it.

The first case to cite *Commonwealth v. Jacobson* followed quickly, with John Mugford losing his appeal in April 1903.[47] When he finally appeared for sentencing in November 1903, the judge fined him ten dollars for his refusal to vaccinate himself and his daughter, and ordered also that he pay court costs. After paying a total of $98.10, health officers approached him outside the courtroom and "offered to vaccinate him free of charge, but before he had time to reply he was pulled away by his attorney."[48] The Board of Health officials did not relinquish their pursuit of Mugford, sending "agents to his home in East Boston and to his store in Somerville."[49] Again he refused and was fined five dollars on a new complaint in December 1903.[50] Mugford probably paid it: Massachusetts state records list one case of vaccination refusal in a Suffolk County municipal court before 30 September 1904. Yet no trials appear in Suffolk County superior courts for either 1904 or 1905, indicating payment of the fine.[51]

State records of criminal prosecutions demonstrate also that the *Jacobson* and *Pear* decision effectively shut down attempts to appeal summons for refusal. Only Suffolk County, home to Cambridge, recorded three cases still pending in superior court (jury trial) for 1904, 1905, and 1906. These cases probably were *Jacobson*, *Pear*, and *Cone*—all awaiting final sentencing after the United States Supreme Court opinion.[52] By 1907, there were no cases of prosecutions for vaccination refusals, probably because no Board of Health had ordered any.

Jacobson v. Massachusetts

After their defeat in the Supreme Judicial Court of Massachusetts, MACVS voted to secure an attorney qualified to argue before the Supreme Court of the United States, even though they believed it unlikely they would prevail.[53] Fortunately for them, one of the most eminent attorneys in the state was available. George Fred Williams—former Democratic congressman for Massachusetts (1891–93) and three-time Democratic nominee for governor of Massachusetts (1895, 1896, and 1897)—had led the Massachusetts state Democratic Party since the early 1890s.[54] By 1903, however, at the age of fifty-one, Williams left the Democrats to form his own party, "The People's Rules."[55] Although this hiatus from Democratic Party politics proved just a temporary blip on a career arc that eventually led him back into its fold, he was at the moment free to take on clients.[56] Sometime after 1897 he had entered into a partnership with Judge James A. Halloran of Norfolk, Massachusetts. The antivaccinationist physician Immanuel Pfeiffer suggested that MACVS employ Williams "to take care of our interest" for the next stage in the appellate process, and the society agreed. By 15 June 1903, Williams had filed a Writ of Error on behalf of his new client, Henning Jacobson, but he filed no appeal for Albert Pear.[57] Neither the society nor any court documents reveal why Pear did not continue in the appeal. Jacobson's original exceptions, however, dealt specifically with the risks of vaccination as well as the constitutional questions posed by both appellants. From the antivaccinationist standpoint, Jacobson's appeal brought together all of the issues whereas Pear's just focused on civil rights.[58]

Born in 1852 in Dedham, Massachusetts, George Fred Williams lost his father, a German ship captain, at an early age.[59] Educated at Dartmouth and in Germany at the University of Heidelberg and the University of Berlin, Williams taught school briefly and then worked as a reporter for the *Boston Globe*. Attending law school in the morning while working afternoons and evenings, he supported his siblings and mother through his newspaper work and by writing a legal reference book, *Williams's Citations of Massachusetts Cases*, regarded in its day as "a standard book of reference for lawyers."[60] Admitted to the bar in 1875, he earned the bulk of his living editing a law digest. A "self-made man in the very best and broadest sense," he epitomized nineteenth-century virtue by acquiring social and intellectual status in Boston through "earnest endeavor, sturdy character, and congenial ability rather than inherited privilege or position."[61] Through travel and study, Williams refined his knowledge of European culture and art, and was regarded as "one of the most fluent and eloquent orators" in both German and English.[62]

Affectionately remembered as "touched in politics with a kind of romanticism which his puzzled opponents called instability," Williams started his political career as a fierce young Republican reformer who fell out with his party over its 1884 presidential candidate, James G. Blaine.[63] Williams and his fellow Mugwumps threw their support to the Democratic candidate, Grover Cleveland, because he pledged to lower tariffs and reform the civil service.[64] Williams, "the dashing young leader of the mugwumps of Massachusetts," joined the Democratic Party and soon was considered the "recognized leader" of the Massachusetts state party organization "on policy principle."[65] Elected to the Massachusetts state legislature in 1889, he made his reputation as a fearless reformer.[66] Williams's "spirited attack on the lobby" in Massachusetts helped him win election to Congress in 1890, where he emerged on the national stage as a junior Democrat renowned for his pluck in standing up to the Speaker of the House of Representatives.[67] An 1895 *New York Times* article admiringly reported, "wherever he has found fraud, corruption, or dishonesty in public places, Mr. Williams has never hesitated to expose it and drive it out."[68]

Although the *New York Times* editor in chief, Charles Ransom Miller, often disagreed with Williams's politics, he still lauded him as a man unusually dedicated to upholding the highest moral and ethical principles no matter what the cost. Intimate friends since their college days, Williams and Miller corresponded and visited frequently throughout their lives.[69] Miller's *New York Times* followed Williams's endeavors closely. One article concluded with this accolade: "Mr. Williams is an eloquent speaker. He uses the choicest and most concise modes of expression. He is a fearless advocate of any cause which he believes to be just. He is a man of distinguished and commanding presence. Personally he is a most charming companion; a witty and fascinating conversationalist, and a 'good fellow' generally. He is very popular with the rank and file of the party, because of his pluck and courage as a fighter and his genial manners."[70]

In 1896, however, Williams perplexed and surprised his political friends. While attending the Democratic National Convention that year as a delegate-at-large

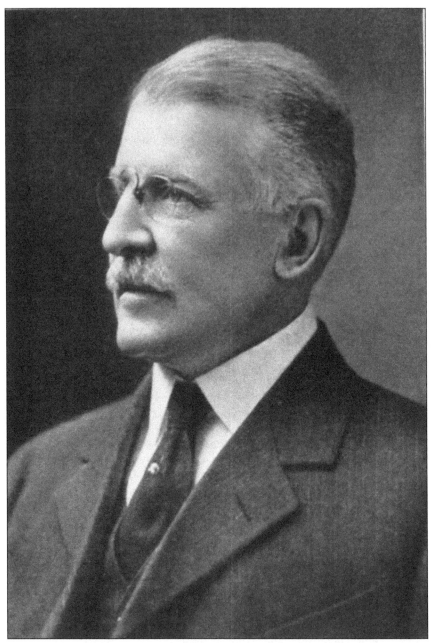

Figure 9.1. George Fred Williams. *The National Cyclopedia of American Biography* (New York: James White and Company, 1943), 30:297.

committed to preserving the gold standard, he "instantaneously converted to free silver," becoming an ardent supporter and confidant of William Jennings Bryan.[71] Williams explained his decision to a reporter as a personal revolt against "the organized band of bloodsuckers of the country," those who put corporate interests ahead of the public interest. "The time has come . . . for a great popular uprising, and I propose to be in it. In taking this step of supporting a silver Democrat, I realize that I am doomed politically in Massachusetts, and that I never shall be forgiven by men who claim to be Democrats. I realize also that these men can punish me socially and financially, but I invite the persecution with a conscientious feeling that I am doing right by voicing the sentiments of an outraged public."[72] True to his prediction, his switch to silver at first "amazed" and then alienated Williams's Democratic colleagues.[73] Nevertheless, "bound to rule or ruin his party," he soon regained his leadership position, running as the Democratic candidate for governor in 1896 and 1897.[74] By 1900 he sat on the Democratic Party National Committee.[75] Williams's control over New England Democrats so impressed his party that it seriously considered him as a running mate for Bryan in the 1900 national election.[76]

Over the next few years, Williams's political views shifted to advocate many progressive reforms. Benjamin Orange Flower of *The Arena* characterized Williams as "one of the leading, if not the leading representative of progressive Democracy in New England."[77] Williams supported William Jennings Bryan's program of "public ownership of railroads, telegraphs and telephones, and the development of a more radical system of government by extending the power of the people over their law-making and law-makers."[78] Yet despite Williams's bitterness about machine politics and the corrupting influence of wealth among the Democrats, he never really gave up on them, except for his brief fling at forming a new party in 1903.

Who better, then, to advocate for the antivaccinationist cause? Williams's radical populism made him very attractive to antivaccinationists who thought of their cause as "a populism of the body."[79] A fixture in Democratic Party politics both at the state and national level, he sat at dinners, attended meetings, and gave speeches at rallies with many leading politicians. He counted William Jennings Bryan and Charles Ransom Miller as close friends. George Fred Williams thus lent the antivaccinationist cause both prestige and credibility before the highest American court.

The case must have appealed to Williams's sensibilities. A principled man, he risked his political career time and again in order to stand true to his beliefs. As a Democratic Party leader, he spoke out against corruption and made enemies when he converted to supporting Bryan's bimetal currency scheme. Later, he would quit an important diplomatic post in Greece just before World War I because he refused to sit in silent witness to massacre and atrocity in Albania, or as one admirer observed, he "resigned his position rather than forfeit the right to champion the cause of the oppressed."[80] A frequent traveler to and from Europe, Williams got caught up in the New York City 1892 cholera quarantine. Although cabin passengers received markedly better treatment than those in steerage, conditions for both deteriorated as food and water ran short at times.[81] Perhaps that experience rendered him sympathetic to antivaccination-ists' arguments about oppressive health officials and policies. Williams probably saw Jacobson as a "little guy" who lacked both money and political connections yet still deserved his day in court, an attitude consonant with an observation that "he never spared himself when he could be of service to others, and his sympa-thies were always on the side of the oppressed."[82]

In his brief to the United States Supreme Court, Williams focused on the Fourteenth Amendment, charging that the compulsory vaccination law vio-lated Jacobson's right to substantive due process. Unlike previous Fourteenth Amendment cases, Jacobson's appeal presented a new permutation of the con-stitutional issues. Did the Fourteenth Amendment protect a citizen's bodily integrity—the most fundamental liberty—from the reach of police power when that person posed no discernible threat to his fellow citizens?

The Supreme Court had not yet considered the constitutionality of gen-eral compulsory vaccination laws. Williams noted that it had skirted the issue in three previous cases, with the most telling comment coming from Justice Rufus Peckham in *The American School of Magnetic Healing v. McAnnulty*, when he acknowledged that "vaccination is believed by many to be a preventive of small-pox, while others regard it as unavailing for that purpose."[83] Williams believed that the Court's recognition of vaccination's controversial status indicated that it ought to consider compulsory laws unreasonable.

Williams next argued that other states and nations did not rely on compul-sory vaccination to control smallpox, especially since "there is a growing ten-dency to resort to sanitation and isolation rather than vaccination." Most states did not compel vaccination: thirty-four states lacked compulsory vaccination stat-utes whereas only eleven states had them. Only thirteen states excluded unvacci-nated children from public schools. Even England had amended its vaccination statutes to accommodate objectors, and other countries "constantly called into question" their vaccination laws.[84]

Even more telling, Williams claimed, people lately greeted compulsory vac-cination with popular outrage, as evidenced by the November 1904 riots in Rio de Janeiro, Brazil. Even the renowned Progressive Wisconsin governor Robert La Follette acknowledged extensive popular distaste for compulsory vaccina-tion: "But I cannot ignore the fact that laws of this character are repugnant to very many good citizens, even among those who are not opposed to vaccination from religious beliefs or prejudices. In some states they have resulted in riots and strife which have outlived the epidemic."[85] Indiana's legislature amended its vaccination laws in 1901 to allow unvaccinated pupils to attend public schools. Minnesota abolished its school vaccination requirement in 1903.[86] Neither uni-versally accepted nor universally applied, compulsory vaccination excited popu-lar outrage, and other states with compulsory vaccination laws had amended or abolished them altogether.

Williams contended that appellate court judges construed health legislation to support compulsory vaccination only under narrowly defined circumstances.

He declared that "apart from a specific legislative act for compulsory vaccination, the courts will not imply the existence of such a police power in the public authorities though vested with the largest authority to protect the public health."[87] In his view, only three cases to date had "considered general compulsory laws," and they demonstrated how carefully the judiciary had deliberated on them, making fine distinctions in order to accommodate those who objected to vaccination.[88] The New York State Court of Appeals, for instance, had rejected the Brooklyn Health Commissioner's quarantine order for vaccination refusals as exceeding the limits of his statutory authority.[89] The Supreme Court of North Carolina supported compulsory vaccination laws, but cautioned that the "legislature did not intend to enforce the law" if "conditions of health might make it dangerous."[90] This court thus acknowledged "due process of law entitled a defendant to offer evidence that vaccination would be injurious to him." Another 1897 Georgia decision upheld an exemption provision in a city vaccination ordinance even though the state law did not provide such an exemption. Williams highlighted these opinions to show judicial sensitivity to the inequities posed by uniform application of vaccination laws and other courts' openness to the idea that the judiciary should serve to arbitrate on exemptions. Williams asserted: "none of these cases are as extreme as the decision in Massachusetts."[91] The Massachusetts trial court denied his client's right to due process by refusing to allow evidence of vaccination's risks.

At this point, Williams brought up the issue of the Fourteenth Amendment and its effect on police power, noting that various court decisions since 1868 had established new limitations to a state's police power. In these opinions courts had declared that statutes designed to protect public health, safety, and welfare must affect public interest, and they must demonstrate that "*the means are reasonably necessary for the accomplishment of the purpose and not unduly oppressive upon individuals.*" Williams italicized this quotation from *Lawton v. Steele,* a famous police power decision, in order to underscore his point that statutes designed to protect health should not injure it. In that opinion Justice Brown noted that "the extent and limits of . . . police power have been a fruitful subject of discussion in nearly every State in the Union." Williams placed Jacobson's appeal in the middle of this national discussion, agreeing that "the state intervenes to secure the personal health, preservation and comfort of the citizen." Yet his case concerned a different type of intervention, one that might harm those the state sought to protect. "But except for compulsory vaccination laws it has not yet undertaken to attack the health of individuals."[92]

Williams did not deny the right of a state to take extreme actions to preserve public health, welfare, and safety. He acknowledged that communities routinely regulated trades, occupations, buildings, animals, corpses, cemeteries, food, water, medicine, and dentistry to protect the public: "The plaintiff in error . . . does not deny that if he or his property be infected with contagious or infectious disease, or if he commits any noxious act, it is the right and duty of the state to defend the rest of the community against him as a public, or even as a private nuisance." Yet Jacobson, "in going about the community, healthy and law-abiding . . . does no injury to the community." Thus Williams declared: "It is not a nuisance for the plaintiff to remain healthy."[93]

Williams understood that police power dealt primarily with prevention—a person or thing did not have to threaten public health or safety at that instant to warrant state intervention—the mere possibility of danger was sufficient. Nevertheless he maintained there were no precedents for imposing police power "upon healthy citizens, merely because as human beings they have the potentiality of contracting contagious diseases." Vaccination instead infected Jacobson with a disease that might harm him and "no constitutional precedent can be found which justifies the exercise of police power to compel a citizen to submit himself to an assault and to inoculation with a disease." Williams contended: "Liberty of the citizen in the very first analysis is immunity of his person from seizure or injury," unless he or she has committed "an offence against the state." He wondered if Jacobson presented such a potential threat, then where would the state stop to prevent or treat all sorts of disease, regardless of the risks entailed? Would it submit citizens "to further experimentation upon our bodies" in the name of public health? Thus he argued that the possibility that Jacobson might contract smallpox "is too small a matter upon which to predicate a criminal penalty."[94]

Williams pointed out that Jacobson did not object to vaccination per se: "It is against the compulsory feature of the Massachusetts law that the plaintiff protests." He explored the senselessness of the compulsory vaccination law and its penalty. If his client happened to get smallpox, "the only possible victims . . . would be those who had themselves failed or refused to be vaccinated." He asserted that the penalty of a one-time five-dollar fine "is too absurd to justify its existence," if by that one payment an individual could then avoid vaccination and thus "continue to be a menace to the public health." If the state repeatedly levied the fine plus court costs, then many Massachusetts citizens "without means of payment" would "stand committed to prison," an outcome that contradicted the lower court's assertion "as to the insignificance of the fine." Also, Williams noted that the law did not apply generally, but instead operated on a strictly local basis for the residents of a specific town or city only. Thus unvaccinated nonresidents could continue to come and go, yet they posed just "as much a menace to the inhabitants" as the unvaccinated resisters.[95]

Williams then reviewed the lower courts' refusal to consider evidence about the possible harmfulness of vaccination—a ruse to introduce the excluded evidence. He emphasized vaccination's novelty as a "surgical operation" that introduced a "disease which does not otherwise afflict humanity." Jacobson had offered "in vain" to provide evidence demonstrating that "suffering and sickness . . . more or less severe" followed all vaccinations, and that he and his son had experienced "great suffering" in previous vaccinations. Furthermore, medical opinion about proper vaccination materials and techniques had varied over the years "and are still a matter of serious difference of opinion." Medical authorities recognized problems with contamination in eminent publications like the *Journal of the American Medical Association*. Vaccination opponents and "many leading medical authorities" claimed that "the proper treatment of epidemic diseases is sanitation and isolation," and he cited Cleveland, Ohio, and Leicester, England, as leading examples for these methods in controlling smallpox. Quoting Justice Oliver Wendell Holmes, Williams asserted that the existence of "actual necessity" limited police power. Ultimately, vaccination presented so many problems and uncertainties that "vaccination is not proved to be a necessary precaution against smallpox." If vaccination could not pass the test of necessity, then making it compulsory amounted to an unreasonable exercise of police power.[96]

But "the law recognized no such defense," and Williams contended that this exclusion not only violated his client's right to due process under the Fourteenth Amendment but also his right to equal protection of the law because this defense *was* available to a certain class of citizens—children. Williams declared that equal protection did not exist "when such a defense is open to parents for the protection of children and is not open to parents themselves." Williams called the exemption of children arbitrary, and the vaccination law itself thus "oppressive and unreasonable" because it clearly acknowledged vaccination's dangers by providing medical exemptions for children but not adults.[97]

Williams also noted that the Massachusetts vaccination law failed equal protection because it did not specify "what constitutes vaccination" but depended on local health authorities' decisions about when and how often to vaccinate. The law did not apply to all citizens equally when one town decided to vaccinate "every year or every month," whereas another required it "once in many years or not at all."[98]

Williams connected his argument to the Civil War amendments, noting their original purpose as "the freedom of the African race and the security and perpetuation of that freedom." Although most of the police power cases brought before the Supreme Court in the years since their passage revolved around issues of unjust state interference with private property, he invited the Court to honor the Fourteenth Amendment's original intention to protect individual liberty. "As the Fourteenth Amendment has so often been appealed to for the protection of property, this plaintiff appeals to it with confidence for the protection of his freedom."[99] Williams hoped to persuade the Supreme Court to interpret the Fourteenth Amendment according to its original intentions to rescue citizens from state infringements on their federal civil rights. Williams presented his client as an individual whose liberty and control over the most intimate aspect of his life—his body—was threatened by the state. By staking out this position, Williams articulated the growing early twentieth-century liberal conception of government that juxtaposed the rights of individual citizens against state police power interests.

Massachusetts State Attorney General Herbert Parker countered Williams's brief with an argument that looked back to a well-regulated society where the idea that "the Legislature has large discretion to determine what personal sacrifice the public health, morals and safety require from individuals is elementary." Citizens were expected routinely to accept a great deal of government regulation of their personal, as well as public, affairs. Attempts to avoid or reject these rules were seen as examples of bad citizenship or civic irresponsibility. Parker depicted Jacobson not as a victim of an overly oppressive state law, but rather as a malcontent who would not accept antivaccinationists' failure to sway the legislature to their way of thinking. Despite Jacobson's many offers to prove the dangers posed by vaccination and his personal history of problems with vaccination, Parker denied that Jacobson had tried to prove that "by his state of health or other circumstance vaccination would be dangerous to him at the time." Instead Parker emphasized Jacobson's disagreement with "the theory of public policy which had guided the Legislature" and charged that he improperly used the courts as a venue to challenge that policy. To ask the Court now to review the law on that basis would usurp the most basic function of the state, police power, "its unquestioned power, to preserve and protect the public health, . . . and . . . to require doubting individuals to yield for the welfare of the community." Refusing to accept this obligation of citizenship gracefully, Jacobson was a shirker who sought to circumvent the will of the people through the courts. Paraphrasing an earlier opinion of Justice John Marshall Harlan, Parker asserted: "If all that can be said of this legislation is that it is unwise or unnecessarily oppressive to people in general, their appeal must be to the Legislature or to the ballot-box, not to the judiciary. . . . It is not a part of the functions of the court to conduct investigations of fact entering into questions of public policy merely to sustain or frustrate legislative will embodied in statutes."[100] Thus however apt George Fred Williams's analysis of the incongruities and perplexities of the Massachusetts vaccination law, that critique properly belonged under the purview of the legislature, not the courts. The only information that Henning Jacobson could have used to defend himself—evidence that his health was too precarious to allow vaccination safely—he failed to offer.

Throughout his brief, Parker touched on the possibility of a defense for Jacobson on medical grounds, even though the law as written offered no such defense. Parker observed other courts had looked favorably on the possibility of using ill health as "a sufficient excuse for . . . non-compliance, since to vaccinate . . . under such conditions would be an arbitrary and unreasonable enforcement of the statute." Clearly anticipating an analysis of the Massachusetts vaccination statute based on reasonableness, Parker contended that the Cambridge vaccination order "was not an undiscriminating rule that every inhabitant of the city must get himself vaccinated before a certain time, notwithstanding his condition of health, . . . but was in the nature of a resolve that all who had not been successfully vaccinated since March 1, 1897, ought to be vaccinated." The vaccination statute "left the matter to the discretion of local authorities" who could chose to apply it so that it did not wreak an undue hardship on those medically unfit for vaccination. Parker reiterated this point in Jacobson's case: "If there were special reasons why the plaintiff in error could not be vaccinated at the time required by the board of health, he should have made them a ground of his refusal; and, if the board neglected to consider them, a defence [sic] to his prosecution."[101]

Why would the attorney general characterize the vaccination order as a resolve that became a legal requirement only when the health department actually demanded vaccination from a specific individual? This way he could argue that the Cambridge Board of Health had the power to consider vaccination on a case-by-case basis, thus absolving it of charges that it did not take individual health considerations into account when it applied the law. This characterization also implied that the police court judges took medical unfitness into account in their consideration of vaccination refusals and allowed defendants extra time to become well enough to withstand the procedure. Parker could argue that Jacobson acted unreasonably when "he arbitrarily refused" vaccination and refute the assertion that the law operated unjustly or unreasonably because it contained no provision for those too sick to stand vaccination.[102]

Parker argued that there was no inequality in the application of the law to Jacobson. If the Cambridge Board of Health had acted in "an arbitrary manner," applying the law only to Jacobson or one class of persons, then they would have violated his Fourteenth Amendment right to equal protection. Parker also asserted that the statute's exception for children "denies to nobody the equal protection of the laws" because the law merely "limits liability to a penalty to persons who have a right to control their own conduct."[103]

Going over the same state court cases that Williams had used to support Jacobson, Parker offered a different perspective of their rulings. All of the vaccination cases where lower courts had ruled against the health boards concerned situations where their vaccination orders "were broader than the authority given by statute." Nevertheless, Parker asserted that state supreme courts had sustained state statutes that granted explicit authority to compel vaccination. Quoting *State v. Hay*, Parker affirmed that this exercise of police power was no different from drafting citizens in time of war: "If a people can draft or conscript its citizens to defend its borders from invasion, it can protect itself from the deadly pestilence."[104] Parker implied here that Jacobson was no different from a cowardly draft dodger who sought to avoid his most fundamental duty, protecting his community in an emergency when it needed him the most.

Harlan's Opinion

Parker and Williams argued their briefs before a Supreme Court presided over by Chief Justice Melville Weston Fuller since 1888.[105] The Fuller Court was noted for its support of the notion that "the law existed above all to protect freedom of contract" and struck down a variety of state laws that sought to regulate businesses.[106] Cases involving laws designed to protect public health were the exception to this rule, and it had no problem ruling in favor of Massachusetts by a majority of seven to two. The opinion, authored by Justice John Marshall Harlan, argued that Jacobson's refusal amounted to a failure to live up to the demands of citizenship. Justices David J. Brewer and Rufus Peckham dissented without comment, so we cannot know precisely the reasons for their objections.

Yet we can look at previous opinions for some insight into their thinking—opinions in which they both connected liberty of contract to substantive due process to support limiting the ability of states to regulate business.

Noted for "opposing firmly the expansion of government regulatory power, state or federal," Brewer "was for the Court of that era the right-wing opposite" of Harlan, with whom he had a history of ideological clashes.[107] Nephew to Supreme Court Justice Stephen J. Field, Brewer sat on the Kansas Supreme Court and then the federal circuit court before his 1890 appointment to the United States Supreme Court. In several opinions on the constitutionality of Kansas prohibition laws, Brewer contended that states could not deprive citizens of their property without compensation. At the United States Supreme Court, he championed liberty of contract and private property rights, stating in an 1892 dissent: "The paternal theory of government is to me odious. The utmost possible liberty to the individual and the fullest possible protection to him and his property, is both the limitation and duty of government."[108] Although his dissent in *Jacobson* was tacit, it does not greatly stretch credulity to imagine that Brewer must have felt a great deal of sympathy for Jacobson's plight and agreed that the state had no business compelling healthy people to acquire the disease of vaccinia.[109]

Justice Peckham likewise "rarely sympathized with the state's use of its police powers," especially when he thought it interfered with individuals' private property rights and their freedom to make contracts.[110] Born and raised in upstate New York, he was a personal friend of Grover Cleveland and quite active in Democratic Party politics before he was elected to the New York Court of Appeals in 1886, partly because he managed to gain the support of Henry George and his single-tax followers. He shared Brewer's distaste for government regulation of business, declaring state price-fixing laws to unduly interfere with "the most sacred rights of property and the individual's liberty of contract."[111] Appointed to the Supreme Court in 1896 by President Cleveland, he "joined a court whose views in many ways resembled his own."[112] Peckham is best known for his opinion in *Allgeyer v. Louisiana* (1897), which "made due process dominant as the doctrine virtually immunizing economic activity from regulation deemed contrary to the laissez-faire philosophy of the day."[113] There, he expanded the meaning of liberty to include "not only the right of the citizen to be free from the mere physical restraint of his person, as by incarceration, but the term is deemed to embrace the right of the citizen to be free in the enjoyment of his faculties; to be free to use them in all lawful ways; to live and work where he will; to earn his livelihood by any lawful calling; to pursue any livelihood or avocation; and for that purpose to enter into all contracts which may be proper, necessary and essential."[114] In another opinion he displayed a certain skepticism about those who claimed to possess sole legitimate medical authority when he characterized controversy over vaccination along with disputes for professional hegemony between homeopaths and AMA regulars as examples of unresolvable competing claims.[115] Since he never articulated why he dissented in *Jacobson*, we cannot exactly know his reasons, but we can guess. At least one scholar of Peckham's life has speculated that "it may be that because liberty, in the original sense of physical restraint, was involved, Peckham was willing to accept the view of Jacobson that the law was 'hostile to the inherent rights of every free man to care for his own body and health in such a way as to him seems best.'"[116]

Chief Justice Fuller assigned the opinion to Justice John Marshall Harlan, who "strongly believed in the exercise of state police power in its proper sphere."[117] Characterized as a "Great Dissenter" both for the frequency of his dissenting opinions and his "almost religious reverence for the Constitution," he is revered today as "the voice crying in the wilderness" for standing up for black Americans' civil rights in dissent after dissent.[118] In 1883, he alone among his Supreme Court brethren supported the constitutionality of the Civil Rights Act of 1875, which had required for all citizens black and white, among other rights, "full and equal enjoyment" of public accommodations like railroad cars, hotels, and theaters.[119] His 1896 dissent in *Plessy v. Ferguson* classically professed: "Our Constitution is color-blind, and neither knows nor tolerates classes among citizens."[120] But, as several legal scholars have commented, this dissent was only treated with great regard after the 1954 *Brown v. Board of Education* decision.[121] One study of Harlan's decisions noted that during his time on the bench and for several generations after his death in 1911, he was considered an eccentric dissenter who "repeatedly protested from the bench against racial discrimination," but not always consistently.[122] Although Progressives held him in high esteem for his dissent from the Supreme Court's rejection of the federal income tax law in 1895 and his antitrust decisions, they also despaired of him for rulings that helped out big companies and railroad corporations. These incongruities led at least one biographer to characterize Harlan as an enigma.[123] For all its importance to public health history, Harlan's biographers give his *Jacobson* opinion scant regard, considering it "a typical Harlan decision," a routine discussion of state police power that barely rates comment.[124] They focus instead on his dissent in another police power case that same year, the infamous *Lochner v. New York* (1905), where a Court reluctant to interfere with business declared that New York could not regulate bakers' hours of labor under its police power because that violated the sanctity of contract.

Harlan's personal history contains profound ironies. Born into a prominent Kentucky slaveholding family, his father a close friend and political ally of Henry Clay, Harlan held to Whig principles of national government throughout his lifetime. A slave owner himself, he supported the Union and fought in the Civil War, but only on the condition that Kentucky remain a slave state. Yet with the collapse of the Whig Party after the war and the passage of the Thirteenth Amendment freeing all slaves, he renounced his support for slavery and joined the Republican Party. He became an associate justice on the United States Supreme Court in 1877 and reined in substantive due process in two important opinions, *Mugler v. Kansas* (1887) and *Powell v. Pennsylvania* (1888). In *Mugler* he held that the states could prohibit the sale of liquor because it clearly posed a danger to public well-being, "brusquely" rejecting Brewer's prior argument at

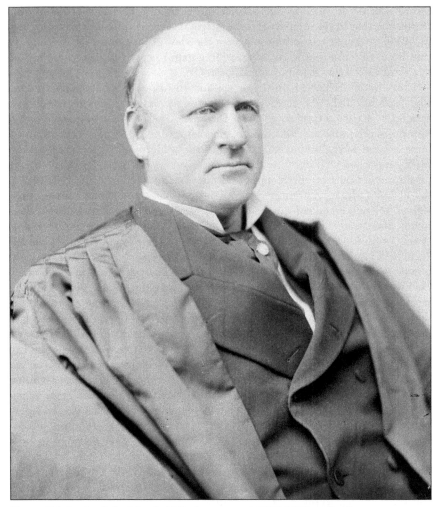

Figure 9.2. Justice John Marshall Harlan, around 1910. Wikimedia Commons.

the state level that owners of these businesses should be compensated for their losses—an opinion that possibly contributed to Justice Brewer's decision to dissent later on *Jacobson*.[125] In *Powell*, he supported Pennsylvania's prohibition of oleomargarine on the theory of its unhealthy properties. In both opinions, Harlan decided the laws were reasonable because they aimed to control harmful substances for the public good.

When Justice Harlan upheld the Massachusetts compulsory vaccination statute, he articulated a long judicial tradition accepting the idea that individual rights must give way to the common good in a well-ordered society. "According to settled principles, the police power of a state must be held to embrace, at least, such reasonable regulations established directly by legislative enactment as will protect the public health and the public safety." The Massachusetts legislature enacted its compulsory vaccination statute with the beneficial intent and perceived necessity to suppress smallpox epidemics and also properly delegated its implementation to local boards of health. "Upon the principle of self-defense, of paramount necessity, a community has the right to protect itself against an epidemic of disease which threatens the safety of its members."[126] Although Harlan never commented on his reasoning in *Jacobson*, he articulated the intellectual context of his notion of police power in a 1900 oration on James Wilson, a founding father whom he much admired. Wilson, along with other political theorists of the early Republic, "vigorously asserted the responsibilities and obligations of government" to create a "well-regulated society" in which "there was no such thing as perfect or absolute liberty."[127] In his lecture, Harlan reiterated this idea when he declared: "No man here is so high that he is above the law." He also located the source of law in the states: "The germinal idea of American liberty is local self-government. . . . To the States we must look primarily for protection in our lives, our liberties and our property. They have rights that are as sacred as the rights of the Nation."[128]

Objecting to Jacobson's complaint that vaccination "is nothing short of an assault upon his person," Harlan famously asserted that the United States Constitution "does not import an absolute right in each person to be, at all times and in all circumstances, wholly freed from restraint. There are manifold restraints to which every person is necessarily subject for the common good." Harlan's elaboration here harked back to older ideas that citizens owed their communities certain duties for the privilege of living in a well-regulated society. He noted that the Constitution of Massachusetts had established "as a fundamental principle" that "the whole people covenants with each citizen, and each citizen with the whole people, that all shall be governed by certain laws for the common good." Nevertheless Harlan demarcated a limit to the reach of police regulations: "There is, of course, a sphere within which the individual may assert the supremacy of his own will, and rightfully dispute the authority of any human government." But he did not elaborate what that "sphere" contained. Instead he presented two crucial examples—quarantine and the military draft—to demonstrate that "the rights of the individual in respect of his liberty may at times, under the pressure of great dangers, be subjected to such restraint, to be enforced by reasonable regulations, as the safety of the general public may demand." Although he admitted that the Fourteenth Amendment protected "the right of a person 'to live and work where he will' . . . yet he may be compelled, by force if need be, against his will and without regard to his personal wishes or his pecuniary interests, or even his religious or political convictions, to take his place in the ranks of the army of his country, and risk the chance of being shot down in its defense."[129] Thus it did not matter whether vaccination posed a real threat to Jacobson's health or whether he consented to it: in epidemics as in war, citizens, willing or not, had to risk, even sacrifice, their lives and livelihoods to protect their communities. In refusing vaccination, Jacobson broke an ancient covenant with his community. He shirked his end of the social contract.

Harlan considered next if the vaccination statute worked as a *reasonable* exercise of police power. Courts could interfere with state legislative enactments only if those laws and regulations failed the test of reason, a test limited to deciding whether the law had "a real and substantial relation" to the protection of public health, morals, or safety. Was compulsory vaccination reasonable? Harlan recognized that while most medical experts supported vaccination, a minority regarded it as dangerous or useless: "the state court knew, as this court knows, that an opposite theory accords with the common belief, and is maintained by high medical authority." Yet only state legislatures could choose between the two views. "We must assume that, when the statute in question was passed, the legislature of Massachusetts was not unaware of these opposing theories, and was compelled, of necessity, to choose between them."[130]

For all his professed deference to the state legislature, Harlan reviewed its reasoning anyway, contending that "the experience of this and other countries whose authorities have dealt with the disease of smallpox" demonstrated compulsory vaccination's "real and substantial relation to the protection of the public health."[131] In order to show that the legislature passed the law with a realistic expectation of controlling smallpox, Harlan resorted to some research. In an extensive footnote, he cited various authorities to show that other countries successfully relied on vaccination to suppress smallpox.[132] He also quoted at length from a New York state appellate case that took judicial notice of "the common belief of the people of this state" that vaccination prevented smallpox.[133] Harlan went to great lengths to show that the Massachusetts legislature had not enacted the law on a whim, but instead reasonably expected that compulsory vaccination would halt the spread of smallpox. Yet he selected only sources and evidence that supported his presumption in favor of vaccination. One of his choices, for instance, explicitly singled out antivaccinationists as "enemies of society."[134] He also ignored evidence about vaccination complications cited by his own sources.[135] Harlan relied only on evidence that supported his argument—he did not attempt to address any facts that might undermine it because he agreed that antivaccination was unreasonable and antivaccinationists were "enemies of society." As far as Harlan was concerned, the antivaccinationists had had their chance. If they could not convince their legislators to provide some exemption for conscientious objectors, then they were out of luck. To appeal to the United States Constitution for due process protection on the basis of their objections to vaccination "invited the court and the jury to go over the whole ground gone over by the legislature" and "practically strip the legislative department of its function to care for the public health and public safety when endangered by epidemics of disease." Jacobson and other antivaccinationists wanted to enjoy the "protection afforded by an organized local government" and yet "defy the will of its constituted authorities."[136] They wanted to enjoy the privileges of citizenship without performing the obligations of citizenship.

Most legal scholars and historians tend to focus on language in *Jacobson* that supports state power to interfere with an individual's control over her or his body.[137] Yet Harlan's opinion also limited this power. First, he decreed a sphere of individual control that would eventually be interpreted as a right to privacy in matters of sexuality and reproduction.[138] Second, he carved out an exception for ill health in the vaccination law where none existed. The research imbedded in Harlan's footnotes shows that he certainly understood that vaccination could pose a significant threat to an individual's health, and even though he chose to play down this medical context when arguing for the law's reasonableness, perhaps it persuaded him to recognize the need for an exception that both the legislature and appellate court had denied. Ironic—considering Harlan's insistence that only legislatures could properly determine that point—that the Massachusetts legislature had heard much testimony about vaccination's potential for harm, yet still refused to amend the law in 1902 to allow just such an exception.

So, despite his regard for the Massachusetts legislature, Harlan essentially amended the statute to provide an exception for ill health by reading it into the law. The law, as he understood it, never intended to give health boards the power to compel vaccination in every circumstance. He postulated "an adult who is embraced by the mere words of the act, but yet to subject whom to vaccination in a particular condition of his health or body would be cruel and inhuman in the last degree." Here Harlan decreed that earlier decisions supported the presumption that "legislatures intended exceptions to its language which would avoid results of this character." Thus he declared that "we are not inclined to hold that the statute establishes the absolute rule that an adult must be vaccinated if it be apparent or can be shown with reasonable certainty that he is not at the time a fit subject of vaccination, or that vaccination, by reason of his then condition, would seriously impair his health, or probably cause his death."[139] With this language Harlan practically wrote in the amendment for an adult unfitness exemption that Massachusetts antivaccinationists had so avidly (and unsuccessfully) sought in 1902. If Harlan had taken notice of the fact that this bill had failed, would he have still concluded that the legislature intended some exemptions in cases of extreme medical hardship? If Pear, who insisted that his health would not permit vaccination, had appealed his case to the United States Supreme Court, would Harlan have upheld his conviction? Note, too, that the first briefs authored by Pickering and Ballard had focused especially on the lack of an exemption for cases of medical unfitness.

Some legal scholars at the time understood this nuance: one law journal editor noted that *Jacobson* "recognizes that the requirement would not be enforceable against a person who was not a fit subject for vaccination."[140] Antivaccinationists made much of this point. Sara Newcomb Merrick wondered, "had a pale, thin, cadaverous man been chosen as the defendant would the decision have been different?" And she believed the decision supported exempting adults for unfitness, warning: "Let vaccinators note this."[141] A leading supporter of vaccination, the physician George Dock, also noticed Harlan's distinction, but thought it would make little difference: "We all know that many unfit people have been vaccinated, sometimes by force, with great brutality, and often with serious or even fatal results. There is no consolation for the parents in such cases to know that they can bring suit for assault."[142] Recently the legal scholar Lawrence Gostin argued: "if there had been evidence that the vaccination would seriously impair Jacobson's health, he may have prevailed in this historic case." Gostin points out that "Jacobson's claim of potential harm was not without merit," noting that Jenner himself described a case of "severe adverse reaction" to vaccination.[143]

Antivaccinationists' legal wrangling over the constitutionality of compulsory vaccination laws had undermined for years health officials' ability to persuade people to get vaccinated. They constituted such a potent disruptive force that their resistance undoubtedly contributed to the tendency of public health officials to tread warily around outright compulsion even when the law supported it. Although the officials involved in *Jacobson* believed in the soundness of vaccination, they were slow to prosecute and used it more for the purposes of demonstration than for any real control of the epidemic. *Jacobson* did not establish compulsory vaccination as the primary method of smallpox control. Public health authorities prosecuted Henning Jacobson to set an example, to discredit the antivaccinationists in general, and to reaffirm their prerogatives. Their determination to enforce compulsory vaccination laws grew from a need to establish public health authority and credibility, not from a desire to actually hunt down and vaccinate every unwilling person. Nagging and nudging people to bare their arms would ultimately prove more effective. Vaccination against smallpox would be normalized as a rite of passage, just one of several immunizations needed for admittance to public schools and universities, the military, or employment of all sorts—that was the true victory they sought.

Henning Jacobson probably never had to get vaccinated. As of 1904, neither the Boston Board of Health nor the Cambridge health department reported any cases of smallpox, and thus the vaccination order would have expired.[144] State records of pending criminal cases report the same three vaccination cases in Middlesex County (in which Cambridge is located) for several years beginning after 1 October 1903 and not disposed before 31 December 1906.[145] The Massachusetts Anti-compulsory Vaccination Society had pledged to pay for Jacobson's defense, but might have needed more time to settle the court costs as well as the fine after the 1905 United States Supreme Court decision. The fact that three cases continue as pending indicates that those of Albert Pear and Frank Cone were linked to the ultimate disposition of Jacobson's case. I assume that they or the Society ultimately paid their fines and costs sometime in 1907 because the cases disappear from the state records that year. I have found no source that discusses the ultimate disposition of these cases.

Henning Jacobson continued to minister to his congregation in Cambridge until his death in 1930. He built a beautiful little church in 1909 that still stands on the corner of Prospect and Broadway in Cambridge. By the 1920s he had cleared all the debts on his church and was well loved by his congregation, one

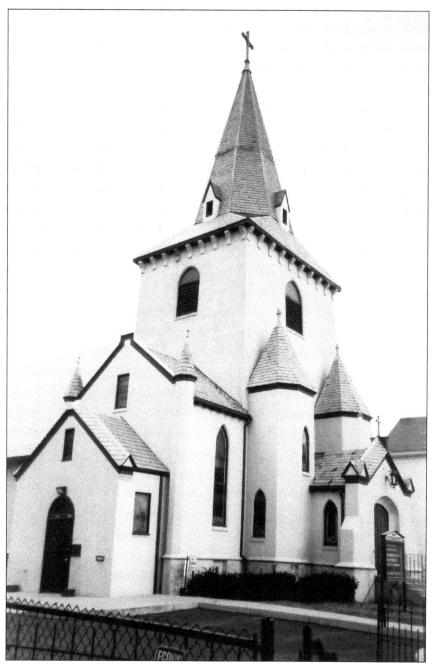

Figure 9.3. Henning Jacobson's church, Augustana Lutheran Church, Cambridge, Massachusetts. Photograph by Karen Walloch.

of whom noted in 1931: "We all know it was not so easy for him to stand up in front of the same faces Sunday after Sunday, year in and year out and preach."[146] For Henning Jacobson, participation in a landmark case of American constitutional law meant little compared to his achievement in building from scratch "a strong congregation" in the face of his congregants' initial spiritual apathy and "a new, fully modern church" in spite of great financial difficulties.[147]

Conclusion

The *Jacobson* decision did not resolve the controversy over vaccination. Lurking in its background is the fact that vaccination had been practiced for over a century, yet smallpox continued to plague American communities because people did not routinely get it done. Although medical societies and health authorities enthusiastically endorsed vaccination, the general population did not seem to regard it with much favor, and information available for Boston and other Massachusetts communities indicates that people seemed to avoid it until compelled or coerced into it by the law or their employers. Parents waited until their children reached school age, and they did not apparently revaccinate at adolescence. The *Jacobson* decision alone did little to change that pattern. In 1909 the *Boston Medical and Surgical Journal* still had to urge people and medical practitioners to vaccinate and revaccinate when the tetanus death of a local child after vaccination reinvigorated public anxiety about school vaccinations.[1]

From its inception, vaccination was never as simple, foolproof, or benign as its proponents claimed. Lauded as a substantial improvement over variolation, which had perpetuated smallpox epidemics throughout the eighteenth century, vaccination was not without its own risks and problems. Smallpox among the vaccinated soon proved early claims of lifelong immunity wrong. Yet people generally did not get vaccinated more than once because they worried that it might induce dangerous diseases or blood poisoning. Even normal vaccination might produce severe discomfort and temporary disability that made it difficult for adults to work. Vaccination also changed a lot over the course of its first one hundred years, as physicians tinkered with various sources for vaccine lymph and tried out all sorts of techniques and instruments.

To make matters worse, every innovation intended to resolve one problem just resulted in other complications. First physicians only reluctantly recognized that arm-to-arm vaccinations could transmit syphilis. Bovine lymph supposedly resolved this issue only to bring new organisms into play. Instead of syphilis, now blood poisoning and infections began to plague a significant number of vaccinations by the 1880s. The addition of the mild antiseptic glycerine supposedly resolved these problems, but lack of effective control over production, storage, and marketing of lymph led to widespread failure and complications from contaminated or outdated batches in 1901 and 1902. Popular outrage at tetanus deaths after vaccination impelled Congress to pass the Biologics Control Act in

1902 to provide for federal licensing and inspection of vaccine establishments that sold their products in interstate commerce.

By the end of the nineteenth century, vaccination had so many problems that it is no wonder that an antivaccination movement welled up in towns and cities across America. Reasonable, literate people like Henning Jacobson, Albert Pear, and John Mugford found very good reasons to oppose vaccination. It is simplistic and inaccurate to describe them or other antivaccinationists as irrational antigovernment cranks. That is rhetoric their opponents used to demean them, and it is a mistake to accept such sentiments at face value. We have an obligation to explore the context of antivaccinatists' arguments and thinking in order to understand why reasonable people would object to a medical innovation that had initially promised so much.

The *Jacobson* decision may have resolved the issue of the constitutionality of compulsory vaccination laws, but it did not stop opposition to vaccination. Undaunted by the adverse ruling, the antivaccination editor Lora Little proclaimed that "the people [are] the only court worth bothering with in matters of this kind," and thus antivaccinationists should work harder to educate the public about vaccination: "Very well; let us . . . go back to the local authority, the State. When we get there, if we find the Legislature sufficiently enlightened, the wrong will be righted."[2] Sara Newcomb Merrick condemned the Supreme Court for "narrowness" in accepting without question so-called commonly held beliefs about vaccination's efficacy. She pointed out that once people had regarded "hanging witches as right and proper, burning at the stake was right also," and Southern states accepted lynchings of African Americans "for a certain crime [as] the best means of protecting the community and stamping out the criminals." Merrick also thought little of Harlan's deference to state legislatures as the representatives of popular opinion: "The Justices presume that the Legislature expressed the 'will of the people' in the passage of its laws. Alas, what a sarcasm! Where have these Justices spent their lives?"[3] With machine politics, cronyism, and lobbyists running rampant in American politics, Merrick was not at all wrong to characterize the Massachusetts legislature as an imperfect instrument to express the public will. In any case, how could any law truly represent the general public when only half the adult population could vote? Observers commented on the overwhelming presence of women at the 1902 legislative hearings on vaccination. If women had had the vote, would the Joint Committee on Public Health have gotten away with killing each and every abolition bill that came its way?

Despite editorials claiming that *Jacobson* "finally and for all time stilled the voices . . . of enemies of the theory of vaccination," antivaccinationists simply continued to work (as they had done for years) against compulsion in their state legislatures.[4] Even as the *New York Times* declared that the ruling "should end the useful life of the societies of cranks formed to resist the operation of laws relative to vaccination," new antivaccinationist societies organized in many states to successfully oppose or amend compulsory laws.[5] Just three years later, for instance, the prominent entrepreneurs John Pitcairn and Charles M. Higgins founded the Anti-vaccination League of America. Although the organization did not achieve a truly national presence, Pitcairn, a wealthy oil, steel, and railroad magnate in Pennsylvania, managed to convince the governor to establish an official commission to study vaccination. Higgins, a Brooklyn ink manufacturer, wrote many pamphlets against vaccination throughout the 1910s and 1920s. Pitcairn's sons later supported the Citizens Medical Reference Bureau (founded in 1919), which worked out of New York City to oppose vaccination laws as well as other manifestations of "state medicine" into the 1940s.[6] Although Lora Little gave up *The Liberator* when she moved to Portland, Oregon, she continued to work to oppose vaccination laws there.[7] James Loyster, an attorney and Republican Party activist in New York State, undertook a "personal crusade" to amend its vaccination law after the death of his son after vaccination in 1914.[8]

Jacobson ultimately made little difference to antivaccinationists—they even seemed to redouble their efforts in the ensuing years. They did not succeed in repealing compulsory vaccination in Massachusetts, but they did succeed in persuading state legislators to tread warily around the subject. In 1907, antivaccinationists disrupted committee hearings on a bill to tighten requirements for exemption from the school vaccination requirement by declaring the proposed legislation "un-American and Russian."[9] The bill sought to restrict the examination for exemption to health department school physicians rather than "regular practicing physicians." Cowed, the public health committee eviscerated the bill's language to retain the status quo, much to the dismay of the *Boston Medical and Surgical Journal*, which declared the bill's "intent is practically lost."[10] Antivaccinationists also threatened legal action when a Rockland schoolteacher sent home children holding exemption certificates "from a certain physician in Boston who takes the ground that no child is a fit subject for vaccination."[11] In 1908 Representative Walter E. Nichols of Boston presented a bill based on a petition of Aurin F. Hill to prohibit compulsory vaccination, but it was defeated overwhelmingly in the state Senate.[12] Bills to prohibit compulsory vaccination and even vaccination altogether appeared in 1909 as well.[13]

The Massachusetts state legislature went back and forth on the issue of compulsory vaccination for years. In 1914 it nearly amended the compulsory vaccination law to allow unvaccinated schoolchildren admission to public schools if their parents opposed vaccination. Bedford's representative was none other than Immanuel Pfeiffer, Jr., son and namesake of the notorious antivaccinationist physician, and he argued passionately for the bill in a long floor debate. Although it passed the Senate, the House rejected the "antivaccination" bill by a vote of 133 to 53.[14] A similar 1916 bill passed in the House by a roll call vote of 127 to 105, although it did not pass in the Senate.[15] In 1917, antivaccinationists tried again, and one town meeting on the measure showed citizens still divided down the middle on compulsory vaccination when they voted "slightly in favor" of abolition.[16] Although the bill did not pass, one year later the state legislature showed its discomfort at increasing vaccination requirements by rejecting another private school vaccination bill.[17] Yet, in 1918, the legislature also limited the exemption to the period during which the examining physician believed vaccination would be dangerous for a child's health.[18] In 1919, although it overwhelmingly refused to consider repeal of the compulsory vaccination law, the state senators again voted against private school vaccination by twenty-six to eleven.[19] And in 1920, the Massachusetts Attorney General issued an opinion that state institutions could vaccinate inmates or patients "against their will"—making explicit a quiet practice of forcible vaccination that formed part of the backdrop for *Jacobson.*[20] Daily involuntary vaccination at the Suffolk County Jail for incoming prisoners, for instance, apparently continued until the attending physician decided it was no longer necessary in July 1903.[21]

The legislature continued to display ambivalence about compulsion in the 1920s. In 1921, the Senate voted sixteen to six to substitute a bill to allow parents to refuse vaccination for their school-age children against an adverse public health committee report, thus allowing the bill the chance of a floor debate and vote, although it did not pass.[22] In 1922, the Massachusetts House of Representatives summarily rejected another bill seeking to impose compulsory vaccination on private school pupils.[23] It was not until 1930 that the state legislature finally passed a bill requiring vaccination in the private schools.[24] Antivaccinationists may not have succeeded in abolishing compulsion, but their continued opposition certainly impeded legislation seeking to tighten the law.

Some leading public health officers shied away from compulsion, preferring persuasion and education. In 1907, Charles V. Chapin, head of the Providence health department in Rhode Island, argued that "men also feel that they should do as they like with their bodies," and noted "it is frequently unwise to attempt such compulsion." He concluded that "the less we appeal to the law the better."[25] The New York state health commissioner Herman Biggs testified in 1915: "I would rather have the sentiment of the community strongly supporting the health authorities without legislation than compulsory legislation and an antagonistic public sentiment."[26] In their view, *Jacobson* may have marked out the potential legal authority health officers might exercise but that decision would not change their day-to-day practice of public health in vaccination. Yet even though these public health leaders counseled restraint and cooperation, unfortunately, other health officials were at times less scrupulous. Boys living at the Newsboys Home, for instance, got "an unexpected Christmas treat" at 2 am, 24 December 1907, when New York City health officers, assisted by a policeman to prevent any escapes, awakened the 225 children with vaccinations whether they wanted them or not.[27]

The *Jacobson* decision emerged out a context of widespread controversy over vaccination—Henning Jacobson did not object to vaccination to make an abstract point about civil liberty. Many people commonly shared his anxieties in the early twentieth century, and for good reasons. Vaccination was a "trying ordeal" that meant lost wages, inconvenience, ugly scars, and discomfort even when it developed along normal lines. And when vaccination went awry, it could result in tragic life-altering events. Occasional death or long-term disability after vaccination may have affected only a few people, but that was enough to create general apprehension about such possibilities, leading many to regard vaccination at best as a necessary evil. They accepted vaccination not because they appreciated its protective benefits but because they *had* to do it to keep their jobs, stay out jail, or avoid paying fines. Coercion, not persuasion, was the mainstay of vaccination campaigns in the first quarter of the twentieth century. And health authorities did not hesitate when it came to forcibly vaccinating the destitute homeless or inmates of asylums, poorhouses, orphanages, jails, and prisons.

The *Jacobson* decision looked back to the ideal of a well-regulated society that emphasized the duties of citizens rather than their rights. Although it also contained language to support the creation of a constitutional right to reproductive privacy, contemporaries glossed over this fact to focus on the potential *Jacobson* presented for justifying eugenics laws. By 1912, at least one legal scholar, noting the passage of laws permitting the sterilization of inmates of insane asylums and state prisons in Indiana (1907), Connecticut (1909), California (1909), and Iowa (1909), argued that police power "certainly enables the state to take some measures to protect itself against the birth of undesirable citizens." Citing *Jacobson*, he asserted that "the operation of vasectomy, at least, is hardly more serious than vaccination," and declared such "statutes are constitutional."[28] Harlan's colleague on the Supreme Court, Oliver Wendell Holmes, Jr., agreed, citing *Jacobson* as the sole precedent for upholding the constitutionality of such legislation in his 1927 *Buck v. Bell* opinion: "The principle that sustains compulsory vaccination is broad enough to cover cutting the Fallopian tubes."[29] American society had to undergo substantial change before the Supreme Court was willing in 1965 to consider the language in Harlan's opinion that supported the right to privacy in *Griswold v. Connecticut*.[30]

Although *Jacobson* provided the constitutional foundation for eugenics laws, only a few states managed to strengthen or pass more compulsory vaccination laws.[31] A 1927 United States Public Health Service study found that only thirteen states had laws authorizing compulsory vaccination, and four actually had laws prohibiting it.[32] Just eleven states had laws or regulations requiring vaccination for admission to public schools.[33] These numbers had barely budged since 1904, when only eleven states had laws authorizing general compulsory vaccination and only thirteen states excluded unvaccinated children from school.[34] Despite support from the United States Supreme Court and the medical establishment, compulsory vaccination remained a contentious issue. One of the legacies of the early twentieth-century antivaccination movement is that although every state eventually established some sort of mandatory immunization law, these laws also provide many avenues to legally opt out of the requirement.[35] Diseases like measles, mumps, and pertussis once thought to be vanquished now pop up with disturbing frequency because some parents refuse to immunize their children, fearing various side effects, just as their predecessors did in 1902. Antivaccinationists may have lost the court battle, but they won the legislative war. The *principle* of compulsion may remain firmly lodged in constitutional law, but no one dares to truly implement it, making the *practice* of compulsion for all intents and purposes void. The failure of the 2003 Bush Administration smallpox vaccination program is a case in point. One legal expert termed it "a public-policy and public-relations disaster" because "the Administration failed to persuade physicians and nurses that the known risks of serious side effects with the vaccine were justified."[36]

Physicians today who want to convince parents to immunize their children should take note of this history. They should treat parents' concerns with real respect, understanding that medical authorities in the past have made overconfident assessments about the safety and efficacy of various vaccines. The history of the antivaccination movement in the early twentieth century shows that labeling people who object to immunizations as stupid, ignorant, or crazy was, and is, a terrible mistake. The public health establishment must honestly address anxiety about vaccine deficiencies and problems rather than demean those who raise objections to immunizations.

Appendix A

Boston Health Department Vaccinations, 1872–1900

Year	Vaccinations	Smallpox cases	Population	Percentage vaccinated
1872–73	17,378	3,367	265,782	6.53
1873–74	485	32	331,395	0.15
1874–75	673	5	341,919	0.20
1875–76	931	3	346,004	0.27
1876–77	1,287	6	350,138	0.37
1877–78	2,078	9	354,322	0.59
1878–79	1,984	0	358,554	0.55
1879–80	2,497	1	362,839	0.69
1880–81	2,841	3	368,190	0.77
1881–82	37,341	65	373,620	10.00
1882–83	1,412	5	379,129	0.37
1883–84	1,577	5	384,720	0.41
1885	6,904	6	390,393	1.77
1886	1,781	1	401,374	0.44
1887	2,044	4	412,663	0.50
1888	3,677	8	424,274	0.87
1889	3,087	10	436,208	0.71
1890	3,323	1	448,477	0.74
1891	4,332	0	457,772	0.95

(continued)

Year	Vaccinations	Smallpox cases	Population	Percentage vaccinated
1892	3,909	0	467,260	0.84
1893	4,332	26	476,945	0.91
1894	129,674	77	486,830	26.64
1895	2,581	0	501,083	0.52
1896	?	0	516,305	
1897	?	10	528,912	
1898	3,282	0	541,827	0.61
1899	?	29	555,057	
1900	?	7	560,892	

Notes: Unless otherwise specified, the vaccination numbers are from the City Physician's Report, in Boston Board of Health Annual Reports. Until 1885, the reporting period was from 1 May to 30 April. I calculated the percentages rounded off to the nearest hundredth. Population figures come from Table XIII, "Population, Deaths, and Death-Rates, per 10,000 Inhabitants, from Nine Infectious Diseases (Consumption Included), in One-Year and Five-Year Groups," in Boston Board of Health, *Thirty-First Annual Report of the Health Department of the City of Boston for the Year 1902* (Boston, 1903), fold-out insert.

1872–73 vaccinations are derived by adding the vaccinations of the medical inspectors (14,977) to the vaccinations reported by the city physician (2,401). They probably vaccinated even more people earlier in 1872, but these are the numbers given in the *First Annual Report.*

Vaccination numbers for 1881–82 are from the city physician and temporary stations combined.

The reporting period changed in 1885 from the fiscal year (1 May to 30 April) to the calendar year (1 January to 31 December) of each year, but the 1885 report covered 1 May 1884 through 31 December 1885.

For 1894, 127,303 vaccinated at special stations from 15 December 1893 to "the spring of 1894," 2,371 at the city physician's office. See Boston Board of Health, *Annual Report of the Health Department for the Year 1894,* 51–52.

Question marks indicate that I have no information in my copies of the Boston Board of Health *Reports* for these years on city vaccinations.

Appendix B

Voting Records for Samuel Durgin's Vaccination Bill before the Massachusetts State Senate

Senators Who Voted for Medical Exemption for Adults on the First Vote

Senator	District	Townships or wards represented
1. Harry C. Foster (R)	3rd Essex	Essex, Gloucester, Hamilton, Ipswich, Manchester, Newbury, Newburyport, Rockport, Rowley, Wenham
2. Archie N. Frost (R)	5th Essex	Andover, Boxford, Lawrence, Methuen, North Andover, Topsfield
3. Alva S. Wood (R)	Middlesex and Essex	Lynn Ward 6, Lynnfield, Middleton, North Reading, Peabody, Saugus, Stoneham, Wakefield, Woburn
4. Albert S. Aspey (R)	2nd Middlesex	Cambridge Wards 1, 2, 4, 5
5. Chester B. Williams (R)	5th Middlesex	Lexington, Lincoln, Marlborough, Medford, Sudbury, Waltham, Wayland, Winchester
6. John T. Sparks (D)	7th Middlesex	Chelmsford, Dracut, Lowell Wards 1–8
7. Willard Howland (R)	1st Suffolk	Boston Ward 1 (East Boston), Chelsea, Revere, Winthrop
8. John A. Sullivan (D)	5th Suffolk	Boston Wards 10, 12 (both South End), 18 (Roxbury)
9. John K. Berry (R)	7th Suffolk	Boston Wards 16, 20, 24 (all Dorchester)
10. Perlie A. Dyar (R)	9th Suffolk	Boston Wards 11 (Back Bay), 19 (West Roxbury), 25 (Roxbury Heights)

(continued)

Senator	District	Townships or wards represented
11. Elisha T. Harvell (R)	1st Plymouth	Abington, Carver, Cohasset, Duxbury, E. Bridgewater, Halifax, Hanover, Hanson, Hingham, Hull, Kingston, Marshfield, Norwell, Pembroke, Plymouth, Plympton, Rockland, Scituate, Whitman
12. David G. Pratt (R)	2nd Plymouth	Bridgewater, Brockton, Lakeville, Marion, Mattapoisett, Middleborough, Rochester, Wareham, W. Bridgewater
13. William A. Nye (RI)	Cape	[Barnstable, Dukes, and Nantucket Counties]: Provincetown, Truro, Wellfleet, Eastham, Orleans, Brewster, Harwich, Chatham, Dennis, Yarmouth, Barnstable, Sandwich, Bourne, Falmouth, Gosnolde, Aquinah, Chilmark, West Tisbury, Tisbury, Edgetown, Oak Bluffs, Nantucket
14. Frank A. Fales (R)	2nd Norfolk	Avon, Bellingham, Brookline, Dedham, Dover, Foxborough, Franklin, Medfield, Medway, Millis, Needham, Norfolk, Norwood, Sharon, Stoughton, Walpole, Wellesley, Westwood, Wrentham
15. Edward C. Holt (R)	1st Bristol	Attleborough, Berkeley, Easton, Mansfield, North Attleborough, Norton, Raynham, Rehoboth, Seekonk, Taunton
16. Andrew H. Morrison (R)	2nd Bristol	Dighton, Fall River, Somerset, Swansea
17. Merrick A. Morse (R)	Franklin/ Hampshire	Amherst, Ashfield, Belchertown, Bernardston, Buckland, Charlemont, Colrain, Conway, Deerfield, Enfield, Erving, Gill, Granby, Greenfield, Greenwich, Hawley, Heath, New Salem, Northfield, Orange, Pelham, Prescott, Rowe, Shelburne, Shutesbury, Sunderland, Ware, Warwick, Wendell, Whately

Senators Who Voted against Adult Exemption on the First Vote

Senator	District	Townships or wards represented
1. Henry S. Fitzgerald (D)	3rd Suffolk	Boston Wards 2, 6, 8
2. William T. Fitzgerald (D)	4th Suffolk	Boston Wards 7, 9, 17
3. Michael J. Sullivan (D)	6th Suffolk	Boston Wards 13, 14, 15
4. Edward Seaver (D)	8th Suffolk	Boston Wards 21, 22, 23
5. Thomas F. Porter (R)	1st Essex	Lynn Wards 1, 2, 3, 4, 5, 7, Nahunt, Swapscott
6. J. Frank Porter (R)	2nd Essex	Beverly, Danvers, Marblehead, Salem
7. Carleton F. How (R)	4th Essex	Amesbury, Georgetown, Groveland, Haverhill, Merrimac, Salisbury, West Newbury
8. Henry R. Skinner (R)	1st Middlesex	Ashland, Framingham, Holliston, Hopkinton, Natick, Newton, Sherbon, Watertown, Weston
9. Leonard B. Chandler (R)	3rd Middlesex	Arlington, Belmont, Somerville
10. George R. Jones (R)	4th Middlesex	Everett, Malden, Melrose
11. Henry C. Bliss (R)	2nd Hampden	Agawam, Chicopee, E. Longmeadow, Granville, Hampden, Holyoke, Longmeadow, Ludlow, Montgomery, Southwick, Tolland, West Springfield, Westfield
12. David Manning	1st Worcester	Worcester Wards 4, 5, 6, 7, 8
13. John P. Munroe (R)	2nd Worcester	Berlin, Bolton, Boylston, Clinton, Harvard, Lancaster, Sterling, West Boylston, Worcester Wards 1, 2, 3
14. Edward F. Blodgett (R)	3rd Worcester	Ashburnham, Athol, Fitchburg, Gardner, Leominster, Lunenburg, Royalston, Westminster, Winchendon
15. George K. Tufts (R)	4th Worcester	Barre, Brookfield, Charlton, Dana, Dudley, Hardwick, Hubbardston, Leicester, New Braintree, North Brookfield, Oakham, Paxton, Petersham, Phillipston, Princeton, Rutland, Southbridge, Spencer, Sturbridge, Templeton, Warren, Webster, West Brookfield

Abstaining Senators on the First Vote

Senator	District	Townships or wards represented
1. Eugene H. Sprague (R)	1st Norfolk	Braintree, Canton, Holbrook, Hyde Park, Milton, Quincy, Randolph, Weymouth
2. John F. Marsh (R)	1st Hampden	Brimfield, Holland, Monson, Palmer, Springfield, Wales, Wilbraham
3. Charles S. Sullivan (D)	2nd Suffolk	Boston Wards 3, 4, 5; Cambridge Ward 3
4. Henry E. Gaylord (R)	Berkshire/ Hampshire	Alford, Becket, Blandford, Chester, Chesterfield, Cummington, Easthampton, Egremeont, Goshen, Great Barrington, Hadley, Hatfield, Huntington, Lee, Lenox, Middlefield, Monterey, Mount Washington, New Marlborough, Northhampton, Otis, Plainfield, Richmond, Russell, Sandisfield, Sheffield, South Hadley, Southhampton, Stockbridge, Tyringham, Washington, West Stockbridge, Westhampton, Williamsburg, Worthington
5. George Z. Dean (R)	Berkshire	Adams, Cheshire, Clarksburg, Dalton, Florida, Hancock, Hinsdale, Lanesborough, New Ashford, North Adams, Peru, Pittsfield, Savoy, Williamstown, Windsor
6. Cornelius R. Day (R)	5th Worcester	Auburn, Blackstone, Douglas, Grafton, Hopedale, Menden, Milford, Millbury, Northborough, Northbridge, Oxford, Shrewsbury, Southborough, Sutton, Upton, Uxbridge, Westborough
7. Herbert E. Fletcher (R)	6th Middlesex	Acton, Ashby, Ayer, Bedford, Billerica, Boxborough, Burlington, Carlisle, Concord, Dunstable, Groton, Hudson, Littleton, Lowell Wards 5 and 9, Maynard, Peperell, Reading, Shirley, Stow, Tewksbury, Townsen, Tyngsborough, Westford, Wilmington
8. Rufus Soule (R): President of the Senate and does not vote	3rd Bristol	Achshnet, Dartmouth, Fairhaven, Freetown, New Bedford, Westport

Vote Arranged by District

Senator	District	Vote 1 (for exemption)	Vote 2 (cancels exemption)
Thomas Porter	1st Essex	No	Yes
J. Frank Porter	2nd Essex	No	Yes
Harry C. Foster	3rd Essex	Yes	Yes*
Carleton F. How	4th Essex	No	No*
Archie N. Frost	5th Essex	Yes	No
Alva S. Wood	Middlesex and Essex	Yes	No
Henry R. Skinner	1st Middlesex	No	Yes
Albert S. Aspey	2nd Middlesex	Yes	No
Leonard B. Chandler	3rd Middlesex	No	Yes
George R. Jones	4th Middlesex	No	Yes
Chester B. Williams	5th Middlesex	Yes	No
Herbert E. Fletcher	6th Middlesex	Abstain	Yes
John T. Sparks	7th Middlesex	Yes	No
Willard Howland	1st Suffolk	Yes	No
Charles S. Sullivan	2nd Suffolk	Abstain	Abstain
Henry S. Fitzgerald	3rd Suffolk	No	Yes
William T. Fitzgerald	4th Suffolk	No	Yes
John A. Sullivan	5th Suffolk	Yes	No
Michael J. Sullivan	6th Suffolk	No	Yes
John K. Berry	7th Suffolk	Yes	No
Edward Seaver	8th Suffolk	No	Yes
Perlie A. Dyar	9th Suffolk	Yes	No
Elisha T. Harvell	1st Plymouth	Yes	No
David G. Pratt	2nd Plymouth	Yes	No
William A. Nye	Cape	Yes	No
Edward C. Holt	1st Bristol	Yes	No
Andrew H. Morrison	2nd Bristol	Yes	Abstain
Rufus Soule	3rd Bristol	Doesn't vote	Doesn't vote
Eugene H. Sprague	1st Norfolk	Abstain	Abstain
Frank Fales	2nd Norfolk	Yes	Abstain
David Manning	1st Worcester	No	Yes
John P. Munroe	2nd Worcester	No	Yes

(continued)

Senator	District	Vote 1 (for exemption)	Vote 2 (cancels exemption)
Edward F. Blodgett	3rd Worcester	No	Yes
George K. Tufts	4th Worcester	No	Abstain
Cornelius R. Day	5th Worcester	Abstain	Abstain
John F. Marsh	1st Hampden	Yes	Abstain
Henry C. Bliss	2nd Hampden	No	Yes
Henry E. Gaylord	Berkshire/ Hampden	Abstain	Yes
George Z. Dean	Berkshire	Abstain	Yes
Merrick A. Morse	Franklin/ Hampshire	Yes	Abstain

* How and Foster pair their votes to cancel each other out on the second vote.

Note: Vote 1: 18 senators vote for Williams's amendment and 15 against it, with 6 abstentions. Vote 2: 14 vote against Porter's cancellation amendment and 17 vote for it, with 8 abstentions. No one changes his position, except Foster and How, who deliberately switch positions to pair their votes, thus neutralizing them. Perlie Dyar of Boston sticks with Williams. Four senators (Marsh, Morrison, Morse, Fales) who first voted with Williams now abstain. Three senators who had abstained from Williams's amendment vote now vote for Porter's cancellation amendment. One senator (Tufts) who had voted against Williams on the first vote, abstains on second vote. From Public Document no. 43, "Number of Assessed Polls, Registered Voters and Persons Who Voted in Each Voting Precinct," *Public Documents of Massachusetts*, vol. 2 (Boston, 1902).

Notes

Introduction

1. James Tobey, *Public Health Law*, 2nd ed. (New York: The Commonwealth Fund, 1939), 89–97. First published as *Public Health Law: A Manual of Law for Sanitarians* (Baltimore, MD: The Williams & Wilkins Company, 1926).

2. Quotation from Kenneth R. Wing, *The Law and the Public's Health*, 4th ed. (Ann Arbor, MI: Health Administration Press, 1995), 24–25. For other important discussions see Wendy E. Parmet, "From Slaughter-House to Lochner: The Rise and Fall of the Constitutionalization of Public Health," *American Journal of Legal History* 40 (1996): 476–505; Parmet, *Populations, Public Health, and the Law* (Washington, DC: Georgetown University Press, 2009), 37–45; Lawrence O. Gostin, *Public Health Law: Power, Duty, Restraint* (New York: The Milbank Memorial Fund, 2000), 61–69; Alan Hyde, *Bodies of Law* (Princeton, NJ: Princeton University Press, 1997), 241–51; Steven M. Fleisher, "The Law of Basic Health Activities: Police Power and Constitutional Limitations," in *Legal Aspects of Health Policy: Issues and Trends*, ed. Ruth Roemer and George McKray (Westport, CT: Greenwood Press, 1980), 3–32; and Lynne Curry, ed., *The Human Body on Trial: A Sourcebook with Cases, Laws, and Documents* (Indianapolis, IN: Hackett, 2002), 51–54 (discussion), 99–112 (documents and opinion).

3. Charles Creighton, "Vaccination," *Encyclopedia Britannica* (Edinburgh: Adam and Charles Buck, 1888): 24:23–30. Creighton was considered one of the foremost English pathologists and medical scholars. He wrote a book critical of Jenner and vaccination, *The Natural History of Cow-Pox and Vaccinal Syphilis* (1887). He also authored the highly respected two-volume *A History of Epidemics in Britain* (Cambridge: Cambridge University Press, 1894). He lost his scientific reputation and career over his opposition to vaccination as well as his criticism of Robert Koch. See E. Ashworth Underwood, "Charles Creighton, the Man and His Work," in Charles Creighton, *A History of Epidemics in Britain*, 2nd ed., with additional material by D. E. C. Eversley, E. Ashworth Underwood, and Linda Ovenall (London: Frank Cass & Co., 1965), 1:43–135.

4. Charles Creighton, "Vaccination: A Scientific Inquiry," *The Arena* 10 (September 1890): 422–40.

5. Alfred Russel Wallace, "Vaccination a Delusion—Its Penal Enforcement a Crime," in Wallace, *The Wonderful Century: Its Successes and Failures* (New York: Dodd, Mead, 1898), 213–315.

6. Herbert Spencer, "Vaccination," in *Facts and Comments* (New York: D. Appleton and Company, 1902), 270–73.

7. See, for instance, John Duffy, *The Sanitarians: A History of American Public Health* (Urbana: University of Illinois Press, 1990), 200; John Duffy, *A History of Public Health*

in New York City, 1866–1966 (New York: Russell Sage Foundation, 1974), 148–54; Donald R. Hopkins, *The Greatest Killer: Smallpox*, reprint of *Princes and Peasants: Smallpox in History* (Chicago: The University of Chicago Press, 1983), with a new introduction by the author (Chicago: University of Chicago Press, 2002), 289–93; James Cassedy, *Charles V. Chapin and the Public Health Movement* (Cambridge, MA: Harvard University Press, 1962), 63; James Cassedy, *Medicine in America: A Short History* (Baltimore, MD: The Johns Hopkins University Press, 1991), 98; and Judith Leavitt, "'Be Safe, Be Sure.': New York City's Experience with Epidemic Smallpox," in *Hives of Sickness*, ed. David Rosner (New Brunswick, NJ: Rutgers University Press, 1995), 104–6. Other older accounts touch on the influence of antivaccination: Dorothy Scanlon, "The Public Health Movement in Boston, 1870–1910," PhD diss., Boston University, 1956, 143; and Wilson G. Smillie, *Public Health: Its Promise for the Future; A Chronicle of the Development of Public Health in the United States, 1607–1914* (New York: The Macmillan Company, 1955), 432. For a popular history that mentions antivaccinatism, see Alan Chase, *Magic Shots: A Human and Scientific Account of the Long and Continuing Struggle to Eradicate Infectious Disease* (New York: William Morrow and Company, 1982), 72–73.

Two important studies of public health in Massachusetts ignored antivaccination. George Whipple's early history of the Massachusetts State Board of Health does not mention either antivaccination or *Jacobson*. George Chandler Whipple, *State Sanitation: A Review of the Work of the Massachusetts State Board of Health*, 2 vols. (Cambridge, MA: Harvard University Press, 1917). Although Barbara Rosenkrantz maintains that the failure to contain the smallpox epidemic of 1901–2 convinced health officials that "protection could only be guaranteed if the state supervised the preparation of vaccine lymph and if qualified physicians performed the vaccination," she does not mention *Jacobson* or the role antivaccinationists played to impel officials to seek control. See Rosenkrantz, *Public Health and the State: Changing Views in Massachusetts, 1842–1936* (Cambridge, MA: Harvard University Press, 1972), 124.

8. Martin Kaufman, "The American Anti-Vaccinationists and Their Arguments," *Bulletin of the History of Medicine* 41 (1967): 463–78.

9. Nadav Davidovitch, "Negotiating Dissent: Homeopathy and Anti-Vaccinationism at the Turn of the Twentieth Century," in *The Politics of Healing: Histories of Alternative Medicine in Twentieth-Century North America*, ed. Robert D. Johnston (London: Routledge, 2004), 11–28. Eberhard Wolff, "Sectarian Identity and the Aim of Integration: Attitudes of American Homeopaths Toward Smallpox Vaccination in the Late Nineteenth Century," in *Culture, Knowledge and Healing: Historical Perspectives of Homeopathic Medicine in Europe and North America*, ed. Robert Jütte, Guenter B. Risse, and John Woodward (Sheffield, England: European Association for the History of Medicine and Health Publications, 1998), 217–50.

10. Judith Leavitt, *The Healthiest City: Milwaukee and the Politics of Health Reform* (Madison: University of Wisconsin Press, 1982), 76–121.

11. Robert D. Johnston, *The Radical Middle Class: Populist Democracy and the Question of Capitalism in Progressive-Era Portland, Oregon* (Princeton, NJ: Princeton University Press, 2003), 177–220, quotation on 178.

12. James Colgrove, "'Science in a Democracy': The Contested Status of Vaccination in the Progressive Era and the 1920s," *Isis* 96 (2005): 182. See also Colgrove, "Between Persuasion and Compulsion: Smallpox Control in Brooklyn

and New York, 1894–1902," *Bulletin of the History of Medicine* 78 (2004): 349–78; and Colgrove, *State of Immunity: The Politics of Vaccination in Twentieth-Century America* (Berkeley: University of California Press, 2006).

13. Arthur Allen, *Vaccine: The Controversial Story of Medicine's Greatest Lifesaver* (New York: W. W. Norton, 2007), 104.

14. Michael Willrich's wonderful history shares some of the historical terrain that I explore here, but strives more to develop a broad narrative of antivaccination activity generally. He discusses the events that led up to *Jacobson*, but does not thoroughly investigate the organization and work of the Massachusetts Anti-compulsory Vaccination Society. See Willrich, *Pox: An American History* (New York: Penguin Press, 2011), 246–336, quotation on 270.

15. Arthur Allen's *Vaccine* mistakenly assumes that antivaccination organizations striving to represent the movement on a national level actually did so. For British antivaccination leagues the most insightful analysis is Nadja Durbach, "'They Might as Well Brand Us': Working-Class Resistance to Compulsory Vaccination in Victorian England," *Social History of Medicine* 13 (2000): 45–62; Durbach, "Class, Gender, and the Conscientious Objector to Vaccination, 1898–1907," *Journal of British Studies* 41 (2002): 58–83; and Durbach, *Bodily Matters: The Anti-Vaccination Movement in England, 1853–1907* (Durham, NC: Duke University Press, 2005). For other important assessments, see Dorothy Porter and Roy Porter, "The Politics of Prevention: Anti-Vaccinationism and Public Health in Nineteenth-Century England," *Medical History* 32 (1988): 231–52; and R. M. MacLeod, "Law, Medicine and Public Opinion: The Resistance to Compulsory Health Legislation, 1870–1907," parts 1 and 2, *Public Law: The Constitutional and Administrative Law of the Commonwealth* (Spring 1967): 107–28, and (Summer 1967): 189–211. See also C. W. Dixon, *Smallpox* (London: J. & A. Churchill, 1962), 282–95, for an early account of English antivaccinationists.

16. See "American Anti-Vaccination League," quoted from the *New York Daily Sun*, 4 October 1879, in *The Vaccination Inquirer and Health Review* 1 (1879–80): 119. See also William Tebb, "Anti-Vaccination in the United States and Canada," *The Vaccination Inquirer* 1 (April 1879–March 1880): 154–57.

17. "How Anti-Vaccinists Are Made," *The Vaccination Inquirer* 24 (April 1902–March 1903): 249.

18. See *Blue v. Beach*, 155 Ind. 121, 56 N.E. 89 (1900). Blue also founded a journal, *Vaccination*.

19. Colgrove also discusses the foundation and work of the Anti-vaccination League of America in *State of Immunity*, 52–53.

20. See Johnston, *Radical Middle Class*, for an extensive account of Little's life and work.

21. Colgrove, *State of Immunity*, 56.

22. Kaufman, "American Antivaccinationists," 466, citing S. R. H. Giles, *Compulsory Vaccination* (Hyde Park, MA: n.p., 1883). The Giles work is a four-page pamphlet held by Countway Library, Harvard University, and it notes publication information simply as Dedham, 1883, with no printer mentioned. S. R. H. Giles was married to Alfred E. Giles, a retired attorney living in Hyde Park, who published *The Iniquity of Compulsory Vaccination* in 1882. She usually used the title "Mrs." before her name and wrote a number of works of poetry. For more information about the couple, see

Andrew Jackson Davis, *Beyond the Valley: A Sequel to the Magic Staff, an Autobiography of Andrew Jackson Davis* (Boston: Colby & Rich, 1885): 246–52.

23. "Anti-Vaccination in the United States," *The Vaccination Inquirer* 24 (1902–3): 218.

24. For instance, England, France, and Sweden all created public health organizations and law that dealt with smallpox on a national level. See Peter Baldwin, *Contagion and the State in Europe, 1830–1930* (Cambridge: Cambridge University Press, 1999). The quotation is from United States Supreme Court Justice John Marshall Harlan's ruling in *Jacobson v. Massachusetts*, 197 U.S. 11 (1905).

25. William J. Silver, "How Utah Won Freedom," *The Liberator* 5 (August 1905): 122. Michael Willrich finds that although leaders of the Church of Latter Day Saints were divided on compulsory vaccination, "decades of political conflict with the U.S. government prepared Utah Mormons to view with distrust any use of government authority to impose scientific beliefs or behavioral mandates upon the public without democratic deliberation." See Willrich, *Pox*, 274–78, for a discussion of Utah anti-vaccinationists in 1900–1901; quotation on 276.

26. Approved by the governor 19 May 1855. Massachusetts Revised Statutes 1855, chapter 414. Arizona, Arkansas, Florida, and Kansas had no law that enabled a board of health to require vaccination. Illinois also did not have a specific law, but boards of health enforced the vaccination of schoolchildren anyway. In 1904, the antivaccination journal *The Liberator* began a series of articles tabulating the various vaccination laws around the nation.

For Arizona, Arkansas, and Florida, see "Vaccination Laws in the United States," *The Liberator* 5 (July 1904): 115. For Kansas, see *The Liberator* 6 (October 1904): 24–25. For Illinois, see *The Liberator* 5 (September 1904): 172. California, New Hampshire, and New Jersey required vaccination as a condition for admission to public school. See "Vaccination Laws in the United States," *The Liberator* 5 (July 1904): 115–16 for CA; *The Liberator* 7 (April 1905): 193–94 for NH and NJ. Although a board of health could order the vaccination of schoolchildren in Indiana, it could not exclude them from school. See *The Liberator* 6 (November 1904): 53.

27. The Illinois State Board of Health, for instance, took advantage of this vagueness until *Potts v. Breen*, 167 Ill. 67 (1897). Other states with similar enabling laws were Alabama, Colorado, Idaho, Maryland, Missouri, Nebraska, and Nevada. See "Vaccination Laws in the United States," *The Liberator* 5 (July 1904): 115–16 [AL, CO], 146 [ID]; *The Liberator* 6 (December 1904): 88 [MD]; *The Liberator* 7 (April 1905): 141 [MO], 193 [NB, NV].

28. For instance, Connecticut's 1888 general vaccination law directed boards of health to adopt measures "they deem proper and necessary to prevent or arrest smallpox," with a five-dollar fine for noncompliance, although a physician's certification of unfitness could exempt an individual. See "Vaccination Laws in the United States," *The Liberator* 5 (August 1904): 145. Other states with specific general compulsory vaccination statutes were Delaware, Georgia, Kentucky, and Maine (but only for paper mill employees). See *The Liberator* 5 (July 1904): 116 [DL]; *The Liberator* 5 (August 1904): 145–46 [GA]; *The Liberator* 6 (October 1904): 25 [KY]; *The Liberator* 6 (December 1904): 88 [ME].

29. Louisiana, Utah, Minnesota, and Wisconsin (Governor La Follette veto) forbade compulsory vaccination. See *The Liberator* 6 (November 1904): 53–54 [LA]; *The*

Liberator 8 (October 1905): 26 [MN]. For Utah, see Silver, "How Utah Won Freedom," 121–22.

30. John Duffy, "School Vaccination: The Precursor to School Medical Inspection," *Journal of the History of Medicine and Allied Sciences* 3 (July 1978): 346. See also Joan Retsinas, "Smallpox Vaccination: A Leap of Faith," *Rhode Island History* 38 (1979): 113–24.

31. See chapter 7.

32. No formal papers or records of the society exist. No one involved in it left any personal papers, correspondence, or manuscripts. Thus I have to rely primarily on published sources for information about the antivaccinationists.

33. Mary Roth Walsh, *"Doctors Wanted: No Women Need Apply": Sexual Barriers in the Medical Profession, 1835–1975* (New Haven, CT: Yale University Press, 1977), 185.

34. James Cassedy estimates that "over a period of some two decades the Massachusetts association probably exerted more influence than any other body upon the development of American municipal and local public health practice." See Cassedy, *Charles V. Chapin*, 85.

35. Johnston, *Radical Middle Class*, 177.

36. See Scanlon, "Public Health Movement in Boston," 167–80.

37. Georgina Feldberg has remarked on the connection between middle-class values and public health regulations in her history of tuberculosis control efforts. See *Disease and Class: Tuberculosis and the Shaping of Modern American Society* (New Brunswick, NJ: Rutgers University Press, 1995), 83. Robert Wiebe applied this connection more generally to Progressive-era politics and reform in *The Search for Order, 1877–1920* (New York: Hill and Wang, 1967), 127–47.

38. Paul Starr, *The Social Transformation of American Medicine: The Rise of a Sovereign Profession and the Making of a Vast Industry* (New York: Basic Books, 1982), 140, argues that the medical profession attained cultural authority by assuming the mantle of science in the late nineteenth century. The diagnostic achievements of bacteriology boosted "the professional claim to special competence" and allowed Progressive reformers to hold up "professional authority as a model of public disinterestedness."

39. *Munn v. Illinois*, 94 U.S. 113 (1877).

40. William J. Novak, *The People's Welfare: Law and Regulation in Nineteenth-Century America* (Chapel Hill: The University of North Carolina Press, 1996), 2.

Chapter One

1. The most comprehensive mid-twentieth-century text on smallpox is Dixon, *Smallpox*. The three types of smallpox—v. major, v. minor, or varioloid—are also categorized according to types of pustules—fulminating (hemorrhagic), confluent, and discrete. Mortality from fulminating (Purpura variolosa) variola major is 100 percent. Confluent variola major has a mortality rate of 20 to 70 percent. Discrete variola major, with no confluent lesions and fewer pustules, has a 0 to 10 percent mortality rate. Dixon, *Smallpox*, 5–56; especially table on 6–7. Almost all cases of variola minor (97.6 percent) tend to be discrete with a low mortality rate, 0 to 10 percent. Varioloid mortality depends on whether the victim is afflicted with v. major or v. minor, with v. major varioloid victims experiencing a mortality rate like that of v. minor, 0–10 percent. Dixon, *Smallpox*, 57–66.

2. John William Moore, "Smallpox," in *Twentieth-Century Practice: An International Encyclopedia of Modern Medical Science By Leading Authorities of Europe and America*, ed. Thomas L. Stedman (New York: William Wood and Company, 1898), 414. Moore was a Fellow of the Royal College of Physicians in Ireland. He edited the *Dublin Journal of Medical Science* and served as Joint Professor of the Practice of Medicine in the School of Surgery of the Royal College of Surgeons in Ireland. He also held appointments at several Dublin hospitals.

3. Moore, "Smallpox," 409.

4. William Osler, *The Principles and Practices of Medicine* (New York: D. Appleton and Company, 1892), 52.

5. Moore, "Smallpox," 413, 417, 415.

6. Osler, *Principles and Practices of Medicine*, 52, 55, 56. See also Moore, "Smallpox," 430 and 431–32.

7. Dixon believes that surviving smallpox confers about ten times the immunity of a primary vaccination. Immunity *lasts* longer, but it does not always last for a lifetime, depending on the vagaries of individual immune systems. Using an 1887 survey of a Sheffield, England, epidemic, he figured that one in one thousand smallpox survivors contracted it again, with a 25 percent mortality rate. See *Smallpox*, 335–36. Yet, recently, two smallpox experts have declared: "Infection with smallpox confers lifelong immunity." See Joel Berman and D. A. Henderson, "Diagnosis and Management of Smallpox," *New England Journal of Medicine* 346 (2002): 1301.

8. J. M. Toner, "A Paper on the Propriety and Necessity of Compulsory Vaccination," *Transactions of the American Medical Association* 16 (1865): 320. Toner figured the frequency at "from 1 in 250 to 1 in 10,000." Toner served as president of the American Medical Association, founded its library in 1868, and was president of the American Public Health Association in 1875. See also Ernest J. Mellish, "Vaccination from the Standpoint of a Surgeon," *American Medicine* 3 (1902): 821, where he acknowledges that "severe second attacks of smallpox itself occur." Additionally, the vaccine producers William C. Cutler and J. F. Frisbie declared that "it is a matter of medical history, often repeated, that smallpox may attack a person twice and sometimes thrice," and give examples, in *Variola and Vaccinia: History and Description* (Boston: New England Vaccine Company, n.d. [1897 from internal references]), 33.

9. Moore, "Smallpox," 467. Italics in original.

10. See Elizabeth Fenn, *Pox Americana: The Great Smallpox Epidemic of 1775–82* (New York: Hill and Wang, 2001). The classic is Alfred W. Crosby, *The Columbian Exchange: Biological and Cultural Consequences of 1492* (Westport, CT: Greenwood, 1972), 35–62. See also Robert T. Boyd, *The Coming of the Spirit of Pestilence: Introduced Infectious Diseases and Population Decline among the Northwest Indians, 1774–1874* (Seattle: University of Washington Press, 1999).

11. Genevieve Miller, *The Adoption of Inoculation for Smallpox in England and France* (Philadelphia: University of Pennsylvania Press, 1957).

12. John B. Blake, "The Inoculation Controversy in Boston, 1721–1722," in *Sickness and Health in America: Readings in the History of Medicine and Public Health*, 2nd ed., rev., ed. Judith Walzer Leavitt and Ronald L. Numbers (Madison: University of Wisconsin Press, 1985), 347–55. Originally published in *The New England Quarterly* 25 (1952): 489–506. See also John B. Blake, *Public Health in the Town of Boston, 1630–1822* (Cambridge, MA: Harvard University Press, 1959), 52–98. Elizabeth Fenn has the

most thorough discussion of inoculation in other colonial towns in *Pox Americana*, 80–103. In addition, Susan Wade Peabody covers the development of law and regulations in "Historical Study of Legislation regarding Public Health in the States of New York and Massachusetts," *Journal of Infectious Diseases*, Supplement no. 4 (February 1909): 1–158. See also Ola Winslow, *A Destroying Angel: The Conquest of Smallpox in Colonial Boston* (Boston: Houghton Mifflin, 1974).

13. George William Winterburn, *The Value of Vaccination: A Non-Partisan Review of Its History and Results* (Philadelphia: F. E. Boericke, Hahnemann, 1886), 18. See also Floyd Crandall, MD, "A Century of Vaccination," *American Medicine* 2 (1901): 896, for a similar judgment.

14. Citing an Epidemiological Society of London report, its authors found a ratio of 71.4 epidemics per 100 years before inoculation in England, a ratio of 84 epidemics per 100 years during inoculation, and a ratio of 24 epidemics per 100 years (prorated) after vaccination. "Report of the Committee on the Value and Necessity of Vaccination and Revaccination for the Eradication of Smallpox," *Transactions of the American Medical Association* 16 (1866): 268.

15. J. F. Marson, *Report of Parliamentary Committee*, 1871, in Winterburn, *Value of Vaccination*, 63.

16. John H. McCollom, "Discussion of Smallpox in Massachusetts," *JMABH* 4 (April 1894): 2.

17. Frank L. Morse, "The Recent Smallpox Epidemic in Massachusetts," *JMABH* 8 (1903–4): 46–64, 47.

18. Jenner's use of "virus" should not be confused with our current understanding of the term. Derrick Baxby cautions that throughout the nineteenth century, "virus" was used to denote a "specific transmissible poison, the nature of which was a mystery." See Baxby, *Jenner's Smallpox Vaccine: The Riddle of Vaccinia Virus and Its Origins* (London: Heinemann Educational Books, 1981), xiii.

19. John Z. Bowers, "The Odyssey of Smallpox Vaccination," *Bulletin of the History of Medicine* 55 (1981): 17–33.

20. Winterburn, *Value of Vaccination*, 20; 25.

21. Joint Special Committee, *Senate . . . No. 155*, Report prepared by C. H. Stedman, chairman (Boston, 1855), 2.

22. Waterhouse as quoted in Blake, *Public Health*, 181. Later medical authorities held this experiment in such high regard a century later that they featured it in a "photographic reproduction of a Boston Board of Health report of the year 1802," *BMSJ* 145 (1901): 445.

23. See John B. Blake, *Benjamin Waterhouse and the Introduction of Vaccination* (Philadelphia: University of Pennsylvania Press, 1957). Also Blake, "Benjamin Waterhouse: Harvard's First Professor of Physic," *Journal of Medical Education* 33 (1958): 771–82.

24. Whitfield J. Bell, Jr., "Dr. James Smith and the Public Encouragement of Vaccination for Smallpox," *Annals of Medical History*, 3rd series, 2 (November 1940): 500–517.

25. Thomas Jefferson to Dr. Coxe, 5 November 1801, in Byrd S. Leavell, MD, "Thomas Jefferson and Smallpox Vaccination," *Transactions of the American Clinical and Climatological Association* 88 (1977): 123–24. By "family" Jefferson probably meant not only biological kin but also the people he owned. See also Whitfield J. Bell, Jr.,

The College of Physicians of Philadelphia: A Bicentennial History (Philadelphia: Science History Publications, 1987), 39.

26. Rush, *Letters*, II, 847; quoted in Bell, *College of Physicians of Philadelphia*, 40.

27. Bell, *College of Physicians of Philadelphia*, 40.

28. "Report of the Committee on the Value and Necessity of Vaccination and Revaccination," 276.

29. See Charles E. Rosenburg's study of the reports and records of dispensaries in New York, Philadelphia, and Boston, "Social Class and Medical Care in 19th-Century America: The Rise and Fall of the Dispensary," in Leavitt and Numbers, *Sickness and Health in America*, 274. First published in *Journal of the History of Medicine and Allied Sciences* 29 (1974): 32–54.

30. Francis Bacon, William A. Hammond, and David F. Lincoln, *Vaccination: A Report Read before the American Social Science Association, at New York, October 27, 1869* (New York: Nation Press, 1870), 14.

31. "The Production of Vaccine Lymph," *BMSJ* 146 (1902): 22.

32. Winterburn, *Value of Vaccination*, 65.

33. Massachusetts State Board of Health, *Thirty-First Annual Report of the State Board of Health of Massachusetts* (Boston, 1900), xiv.

34. Morse, "Recent Smallpox Epidemic," 49, 51.

35. Samuel W. Abbott, "Vaccination and Its Results," *JMABH* 4 (1894): 21.

36. See for instance, Massachusetts State Board of Health, "Vaccinations Performed at Public Cost, 1901," *Thirty-Third Annual Report of the State Board of Health of Massachusetts* (Boston, 1902), 558.

37. Samuel W. Abbott, "Legislation with Reference to Smallpox and Vaccination," *BMSJ* 147 (1902): 268.

38. See for instance, William Howard, *Public Health Administration and the Natural History of Disease in Baltimore, Maryland, 1797–1920* (Washington, DC: The Carnegie Institution, 1924), 277–96. Issac D. Rawlings, *The Rise and Fall of Disease in Illinois*, 2 vols. (Springfield, IL: State Department of Public Health, 1927), 1:49–51, 307–20. Phillip D. Jordan, *The People's Health: A History of Public Health in Minnesota to 1948* (St. Paul: Minnesota Historical Society, 1953). Duffy, *A History of Public Health in New York City, 1625–1866* (New York: Russell Sage Foundation, 1968); and Duffy, *A History of Public Health in New York City, 1866–1966*. Duffy also found that inspectors routinely discovered large percentages of unvaccinated students in New York City, Chicago, and New Orleans. See Duffy, "School Vaccination," 344–55. Stuart Galishoff concludes that in Newark, New Jersey, "vaccination as first practiced had too many pitfalls to gain universal acceptance." See Galishoff, *Newark: The Nation's Unhealthiest City, 1832–1895* (New Brunswick, NJ: Rutgers University Press, 1988), 143–62, quotation on 145. Judith Walzer Leavitt documents how continued resistance to vaccination wrought havoc for successive health officers in Milwaukee, Wisconsin, during the nineteenth century. See Leavitt, *Healthiest City*, 76–121.

39. Winterburn, *Value of Vaccination*, 117.

40. William R. Lawrence, *History of the Boston Dispensary* (Boston: John Wilson and Son, 1859), citing statistics from the New York Dispensary, 10. See also Rosenburg, "Social Class," 284 (note 9).

41. P. Brouardel, "Vaccina," in Stedman, *Twentieth-Century Practice*, 520. Brouardel was Professor of Medical Jurisprudence and Dean of the Faculty of Medicine at the

University of Paris. He also held an appointment as physician to the Hôpital de la Charité.

42. Toner, "A Paper," 319, 322.

43. "Report of the Committee on the Value and Necessity of Vaccination and Revaccination," 272.

44. James F. Hibberd, "Propositions concerning Vaccination," *Public Health Papers and Reports* 8 (1882): 123.

45. Samuel Abbott, *The Past and Present Condition of Public Hygiene and State Medicine in the United States* (Boston: Wright & Potter, 1900), 27. Abbott gave no evidence to back up this assertion.

46. Brouardel, "Vaccina," 524.

47. Moore, "Smallpox," 465.

48. Mellish, "Vaccination," 821, 822.

49. Toner, "A Paper," 313, 317.

50. "Report of the Committee on the Value and Necessity of Vaccination and Revaccination," 276.

51. Allan McLane Hamilton and Bache McE. Emmett, "Small-Pox and Other Contagious Diseases," in *A Treatise on Hygiene and Public Health*, ed. Albert H. Buck (New York: William Wood & Company, 1879), 524, 527.

52. Hibberd, "Propositions concerning Vaccination," 124.

53. Eugene Foster, "Report of the Committee on Compulsory Vaccination; also, a Supplementary Report on the Efficiency and Safety of Vaccination," *Public Health Papers and Reports* 9 (1883): 243.

54. Henry B. Baker, MD, "Vaccination versus Compulsory Vaccination," *The American Lancet*, new series, 14 (1890): 281, 283.

55. C. S. Lindsley, MD, letter reprinted in Clark Bell, "Compulsory Vaccination: Should It Be Enforced By Law?" *JAMA* 28 (1897): 50.

56. A. Walter Suiter, "Report of the Committee on Cause and Prevention of Infectious Diseases," *Public Health Papers and Reports* 16 (1901): 70.

57. Scanlon, "Public Health Movement in Boston," 20–42.

58. Gert H. Brieger, "Sanitary Reform in New York City: Stephen Smith and the Passage of the Metropolitan Health Bill," in Leavitt and Numbers, *Sickness and Heath in America*, 399–413. First published in *Bulletin of the History of Medicine* 40 (1966): 407–29.

59. Blake, *Public Health*, 182.

60. See Lawrence, *History of the Boston Dispensary*, 48–49 (1803 recommendation), 183 (mention of vaccination); and Robert W. Greenleaf, *An Historical Report of the Boston Dispensary for One Hundred and One Years, 1796–1897* (Brookline, MA: The Riverdale Press, 1898), 20 (1803 recommendation). Unfortunately neither of these histories provides data on vaccinations, although they are quite specific about other medical and prescription services.

61. Blake, *Public Health*, 182–83.

62. Walter L. Burrage, *A History of the Massachusetts Medical Society with Brief Biographies of the Founders and Chief Officers* (Norwood, MA: The Plimpton Press, 1923), 90, quoting an 1808 Massachusetts Medical Society report on vaccination.

63. Blake, *Public*, see discussion 183–90, quotation on 187. Medical fees in general were probably far beyond the means of the lower classes in the mid-nineteenth

century. In 1855, for instance, the Boston Medical Association set fees of $1.50 to $2.00 for a medical visit, with a night visit costing anywhere from $3.00 to $8.00. See "Boston Medical Association," *BMSJ* 51 (1855): 326.

64. Lemuel Shattuck, *Report of a General Plan for the Public and Private Health, Devised, Prepared and Recommended by the Commissioners Appointed under a Resolve of the Legislature of Massachusetts, relating to a Sanitary Survey of the State* (1850; reprint, New York: Arno Press, 1972), 180. Shattuck started his career as a schoolteacher and later became a bookseller and publisher. In 1837 he devised a plan for arranging, printing, and preserving Boston city documents. In 1841, he published a system for recording genealogical facts and helped convince the legislature to pass a law requiring the registration of births and deaths in Massachusetts. In 1845 he completed a sanitary survey of Boston and lobbied for funds for a sanitary commission to undertake a similar survey of the state. Although his *Sanitary Survey* outlined a state system of public health, the legislature did nothing to further it for over twenty years except to pass the compulsory vaccination law. See Whipple, *State Sanitation*, 1:30. Perhaps indicative of this transition to private sources is that vaccine lymph was first advertised for sale in Boston in an 1835 issue of the *Boston Medical and Surgical Journal*. See "Production of Vaccine Lymph," 22.

65. Blake, *Public Health*, 191 (note 46), referring to *Acts and Resolves* 1838, chapter 138. The Medical Society might have believed that vaccination had practically eliminated smallpox, thus obviating the need for any special measures against it. It might also have had something to do with repealing the old inoculation regulations.

66. Shattuck, *Report of a General Plan*, 180.

67. Ibid., 181.

68. J. H. McCollom, "Deaths from Smallpox in Boston for Forty Years—1852–1871, and 1874–1893," *JMABH* 4 (April 1894): 6–7.

69. "Medical Miscellany," *BMSJ* 51 (1854): 267.

70. Untitled editorial, *BMSJ* 51 (1854): 406. Dr. J. V. C. Smith, senior editor until the end of 1854, probably wrote this editorial. Elected mayor of Boston, he relinquished his position to Drs. William W. Morland and Francis Minot, who both wrote the editorials for 1855. Morland also acted as secretary for the Boston Society for Medical Improvement. See "Proprietor's Note," *BMSJ* 51 (1855): 547.

71. Untitled editorial, *BMSJ* 51 (1855): 486.

72. Joint Special Committee, *Senate . . . No. 155*, 3.

73. Peabody, "Historical Study of Legislation," 50.

74. "An Act to Secure General Vaccination," *Acts* 1855, chapter 414, 812–13.

75. "Smallpox and Vaccination—Mr. Shattuck's Memorial," *BMSJ* 54 (1856): 265.

76. F. S. A., "Compulsory Vaccination," letter to the editor dated June 1856, *BMSJ* 54 (1856): 378.

77. Scanlon, "Public Health Movement in Boston," 23. I use 250,000 as the population for 1869, based on an 1871 total of 258,000 given in Scanlon, from Boston, City Document no. 34, *Annual Report of the City Physician* (Boston, 1870).

78. Massachusetts State Board of Health, "Health of Towns," *Second Annual Report of the State Board of Health of Massachusetts* (Boston, 1871), 55–56.

79. Massachusetts State Board of Health, *Thirty-First Annual Report* (1900), xiv.

80. Massachusetts State Board of Health, "Health of Towns," *Second Annual Report* (1871), 82 (Worcester), 7 (Holyoke).

81. Massachusetts State Board of Health, *Third Annual Report of the State Board of Health of Massachusetts* (Boston, 1872), 301.

82. Ibid., 300. French Canadians had a long history of resistance to vaccination and troubles with vaccination complications. William Osler declared that starting in the 1870s, "a great deal of feeling had been aroused among the French Canadians by the occurrence of several serious cases of ulceration, possibly of syphilitic disease, following vaccination; and several agitators, among them a French physician of some standing, aroused a popular and wide-spread prejudice against the practice. There were indeed vaccination riots." Osler, *Principles and Practice of Medicine*, 64. See also Michael Bliss, *Plague: A Story of Smallpox in Montreal* (Toronto: HarperCollins, 1991).

83. Massachusetts State Board of Health, *Third Annual Report* (1872), 301–2.

84. Boston Board of Health, "Report of the City Physician," *First Annual Report of the Board of Health of the City of Boston* (Boston, 1873), 26.

85. Boston Board of Health, "Rules and Regulations of the Board of Health," *First Annual Report* (1873), 8.

86. Massachusetts State Board of Health, *Fifth Annual Report of the State Board of Health of Massachusetts* (Boston, 1874), 480. Emphasis in the original.

87. Massachusetts State Board of Health, *Thirty-First Annual Report* (1900), ix, xix.

88. Advertisement, *BMSJ* 51 (1854), back page.

89. "Police Physicians," Editorial, *BMSJ* 51 (1855): 324.

90. Boston Board of Health, City Document no. 84, "Report of the City Physician," *First Annual Report* (1873), 25.

91. Boston Board of Health, City Document no. 67, "Vaccination," in *Fifth Annual Report of the Board of Health of the City of Boston* (1877), 13–14.

92. Boston Board of Health, *Thirtieth Annual Report of the Health Department of the City of Boston for the Year 1901* (Boston, 1902), 45.

93. Boston Board of Health, City Document no. 84, "Medical Inspectors," *First Annual Report* (1873), 12–13.

94. Boston Board of Health, "Report of the City Physician," in *First Annual Report* (1873), 25.

95. Boston Board of Health, "Report of the City Physician," *Second Annual Report of the Board of Health of the City of Boston* (Boston, 1874), 53. Population was 273,755, from Scanlon, "Public Health Movement in Boston," 55.

96. Boston Board of Health, "Report of the City Physician," *Second Annual Report* (1874), 53.

97. Boston Board of Health, "Medical Inspectors," *First Annual Report* (1873), 13.

98. Boston Board of Health, "Report of the City Physician," *Second Annual Report* (1874), 53–54. City Physician Samuel A. Green vaccinated 1, 519 inmates out of a total jail population of 3,227 prisoners.

99. Boston Board of Health, "Report of the City Physician," *Third Annual Report of the Board of Health of the City of Boston* (Boston, 1875), 106 (1 May 1874 through 30 April 1875).

100. Boston Board of Health, *Tenth Annual Report of the Board of Health of the City of Boston* (Boston, 1882), "Vaccination," 33–34; "City Physician's Report," 72; "Cases reported," 30.

101. Boston Board of Health, *Tenth Annual Report* (1882), 37–38.

102. Charles L. Webster, MD, "Some Proofs That Vaccination Prevents and Mitigates Smallpox," *Cleveland Medical Journal* 6 (1901): 137.

103. Boston Board of Health, "Report of the City Physician," in *First Annual Report* (1873), 25. The City Physician's report covers May 1872 through 30 April 1873. He commented, "until the present year [1873] it has not been the duty of the City Physician to re-vaccinate applicants." That year he revaccinated 203, then 29 (1873–74), 10 (1874–75), 6 (1875–76), 6 (1876–77). After 1877, the city physician no longer differentiates, but my guess is that the numbers of revaccination remain tiny.

104. Massachusetts State Board of Health, *Twenty-Fifth Annual Report of the State Board of Health of Massachusetts* (Boston, 1894), ix.

105. Boston Board of Health, *Annual Report of the Health Department for the Year 1893* (Boston, 1895), 40.

106. Ibid.

107. Massachusetts, *Acts* 1894, chapter 515. I will discuss this amendment in more detail in following chapters.

108. Rosenburg, "Social Class," 282.

109. Boston Board of Health, "Smallpox," in *Ninth Annual Report of the Board of Health of the City of Boston for the Financial Year 1880–81* (Boston, 1881), 26.

110. For comments about limited hours and inability to keep up with demand in 1881–82, see Boston Board of Health, "Vaccination," *Tenth Annual Report* (1882), 34.

111. Boston Board of Health, *Annual Report of the Health Department for the Year 1893*, 40.

112. Boston Board of Health, *Annual Report of the Health Department for the Year 1894* (Boston, 1896), 50–52.

113. See appendix A for Boston Health Department vaccinations, 1872–1900. Boston's population grew from 273,755 to 560,892 by 1900. For city physician vaccinations, see Boston Board of Health, "A Tabular Statement of the Vaccinations at the City Physician's Office from the Year Ending April 30, 1873, to the Year Ending Dec. 31, 1887 (inclusive)," in *Sixteenth Annual Report of the Board of Health of the City of Boston for the Year 1887* (Boston, 1889), 63. Population for 1887 on 3.

Chapter Two

1. Cutler and Frisbie, *Variola and Vaccinia*, 35.

2. Ibid.

3. Bacon, Hammond, and Lincoln, *Vaccination*, 5, quoting Jenner.

4. Edward Cator Seaton, MD, "Vaccination," in *A System of Medicine*, vol. 1, ed. J. Russell Reynolds (Philadelphia: Henry C. Lea's Son & Co., 1880), 160. Seaton also wrote *The Handbook of Vaccination*, which many nineteenth-century physicians regarded as the most comprehensive text on vaccination. Reynold's *System* was a standard medical textbook in the nineteenth century intended for teaching and reference. American physicians writing about vaccination invariably refer to both Seaton and J. F. Marson, who wrote an article on smallpox for the text. First published in England in 1866, this popular textbook was republished in 1870, 1871, 1876, and 1878 before the American edition debuted in 1880. Seaton's article originally appeared in the 1866 English edition.

5. Seaton, "Vaccination," 159.

6. Winterburn, *Value of Vaccination*, 28–29.

7. Brouardel, "Vaccina," 517.

8. Mellish, "Vaccination," 820.

9. Cutler and Frisbie, *Variola and Vaccinia*, 39, 36. Definitions in parentheses from Mikel A. Rothenberg, MD, and Charles F. Chapman, *Dictionary of Medical Terms for the Nonmedical Person*, 3rd ed. (Hauppauge, NY: Barron's Educational Series, 1994), 430, 279.

10. Brouardel, "Vaccina," 531.

11. Sidney D. Wilgus, "A Case of Generalized Vaccinia with Unusual Complications," *American Medicine* 3 (1902): 501.

12. Seaton, "Vaccination," 161.

13. J. F. Marson, "Smallpox," in Reynolds, *A System of Medicine*, 1:152. American practitioners regarded Marson highly. J. M. Toner declared his "experience in small-pox is scarcely equaled by any living practitioner" in "A Paper," 327. Toner misspells Marson's name as "Marston."

14. Massachusetts State Board of Health, *Twenty-Fifth Annual Report* (1894), xii.

15. Moore, "Smallpox," 470.

16. Seaton, "Vaccination," 161.

17. Henry Austin Martin, "Anti-Vaccinism," *North American Review* 134 (April 1882): 374.

18. Osler, *Principles and Practice of Medicine*, 61. At the time, Osler served as physician-in-chief at the Johns Hopkins Hospital and as medical professor at the Johns Hopkins University medical school.

19. Brouardel, "Vaccina," 534.

20. Seaton, "Vaccination," 161.

21. Winterburn, *Value of Vaccination*, 34.

22. Osler, *Principles and Practice of Medicine*, 61.

23. Brouardel, "Vaccina," 527.

24. Cutler and Frisbie, *Variola and Vaccinia*, 35.

25. Ibid., 36.

26. Erysipelas is an "acute skin disease, caused by infection with bacteria of genus *streptococcus* (esp. *Streptococcus pyogenes*) and characterized by redness, swelling, fever, pain and skin lesions. Treatment is by antibiotics." Rothenberg and Chapman, *Dictionary of Medical Terms*, 172.

27. John H. McCollom, MD, "Vaccinations: Accidents and Untoward Effects," *BMSJ* 147 (1902): 203.

28. Winterburn, *Value of Vaccination*, 42–43.

29. Derrick Baxby, *Vaccination: Jenner's Legacy* (Berkeley, England: The Jenner Educational Trust, 1994), 10.

30. Derrick Baxby, *Jenner's Smallpox Vaccine*, 165–78. See also Edgar M. Crookshank, *The History and Pathology of Vaccination: A Critical Inquiry*, 2 vols. (London: H. K. Lewis, 1889), 1:373–418.

31. Baxby, *Jenner's Smallpox Vaccine*, 131.

32. Baxby, *Vaccination*, 10.

33. Baxby, *Jenner's Smallpox Vaccine*, 132.

34. John Badcock, *A Detail of Experiments confirming the Power of Cow Pox to Protect the Constitution from a Subsequent Attack of Small Pox* (Brighton, 1845), in Crookshank, *History and Pathology of Vaccination*, 2:515–16. Italics in original.

35. Dixon, *Smallpox*, 119.

36. See John Baron, chairman, *Report of the Vaccination Section of the Provincial Medical and Surgical Association*, reprinted from *Transactions of the Provincial Medical and Surgical Association* 8 (1840), in Crookshank, *History and Pathology of Vaccination*, 2:451–67. In 1939 the British scientist Alan Downie proved that vaccinia was not the same virus as cowpox, nor was it attenuated smallpox. Dixon, *Smallpox*, 120.

37. "Report of the Committee on the Value and Necessity of Vaccination and Revaccination for the Eradication of Smallpox," *Transactions of the American Medical Association* 16 (1866): 270.

38. Derrick Baxby notes that cows are not natural reservoirs for cowpox; rather it is a human infection conveyed to milk cows through handling the teats. Several other teat infections cause cowpox-like pustules: they are termed "spurious cowpox" because lymph drawn from these pustules does not induce vaccinia. See *Jenner's Smallpox Vaccine*, 166–78. Cyril Dixon also noted "confusion in terminology" about Jennerian and spurious cowpox. He asserts that "Jennerian cowpox appeared to be fairly common in the early nineteenth century" but later "writers frequently referred to the disease as being less common than previously." Dixon, *Smallpox*, 160. Quoted material from Badcock, *A Detail of Experiments*, 516.

39. Seaton, quoting Robert Ceeley in "Vaccination," 173 n. 1.

40. Crookshank, *History and Pathology of Vaccination*, 1:367. Italics in the original.

41. Baxby, *Jenner's Smallpox Vaccine*, 181, quoting John Estlin, who developed this vaccine, in a letter to the *Medical Gazette*; also reprinted in Crookshank, *History and Pathology of Vaccination*, 2:328–29.

42. Crookshank, *History and Pathology of Vaccination*, 1:370.

43. Badcock, *A Detail of Experiments*, 520.

44. Dixon, *Smallpox*, 119.

45. Ephraim Cutter, "Partial Report on the Production of Vaccine Virus in the United States," *Transactions of the American Medical Association* 23 (1872): 201–3. My thanks to John Buder for pointing out this source.

46. Baxby, *Jenner's Smallpox Vaccine*, 156. Quotation from Winterburn, *Value of Vaccination*, 38–39.

47. Cutter, "Partial Report on the Production of Vaccine Virus," 200–201, quoting a letter dated February 1860, originally published in the *Boston Medical and Surgical Journal*.

48. Ibid., 206.

49. Winterburn, *Value of Vaccination*, 42.

50. Dixon, *Smallpox*, 119.

51. Martin, "Anti-Vaccinism," 369.

52. Samuel W. Abbott, letter reprinted in Bell, "Compulsory Vaccination," 51.

53. Editorial, "Production of Vaccine Lymph," 24.

54. Report of Lt. Col. John J. Milhau, in Cutter, "Partial Report on the Production of Vaccine," 208–11.

55. Cutter, "Partial Report on the Production of Vaccine," 219–20.

56. Winterburn, *Value of Vaccination*, 39.

57. "The Source of Vaccine," Queries and Minor Notes, *JAMA* 40 (1903): 999–1000.

58. Brouardel, "Vaccina," 507, 511.

59. Seaton, "Vaccination," 162. Italics in original.

60. Ibid., 163.

61. Crookshank, *History and Pathology of Vaccination*, 1:371.

62. John B. Buist, *Vaccinia and Variola: A Study of Their Life History* (London: J. & A. Churchill, 1887), 3.

63. Seaton, "Vaccination," 163.

64. Buist, *Vaccinia and Variola*, 4.

65. Baxby, *Vaccination*, 21.

66. Toner, "A Paper," 323.

67. Bacon, Hammond, and Lincoln, *Vaccination*, 7.

68. Cutter, "Partial Report on the Production of Vaccine," 210.

69. Hartshorne, editorial aside, in Reynolds, *A System of Medicine*, 163.

70. Charles V. Chapin, *Municipal Sanitation in the United States* (Providence, RI: Snow & Farnham, 1901), 580.

71. Bacon, Hammond, and Lincoln, *Vaccination*, 7.

72. Boston Board of Health, *First Annual Report* (1873), 13. Fifty-five percent of 10,546 vaccinations.

73. Toner, "A Paper," 324.

74. Editorial, "Production of Vaccine Lymph," 22.

75. Ibid., 22 n. 3.

76. Winterburn, *Value of Vaccination*, 52, 51.

77. George Dock, "Vaccination," in *Modern Medical Practice: Its Theory and Practice*, ed. Sir William Osler and Thomas McCrae (Philadelphia, PA: Lea & Febiger, 1913), 828. Dock held both the chair of medicine and pathology at the University of Michigan from 1899 to 1908, and then moved on to become professor of clinical pathology at Tulane University.

78. Toner, "A Paper," 325.

79. Seaton, "Vaccination," 165.

80. Moore, "Smallpox," 471.

81. Seaton, "Vaccination," 165.

82. Winterburn, *Value of Vaccination*, 53.

83. Massachusetts State Board of Health, *Twenty-Fifth Annual Report* (1894), xiii.

84. George Dock, "The Works of Edward Jenner and Their Value in the Modern Study of Smallpox," *The New York Medical Journal* 76, part 2 (1902): 983. In 1913 he still criticized his colleagues for abrading too deeply and creating a thicker scab that "not only interferes with the development of the normal vesicle, but is irritating and induces rubbing or scratching, which promote secondary infection." See Dock, "Vaccination," 831.

85. Dixon, *Smallpox*, 131.

86. Toner, "A Paper," 328.

87. Seaton, "Vaccination," 163.

88. W. F. Elgin, "Comments in Discussion of Papers of Dr. Bryce and Dr. Bernaldez," *Public Health Papers and Reports* 27 (1902): 341.

89. Samuel Durgin, "Comments in Discussion of Papers of Dr. Bryce and Dr. Bernaldez," *Public Health Papers and Reports* 27 (1902): 340.

90. Dr. David P. Austin, remarks following Frank S. Fielder, "What Constitutes Efficient Vaccination?" Report of Papers Read at the New York County Medical Association, 17 March 1902, *JAMA* 38 (1902): 959.

91. Eugene Darling, "Vaccination: The Technique," *BMSJ* 147 (1902): 202.

92. Toner, "A Paper," 326. Physicians seemed to worry exclusively about using shields to protect the vaccinated person from contaminating his or her vaccination with dirt. I have as yet seen no discussion in any of my sources where they used shields to protect others from contact with the vaccination site, and thus inadvertent vaccination in inconvenient places.

93. Cutler and Frisbie, *Variola and Vaccinia*, 53.

94. Darling, "Vaccination," 202.

95. Paul Burrows, *Organized Medicine in the Progressive Era: The Move toward Monopoly* (Baltimore, MD: The Johns Hopkins University Press, 1977), 14–28 on McCormack, quotation on 27; and J. N. McCormack, "The Value of State Control and Vaccination in the Management of Smallpox," *JAMA* 38 (1902): 1435.

96. "Vaccine Virus," advertisement for Codman & Shurtleff, *JMABH* 4 (April 1894), unnumbered last page.

97. Edward W. Watson, "Some Experiences in Vaccination," *American Medicine* 2 (1901): 683.

98. D. B. McKinley, letter, *Medical Talk for the Home* 2 (1901): 276.

99. Mellish, "Vaccination," 820.

100. See, for instance, Judson Daland advising his colleagues in late 1901 to apply "one of the ordinary shields" to protect a vaccination. Dr. Judson Daland, "The Technique, Value and Object of Vaccination," Report of a Paper Read before the North Branch of the Philadelphia County Medical Society, 20 December 1901, *JAMA* 38 (1902): 268.

101. C. P. Franklin, "Vaccination Shield," *American Medicine* 3 (1902): 57–58. See also C. P. Franklin, "Vaccination Shield," *JAMA* (1901): 1691.

102. Dock, "Works of Edward Jenner," 931. It is unlikely this practice continued for long in the United States because physicians and the AMA would have complained loudly about the impropriety and competition lay vaccination represented. So far I have found no such discussion in any medical journal.

103. Peter H. Bryce, "Vaccinal Immunization from the Health Officer's Standpoint," *Public Health Papers and Reports* 27 (1902): 179.

104. Heman Spalding, "Some Facts about Vaccination," *JAMA* 39 (1902): 906.

105. Mellish, "Vaccination," 820.

106. "Report of Committee on the Relative Immunizing Value of Human and Bovine Vaccine Virus," *BMSJ* 148 (1903): 41.

107. Medical News, Minnesota, "Smallpox at Argyle," *JAMA* 44 (1905): 1125.

108. McKinley, letter, 277.

109. Darling, "Vaccination," 202.

110. Dr. J. H. McCollom, remarks in discussion following Darling's "Vaccination," 203.

111. Dock, "Works of Edward Jenner," 983.

112. Stephen C. Martin, "A Pregnant Cause of Failure in Vaccination," *BMSJ* 120 (1889): 398.

113. Cutler and Frisbie, *Variola and Vaccinia*, 53.

114. J. W. Keath, "The Proper Method of Vaccination," *JAMA* 38 (1902): 526.

115. Winterburn, *Value of Vaccination*, 53.

116. Osler, *Principles and Practice of Medicine*, 64.

117. Editorial, "The Choice of a Site for Vaccination," *JAMA* 35 (1900): 503.

118. Daland, "The Technique, Value and Object of Vaccination," 268.

119. Mellish, "Vaccination," 820. For the case, see F. H. Russell, "A Case of Fatal Vaccination Infection Which Resembled Appendicitis," *JAMA* 38 (1902): 34–35.

120. Cutler and Frisbie, *Variola and Vaccinia*, 53.

121. Moore, "Smallpox," 471.

122. Brouardel, "Vaccina," 551.

123. Darling, "Vaccination," 202.

124. Winterburn, *Value of Vaccination*, quoting Edward Ballard, *On Vaccination: Its Value and Alleged Dangers: A Prize Essay* (London: Longmans, Green, 1868), 93.

125. Seaton, "Vaccination," 178–82. Quotation on 181.

126. Ibid., 182.

127. Jonathan Hutchinson, *Illustrations of Clinical Surgery*, 2 vols. (London: J. & A. Churchill, 1878–88), 114–33.

128. Philip Mortimer, "Robert Cory and the Vaccine Syphilis Controversy: A Forgotten Hero?" *Lancet* 367 (2006): 1112–15.

129. Hutchinson noted that "until my original papers were published almost the whole British profession was incredulous on this point." *Illustrations*, 133. See also Seaton, "Vaccination," 178–81; and Dock, "Vaccination," 828. George Winterburn noted in 1886 that "the existence of vaccinal-syphilis was until recently most strenuously denied." *Value of Vaccination*, 119. For a continental European perspective on the syphilis controversy, see Brouardel, "Vaccina," 539–45. Despite the evidence, some British physicians believed that if vaccinators took care to ascertain the donor's health history, humanized lymph was safe. Cory acquired syphilis because he had violated the so-called primary rule (to take no vaccinifer not obviously healthy), according to John C. McVail, *Vaccination Vindicated: Being an Answer to the Leading Anti-Vaccinators* (London: Cassell & Company, 1887), 133.

130. Hopkins, *Greatest Killer*, 88.

131. Winterburn, *Value of Vaccination*, 129–31.

132. McCollom, "Vaccinations," 203.

133. Toner, "A Paper," 323.

134. Osler, *Principles and Practices of Medicine*, 63.

135. Massachusetts State Board of Health, *Twenty-Fifth Annual Report* (1894), xiii.

136. M. J. Rosenau, "Dry Points versus Glycerinated Virus, from a Bacteriological Standpoint," *American Medicine* 3 (1902): 637. See also Brouardel, "Vaccina," 547, for a discussion of the numbers of vesicles cultivated on the typical calf.

137. Editorial, "Production of Vaccine Lymph," 23.

138. The proprietors of the New England Vaccine Company advised lymph collection precisely in terms of *hours* rather than days after the initial vaccination of a cow. See Cutler and Frisbie, *Variola and Vaccinia*, 49.

139. Editorial, "The Relative Immunizing Value of Human and Bovine Vaccine Virus," *BMSJ* 148 (1903): 24.

140. Editorial, "Production of Vaccine Lymph," 22, citing the surgeon John J. Milhau in *Medical and Surgical History of the War*, vol. 3 (Washington, DC: Government Printing Office, 1875–88), 634.

141. Massachusetts State Board of Health, *Fourth Annual Report of the State Board of Health of Massachusetts* (Boston, 1873), 3.

142. Advertisement for Dr. J. B. Fisher & Co., in *Fourth Annual Announcement of the Woman's Hospital Medical College of Chicago, Illinois* (Chicago: Fergus Printing Company, 1873). My thanks to Eve Fine for providing this source. Capitalization in the original.

143. Winterburn, *Value of Vaccination*, 51–52.

144. Massachusetts State Board of Health, *Twenty-Fifth Annual Report*, xii.

145. Chapin, *Municipal Sanitation in the United States*, 580.

146. Winterburn, *Value of Vaccination*, 52.

147. Cutler and Frisbie, *Variola and Vaccinia*, 49.

148. Winterburn, *Value of Vaccination*, 52.

149. Abbott, "Vaccination and Its Results," 23.

150. McCormack, "Value of State Control and Vaccination," 1435.

151. Martin, "Anti-Vaccinism," 375.

152. "Dr. Martin's Vaccine Virus," advertisement, *JMABH* 4 (April 1894), back cover.

153. Hopkins, *Greatest Killer*, 268.

154. New England Vaccine Co., "Vaccine Virus," advertisement, *JMABH* 4 (April 1894), back of front cover.

155. This advertisement, placed by the Boston druggist Otis Clapp & Son, ran in every issue of the homeopathic *New England Medical Gazette* from 1900 to 1902. See, for example, *New England Medical Gazette* 35 (August 1900).

156. "Vaccine Virus. Codman & Shurtleff," advertisement, *JMABH* 4 (April 1894), last page.

157. D. H. Beckwith, MD, "Vaccination" (Pittsburgh, PA: Stevenson & Foster, 1882), 5. Transcript of a talk given before the American Institute of Homeopathy, Indianapolis, IN, June 1882.

158. Ibid., 7.

159. Dr. T. S. Hopkins, Thomasville, GA. From the National Board of Health *Bulletin*, Washington DC, March 4, 1882, quoted in Winterburn, *Value of Vaccination*, 51.

160. Cutler and Frisbie, *Variola and Vaccinia*, 49.

161. "Report of the Examination of Vaccines by the Pennsylvania State Board of Health," Table of Vaccines, Showing Number of Bacteria to Each Vaccination, *American Medicine* 3 (1902): 136.

162. Mellish, "Vaccination," 821.

163. W. F. Elgin, "Some Facts That Physicians Should Know in Reference to Vaccine and Vaccination," Paper Read at the Semiannual Meeting of the Medical and Chirurgical Faculty at Annapolis, MD, 27–28 September 1906, 4. Vaccination file, Ebling Library, University of Wisconsin–Madison. Glycerin, also spelled "glycerine," is a "sweet, colorless preparation of glycerol used [today] as a moisturizing agent for chapped skin; in suppositories; and as a sweetening agent in drugs." Rothenberg and Chapman, *Dictionary of Medical Terms*, 209. How glycerin worked to

kill microorganisms is a mystery. Nevertheless, physicians and bacteriologists in the 1890s believed that glycerin worked to slowly kill or suppress the growth of extraneous bacteria in vaccine lymph and they thought it somehow weakened or killed the vaccinia virus if left to cure too long.

164. "Report of the Examination of Vaccines By the Pennsylvania State Board of Health," 136.

165. Mellish, "Vaccination," 821.

166. Webster, "Some Proofs," 141.

167. Cutler and Frisbie, *Variola and Vaccinia*, 51.

168. W. F. Elgin, MD, "Influence of Temperature on Vaccine Virus," *Public Health Papers and Reports* 27 (1901): 80, 83.

169. Elgin, "Some Facts," 7.

170. H. D. Geddings, in discussion of report on "Conference of State and Provincial Boards of Health of North America," *JAMA* 39 (1902): 1203.

171. Dr. C. W. Wooldridge, in discussion following Webster, "Some Proofs," 139. Italics in original.

172. Darling, "Vaccination," 201.

173. Rosenau, "Dry Points versus Glycerinated Virus," quotations on 639, 637, and 639.

174. M. J. Rosenau, MD, *The Bacteriological Impurities of Vaccine Virus: An Experimental Study*, Hygenic Laboratory Bulletin no. 12 (Washington, DC: Government Printing Office, 1903).

175. Abbott, "Vaccination and Its Results," 23. Abbott served as secretary from 1886 to 1905.

176. Massachusetts, *Acts of 1894*, chapter 355.

177. H. P. Walcott remarks on free distribution of antitoxin and vaccine lymph, *JMABH* 12 (1902): 130. Walcott served as chairman from 1886 to 1914.

178. George Groff, "Vaccine Production and Vaccination," *American Medicine* 2 (1901): 907–8, 907. Groff served also as First Secretary of the Superior Board of Health of Porto Rico and as an anatomy and physiology professor at Bucknell University.

179. Theobald Smith, MD, "The Preparation of Animal Vaccine," *BMSJ* 147 (1902): 197–201, 197.

180. "No More Anti-Toxin," *Boston Evening Transcript*, July 2, 1902, 1.

181. H. K. Mulford Company, advertisement, *Cleveland Medical Journal* 1 (1902), three pages, no page number.

182. Editorial, "Production of Vaccine Lymph," 25.

183. Peter H. Bryce, MD, "Discussion of Papers of Dr. Bryce and Dr. Bernaldez," *Public Health Paper and Reports* 27 (1902): 342.

184. Mellish, "Vaccination," 821.

185. Editorial in the *St. Paul Medical Journal*, quoted in "Editorial Echoes," *American Medicine* 3 (1902): 6.

186. Salvador Garciadiego, "The Only Certain Prophylaxis against Smallpox Is Human Vaccine Which, If Well Inoculated, Does Not Transmit Infectious Contagious nor Diathetic Disease," *Public Health Papers and Reports* 26 (1901): 84–86; Francisco De Bernaldez, "Human Vaccine as a Prophylactic of Smallpox: Its Advantages and Disadvantages," *Public Health Papers and Reports* 26 (1901): 87–91; and Eduardo

Liceaga, "The Jenner Vaccine Well Preserved and Carefully Propagated Is a Permanent Preservative against Smallpox," *Public Health Papers and Reports* 26 (1901): 92–97. See also Francisco De Bernaldez, "Remarks Intended to Show the Innocuous Character of Humanized Vaccine as a Preventative of Smallpox," *Public Health Papers and Reports* 27 (1902): 182–83.

187. Bryce, "Discussion of Papers of Dr. Bryce and Dr. Bernaldez," 341.

188. Chapin, *Municipal Sanitation in the United States*, 580 n. 4.

189. McCormack, "Value of State Control and Vaccination," 1434.

190. "Glycerinated Virus versus Dried Vaccine Virus," Editorial, *JAMA* 38 (1902): 1306.

191. Chapin, *Municipal Sanitation in the United States*, 582.

192. "Report of Committee on the Relative Immunizing Value," 41.

193. Massachusetts, *Acts of 1894*, chapter 355. Chapin, *Municipal Sanitation in the United States*, 581.

194. George Dock, MD, "Vaccine and Vaccination," *The Johns Hopkins University Bulletin* 15 (April 1904): 16.

195. Novak, *People's Welfare*, 1.

196. See chapter 4 for more discussion about the tetanus deaths and their effect on public anxiety about vaccination.

197. Federal Act of 1 July 1902, 32 Stat. L., 728. See Jonathan Liebenau, *Medical Science and Medical Industry: The Formation of the American Pharmaceutical Industry* (Baltimore, MD: The Johns Hopkins University Press, 1987), 79–90, for a discussion of how these incidents touched off an intense debate over culpability between two rival producers, H. K. Mulford and H. M. Alexander. See also J. M. Greene, "A Great Medical Scandal," *The Animals' Defender* 7 (November 1902): 28–29, for a discussion of the "mud-slinging" attacks between Mulford and other producers.

198. The Boston physician T. Talbot remarked in 1882 that when an 1873 petition for state supervision came before the public health committee, "a few persons personally interested in the production of bovine virus, opposed this petition so strongly that they got an adverse report from committee." See Beckwith, "Vaccination," 31.

199. Dr. Davenport, discussion following remarks of Dr. Walcott, *JMABH* 12 (October 1902): 138.

200. Mr. Coffey, reading an excerpt from a letter Canning sent to the *Boston Evening Transcript* sometime before 24 July 1902, discussion following remarks of Dr. Walcott, *JMABH* 12 (October 1902): 135.

201. Remarks of Dr. Walcott, *JMABH* 12 (October 1902): 129. Walcott hesitated for years to ask for legislation to fund antitoxin production because it involved making a remedy and distributing it for free, thus interfering with private enterprise. He relied on the regular appropriation from 1894 to 1903 to quietly fund antitoxin manufacture. See Rosenkrantz *Public Health and the State*, 114. Samuel Durgin, not Walcott, raised the issue of state production and distribution of free vaccine lymph time and again with the state legislature.

202. Massachusetts State Board of Health, *Thirty-Third Annual Report* (1902), xvi. Emphasis in the original.

203. Smith, "Preparation of Animal Vaccine," 200.

204. A. E. Miller, remark during a discussion of free distribution of antitoxin and vaccine lymph at the July 1902 quarterly meeting, *JMABH* 12 (1902): 133–34.

205. "Quarantine Question," Letter to the editor signed Pro Bono Publico, *Cambridge Chronicle*, 16 August 1902, 7.

206. Dr. Stevens, discussion during the July 1902 quarterly meeting of the Massachusetts Association of Boards of Health, *JMABH* 12 (1902): 137.

207. Commonwealth of Massachusetts, "April 14, 1902," *Journal of the Senate for the Year 1902* (Boston, 1902), 609. Durgin took the lead in procuring official funding for a state-run vaccine plant. He authored the bill and personally petitioned for it. See Rosenkrantz, *Public Health and the State*, 114, for Walcott's views. She ignores Durgin's role in her narrative, possibly because she did not look at legislative documents that clearly reveal Durgin as the prime mover on this legislation, a role contemporaries acknowledged at the time. See "Medical Legislation of 1903," *BMSJ* 149 (1903): 109–10.

208. Dr. Durgin, discussion following remarks of Dr. Walcott, *JMABH* 12 (October 1902): 136. Others also believed that druggists on the Public Health Committee had killed the bill. Lora Little reported on an article in the *Boston Record*, 21 April 1903, making a similar claim; see "Bills Killed By Druggists," *The Liberator* 3 (June 1903), 251.

209. "A Loathsome Danger," *Boston Daily Advertiser*, 25 April 1902, 4. Durgin may have had a hand in leaking this story to the press in order to stir up public support for state funding of vaccine production. A Boston paper agreed: "the bill was killed in committee, in the interest of the drug trade, it is said, the majority of the members being druggists." See "No More Anti-Toxin," *Boston Evening Transcript*, 2 July 1902, 1. Durgin had added a request for state funding of vaccine lymph production to the annual request for antitoxin funds. The whole bill thus failed on the vaccine question. Even the antivaccinationist Joshua D. Small observed that "the druggists maintain a strong lobby at the state house," a lobby "used to prevent Dr. Durgin's bill being introduced into the legislature." See Joshua D. Small, "Anti-Vaccination Department," *Our Home Rights* 2 (January 1903): 19.

210. The bill, S. 367, passed on 23 June 1903. See Commonwealth of Massachusetts, "Bills Enacted and Resolves Passed," *Journal of the Senate for the Year 1903* (Boston: Wright & Potter Printing Co., 1903), 1140. For Durgin's efforts and his opposition, see "Medical Legislation of 1903," 109–10.

211. Dr. Durgin, discussion during the July 1902 quarterly meeting of the Massachusetts Association of Boards of Health, *JMABH* 12 (1902): 136.

Chapter Three

1. S. H. Durgin, "Vaccination and Smallpox," *BMSJ* 146 (1902): 114. The article is a transcription of a talk he gave on 2 December 1901 before the Boston Society for Medical Improvement. See *BET*, 3 December 1901, 1.

2. Moses King singles out the smallpox epidemic as the trigger for reform. See *King's Handbook of Boston* (Boston: Moses King Corporation, 1889), 223.

3. Scanlon, "Public Health Movement in Boston," 46.

4. Biographical information based on "Samuel Holmes Durgin," *The National Cyclopedia of American Biography* (New York: James T. White & Co., 1906): 574. Durgin had a very long life (26 July 1839–3 June 1931), was twice married, and enjoyed

a pleasant retirement of travel after 1912. See "Samuel H. Durgin Dies at Age of 91," *BET*, 6 March 1931, 1. See also George A. Babbitt, "Retirement of Dr. Samuel Holmes Durgin from the Boston Board of Health," *American Journal of Public Health* 2 (May 1912): 384–85.

5. "Mayor Prince and the Board of Health," Editorial, *BMSJ* 75–76 (1877): 659. See Scanlon, "Public Health Movement in Boston," 38–48, for discussion of the creation of Boston's Board of Health in 1873.

6. Quotation from Whipple, *State Sanitation*, 1:16. See also Scanlon, "Public Health Movement in Boston," 76 n. 116.

7. See, for instance, Cassedy, *Charles V. Chapin*; Judith Walzer Leavitt, *Typhoid Mary: Captive to the Public's Health* (Boston: Beacon Press, 1996); and Nancy Tomes, *The Gospel of Germs: Men, Women, and the Microbe in American Life* (Cambridge, MA: Harvard University Press, 1998).

8. Chapin, *Municipal Sanitation in the United States*, 31.

9. Ibid., 36. See also his tribute to Durgin, "Doctor Samuel H. Durgin," *American Journal of Public Health* 2 (May 1912): 357–58. Durgin earned $4,500 per year. Only New York City ($6,000), Chicago ($5,000), and New Orleans ($5,000) paid more. Buffalo, New York, paid its health commissioner $4,000, but after that the salaries drop off quickly.

10. "Samuel H. Durgin" listing at 845 Boylston Street in *The Boston Directory* (Boston: Sampson, Murdock, Co., 1902), 2037. For Back Bay quotations, see Edwin M. Bacon, *Boston: A Guide Book to the City and Vicinity* (Boston: Ginn and Company, 1922 [1903]), 74–76.

11. "Wife of Dr. Durgin," Obituary for Mary Bradford Durgin, *BET*, 26 November 1906. For information about Trinity Church, see *King's Handbook of Boston*, 172–75.

12. "Samuel Holmes Durgin," *Medical Directory of Greater Boston* (Boston: Boston Medical Publishing Co., 1906), 88–89. "Samuel H. Durgin Dies at Age of 91," 1.

13. Scanlon, "Public Health Movement in Boston," 76–77.

14. The *Journal of the Massachusetts Association of Boards of Health* eventually became the *American Journal of Public Health*. First established in 1901, in 1904 it became the *American Journal of Public Hygiene and Journal of the Massachusetts Association of Boards of Health*. In 1910 it changed its name again to become the *American Journal of Public Hygiene*. In 1911 it became the *American Journal of Public Health*.

15. C.-E. A. Winslow, "A Half-Century of the Massachusetts Public Health Association," *American Journal of Public Health and The Nation's Health* 30 (April 1940): 327.

16. Winslow, "A Half-Century," 327. The ship was most likely the *Kansas*, which arrived from Liverpool on 15 January 1902 with one smallpox death at sea. Everyone was put into quarantine, but the vessel was allowed to leave for its return trip after only six days. When it arrived back at Liverpool, it had eight smallpox cases on board. Durgin received a bit of criticism for this decision. See "Eight Cases on Board," *BG*, 7 February 1902, 4.

17. Sam Bass Warner, Jr., *Streetcar Suburbs: The Process of Growth in Boston, 1870–1900*, 2nd ed. (Cambridge, MA: Harvard University Press, 1978 [1962]), quotation on 2. See also Albert Benedict Wolfe, *The Lodging House Problem in Boston* (Boston: Houghton, Mifflin, 1906).

18. Robert Woods and Albert J. Kennedy, *The Zone of Emergence*, ed. Sam Bass Warner, Jr. (Cambridge, MA: Harvard University Press, 1962), 55. The research for *Zone* was done between 1907 and 1914 at the behest of Kennedy and Woods, both important social workers in Boston, but never published until 1962. Each chapter consists of a detailed socioeconomic-political-cultural study of each Boston and Cambridge district.

19. Woods and Kennedy, *Zone of Emergence*, 40.

20. Thomas B. Shea, "Smallpox and Vaccination," *JMABH* 12 (April 1902): 19.

21. Boston Board of Health, *Thirtieth Annual Report for 1901*, 44.

22. "Six New Cases of Smallpox," *BET*, 14 October 1901, 2. Smallpox takes twelve days to incubate, whereas vaccination takes just nine to produce immunity. See Cutler and Frisbie, *Variola and Vaccinia*, 47.

23. "Six New Cases of Smallpox," 2.

24. "Smallpox in Boston," *BET*, 19 August 1901, 5.

25. Boston Board of Health, *Thirtieth Annual Report for 1901*, 45.

26. "Smallpox in Boston," 5.

27. Quotations from "No New Cases of Smallpox," *BET*, 20 August 1901, 1; "A Smallpox Epidemic," *BET*, 3 September 1901, 1. See also "Smallpox in Boston," 5; "More Smallpox Cases," *BET*, 28 August 1901, 8; "Another Case of Smallpox," *BET*, 29 August 1901; "Two More Smallpox Cases," *BET*, 31 August 1901; "Two More Smallpox Patients," *BET*, 4 September 1901, 2; and "Roxbury People Aroused," *BET*, 6 September 1901, 2.

28. "Roxbury People Aroused," 2.

29. Boston Board of Health, *Thirtieth Annual Report for 1901*, 53.

30. "Roxbury People Aroused," 2.

31. "Five Schools Closed," *BET*, 11 September 1901, 10; and "City Schools Opened: Few Cramped for Room," *BP*, 12 September 1901. See also "No School for Roxbury Pupils," *BP*, 11 September 1901; and "The Smallpox Situation in Boston," *BMSJ* 145 (1901): 286–87.

32. Dr. Palmer's remarks in discussion of isolation hospitals, *JMABH* 12 (October 1902): 149.

33. "New Cases Recorded," *BET*, 11 November 1901, 1.

34. Massachusetts State Board of Health, circular issued June 1900, in *Thirty-Second Annual Report of the State Board of Health of Massachusetts* (Boston, 1901), xxi.

35. "Plucky Nurse Girl in Medford Pesthouse," *BP*, 13 September 1901.

36. Draper testimony before the Joint Public Health Committee hearing on abolition of compulsory vaccination bill, in "More Protest against Repeal of Law," *BG*, 3 February 1902, 4.

37. Samuel H. Durgin, "Discussion of Papers of Drs. Doty and Iglesias," *Public Health Papers and Reports* 26 (1901): 248. Durgin was defending A. H. Doty's contention that in his "experience of twenty years" with the New York City health department he had observed that "infectious diseases are not commonly transmitted in the clothing actually worn by well persons." See A. H. Doty letter in the discussion, 252.

38. H. M. Bracken, "Discussion of Papers of Drs. Doty and Iglesias," *Public Health Papers and Reports* 26 (1901): 244.

39. Moore, "Smallpox," 400.

40. Testimony of Dr. Reginald H. Fitz, Joint Committee on Public Health hearing on compulsory vaccination, reported in "Compulsory Vaccination," *BET*, 31 January 1902, 6. See also *BG*, 1 February 1901, 4. Fitz coined the term "appendicitis" and recommended surgical treatment for it. He was regarded as one of the top physicians in America. See Morris Vogel, *The Invention of the Modern Hospital: Boston 1870–1900* (Chicago: University of Chicago Press, 1980), 61–2.

41. Shea testimony before the Joint Public Health Committee hearing on compulsory vaccination in "Compulsory Vaccination," *BET*, 31 January 1902, 6; and "Vaccination Opposed," *BET*, 4 February 1902, 3.

42. "Vaccination Opposed," 3.

43. "Smallpox Scourge," *CC*, 21 June 1902, 4.

44. "Mayor McNamee Scores a Point," *CC*, 12 July 1902, 1, 4.

45. "The Revival of Smallpox," *CC*, 12 July 1902, 4.

46. "Three Strong Letters against Quarantining," *CC*, 19 July 1902, 1.

47. Mr. Bodwell's remarks in discussion of infectious diseases, *JMABH* 12 (October 1902): 160.

48. "Every Precaution at Wakefield," *BET*, 9 October 1901, 9.

49. "One Death in Malden," *BER*, 13 February 1902, 2.

50. "Pfeiffer Case Excites Bedford," *BER*, 17 February 1902, 8.

51. "Six New Cases of Smallpox," *BET*, 14 October 1901, 2.

52. Massachusetts State Board of Health, *Thirty-Fourth Annual Report of the State Board of Health of Massachusetts* (Boston, 1903), 580.

53. Dr. Gardner T. Swartz [possibly Swarts, because he is listed with both spellings], comments following Thomas B. Shea's talk, "Smallpox and Vaccination," *JMABH* 12 (April 1902): 38–41, 41.

54. James C. Coffey, comments following Thomas B. Shea's talk, "Smallpox and Vaccination," *JMABH* 12 (April 1902): 41–46, 43.

55. Samuel H. Durgin and James Coffey, remarks in discussion of infectious diseases, *JMABH* 12 (October 1902): 159–60.

56. Alice M. Adams, Letter to the Editor, *BG*, 29 November 1901, quoted in Joseph M. Greene, "The Vaccination Scourge," *The Animals Defender* 7 (January 1902): 23.

57. "One Case Was Fatal," *BET*, 28 October 1901, 1.

58. "Seven New Cases," *BET*, 29 October 1901, 3.

59. Samuel Durgin, answering questions at a meeting of the Massachusetts Association of Boards of Health, 30 January 1902, *JMABH* 12 (April 1902): 48.

60. "Smallpox in Egleston Square," *BET*, 1 November 1901, 9.

61. "Health Board Urges All to Be Vaccinated," *BP*, 19 November 1901, 4.

62. "Dr. Durgin Warns as to Spread of Smallpox," *BP*, 30 October 1901, 8.

63. Morse, "Recent Smallpox Epidemic," 47. Morse noted that Massachusetts had 5,606 cases with 1,029 deaths over the course of thirteen months in 1872–73, an 18.4 percent death rate. Boston experienced a slightly higher death rate of 28.4 percent in 1872 and 27.3 percent in 1873. See Boston Board of Health, Table XII, "Cases Reported, and Deaths from Smallpox, Diphtheria, Scarlet Fever, Typhoid Fever, and Measles, with Percentages," *Thirty-First Annual Report of the Health Department of the City of Boston* (Boston, 1903), 13.

64. Joseph E. Duxbury, "Variola, or Smallpox," *BMSJ* 146 (1902): 165.

65. "The Argument Relative to Vaccination," *BMSJ* 145 (1901): 632.

66. Charles Good, "The Vexed Question of Vaccination," *American Medicine* 2 (1901): 778.

67. Frederick H. Dillingham, "Some Observations in Regard to Smallpox," *American Medicine* 4 (1902): 493–98, 493.

68. See Willrich, *Pox*, 41–76, for a description of Marine Hospital Service work during this pandemic in the southern states.

69. "Dr. Durgin Warns as to Spread of Smallpox," 8.

70. "The Diagnosis of Smallpox," Editorial, *JAMA* 34 (1900): 368–69; T. J. Happel, "Pseudo (?) or Modified (?) Smallpox," *JAMA* 35 (1900): 600–607; Happel, "A Further Study of Pseudo, or Modified Smallpox (?)," *JAMA* 37 (1901): 295–98; H. M. Bracken, "Pseudo, Modified, or True Smallpox—Which Is It?" *JAMA* 35 (1900): 608–10; Jay F. Schamberg, "The Diagnosis of Smallpox," *American Medicine* 2 (1901): 899–903; Heman Spalding, "Differential Diagnosis between Chickenpox and Smallpox," *JAMA* 36 (1901): 497–500; Albert Soiland, "Notes on One Hundred and Fifty Cases of Smallpox in Private Practice," *JAMA* 37 (1901): 912–13; Jay F. Schamberg, "The Diagnosis of Smallpox," *JAMA* 38 (1902): 215–17; J. D. Brummall, "The Epidemic of So-Called Smallpox," *American Medicine* 3 (1902): 180; Duxbury, "Variola, or Smallpox," 165–67; "The Early Recognition of Smallpox," Editorial, *JAMA* 39 (1902): 83–84; John T. Bullard, "Smallpox: Its Diagnosis," *BMSJ* 147 (1902): 207–10; Frederick H. Dillingham, "Some Observations in regard to Smallpox," *American Medicine* 4 (1902): 493–98; John C. Hancock, "Some Aspects of the Present Smallpox Epidemic," *Medicine* 8 (1902): 807–18; and William L. Somerset, "The Course and Diagnosis of Variola—Based on Its Last Outbreak in New York City," *New York Medical Journal and Philadelphia Medical Journal* 78 (1903): 989–91.

71. Happel, "Pseudo (?) or Modified (?) Smallpox"; Bracken, "Pseudo, Modified, or True Smallpox"; and Happel, "A Further Study of Pseudo, or Modified Smallpox (?)."

72. Among the papers read were Heman Spalding, "Diagnosis of Mild and Irregular Smallpox as Found in the Present Outbreak in the United States," *JAMA* 37 (1901): 302–5; W. L. Beebe, "Smallpox—Old and New," *JAMA* 37 (1901): 299; Frederick Leavitt, "The Distinguishing Characteristics between Mild Discrete Smallpox and Chicken-Pox," *JAMA* 37 (1901): 305–7; H. M. Bracken, "Variola," *JAMA* 37 (1901): 307–10; and discussion of these papers in *JAMA* 37 (1901): 310–14.

73. "Under Grave Disadvantages," *BET*, 9 November 1901, 3; see also "Filling Smallpox Hospital," *BET*, 8 November 1901, 3, for reports of misdiagnosis.

74. "Two New Cases," *BET*, 12 November 1901, 5.

75. Case 1, "Record of Visits Made to 75 Cities and Towns By the Medical Inspector, for the Purpose of Investigating 107 Cases Suspected of Being Small-pox, during 1901," *Thirty-Third Annual Report of the State Board of Health of Massachusetts for the Year 1901* (Boston, 1902), 592.

76. "Under Grave Disadvantages," 3.

77. "Health Board Urges All to Be Vaccinated," 4. Over a year later, he would attribute most of the difficulty he encountered in containing the epidemic to "a large number of mild, unrecognized cases of smallpox . . . going about from place to place" coupled with "a large percentage of unprotected people exposed to these unrecognized cases." Boston Board of Health, "Smallpox," *Thirty-First Annual Report for 1902*, 36.

78. C. S. Carr, "Smallpox Quarantine," *Medical Talk for the Home* 3 (August 1902): 393.

79. See Leavitt, *Healthiest City*, 76–121.

80. See Charles Rosenburg, *The Care of Strangers: The Rise of America's Hospital System* (New York: Basic Books, 1987); Rosemary Stevens, *In Sickness and in Wealth: American Hospitals in the Twentieth Century* (New York: Basic Books, 1989), 3–80; and Vogel, *Invention of the Modern Hospital.*

81. "Pest-houses," in "American News and Notes," *American Medicine* 3 (1902): 377.

82. "More Smallpox Hospitals," Editorial, *Boston Traveler*, 11 January 1902, reprinted in Immanuel Pfeiffer, "Dr. Pfeiffer's Statement," *Our Home Rights* 2 (February–April 1902): 36. Joseph M. Greene identifies the source of the editorial in his "Notes on Vaccination," *The Animals' Defender* 7 (February 1902): 12.

83. Michael Kelly, "Smallpox: Its Medical Treatment," *BMSJ* 147 (1902): 237.

84. Massachusetts Medical Society Meeting, 10 June 1902. Discussion following Kelly, "Smallpox," 240.

85. "Under Grave Disadvantages," 3.

86. "Smallpox Record Grows," *BET*, 18 November 1901, 14; also "Mrs. G. A. Flynn a Victim," *BG*, 19 November 1901, 14.

87. "Health Board Urges All to Be Vaccinated, 4.

88. "Smallpox Record Grows," 14.

89. Boston Board of Health, *Thirtieth Annual Report for 1901*, 44.

90. Quoted material in "Smallpox Record Grows," 14; See also "Virus Squad Out," *BG*, 18 November 1901, 7. For forcible vaccination, see "Tramps Object to Vaccination," *BP*, 26 January 1902, 8; and Joseph M. Greene, "Facts about Vaccination," *The Animals' Defender* 7 (December 1901): 23. See chapter 8 below for a complete description of forced vaccinations during health department vaccination sweeps in 1901–2.

91. "Don't Get Scared," *BP*, 22 November 1901, 6.

92. "Smallpox Record Grows," 14.

93. "Twenty New Cases," *BET*, 26 November 1901, 2.

94. "New Cases Reported," *BET*, 19 November 1901, 1.

95. "Six New Smallpox Cases," *BP*, 8 December 1901; also "Lull in Vaccination," *BG*, 8 December 1901, 2.

96. Boston Board of Health, *Thirtieth Annual Report for 1901*, 45; quotation from "Smallpox Decreasing," *BG*, 26 December 1901, 2. This law, passed originally in 1855, authorized local boards of health to require vaccination and revaccination whenever they deemed it necessary of all city or town inhabitants under penalty of a five-dollar fine. The state board of health did not have such authority to demand vaccination—only local boards could call for a general compulsory vaccination. As of 1901, the law had been amended just once to allow for the exemption of children certified by a physician as too weak for vaccination. Revised Statutes of Massachusetts, 1855, chapter 414; 1894, chapter 515.

97. Cambridge Board of Health, "Report," in *Annual Reports Made to the City Council for the Year 1902* (Cambridge, 1903), 641–63, 642.

98. "Smallpox Rate Small," Editorial, *CC*, 18 January 1902, 5; and Boston Board of Health, *Thirtieth Annual Report for 1901*, 44.

99. Spencer was born in North Kingston, Rhode Island, on 4 February 1833. He died 19 January 1903 of a heart attack. See "E. Edwin Spencer," *JAMA* 40 (1903): 392; and "Dr. E. Edwin Spencer Dies Very Suddenly," *CC*, 24 January 1903, 3.

100. At the time Spencer attended the Eclectic Medical Institute, the school possessed both a distinguished faculty and impressive building but tottered on the verge of institutional disintegration when rival factions openly warred for control of the school. See Ronald L. Numbers, "The Making of an Eclectic Physician: Joseph M. McElhinney and the Eclectic Medical Institute of Cincinnati," *Bulletin of the History of Medicine* 47 (1973): quotes on 157, 155. My thanks to Ron Numbers for providing this source and welcome enlightenment about the history of eclecticism. Also see John S. Haller, *Medical Protestants: The Eclectics in American Medicine, 1825–1939* (Carbondale: Southern Illinois University Press, 1994); William G. Rothstein, *American Physicians in the Nineteenth Century: From Sects to Science* (Baltimore, MD: The Johns Hopkins University Press, 1972); and Rothstein, "The Botanical Movements and Orthodox Medicine," in Gevitz, *Other Healers*, 47–51. For older accounts, see Frederick C. Waite, "American Sectarian Medical Colleges before the Civil War," *Bulletin of the History of Medicine* 19 (1946): 148–66; and Alex Berman, "Neo-Thomsonianism in the United States," *Journal of the History of Medicine* 11 (1956): 133–55.

101. Worcester Medical Institution was founded in 1850 as an eclectic medical college in Worcester, Massachusetts. See Isabel R. A. Currier, "A Worcester College That Grew Up in Waltham," *Worcester Sunday Telegram*, 10 December 1933, citing Charles Nutt, *History of Worcester and Its People*, 4 vols. (New York: Lewis Historical Publishing Co., 1919). Dr. Robert Walker Geddes was Spencer's brother-in-law, married to his sister, Alice.

102. "Dr. E. Edwin Spencer Dies Very Suddenly," 3. See also obituary notices in *The Eclectic Review* 6 (1903): 32, 54–55.

103. "A Good Chance for an Example," Editorial, *CC*, 24 January 1903, 2.

104. "Dr. E. Edwin Spencer Dies Very Suddenly," 3.

105. William Rodman Peabody, Letter, *CC*, 24 January 1903, 3. See "Only Two Members of the Board of Health," *CC*, 8 February 1902, 9, 13, for identification of Peabody's profession and story about the expiration of his term on the Board of Health.

106. Peabody, Letter, *CC*, 24 January 1903, 3. See also Dr. Farnham, Letter, *CC*, 24 January 1903, 3.

107. Spencer probably was vaccinated, although he never specifically mentioned that he was. He always strongly supported vaccination. He also was recently widowed, losing his wife, Annie E. C. White, in January 1901. See Almira Larkin White, ed., *White Family Quarterly: An Illustrated Genealogical Magazine*, 3 vols. (Haverhill, MA: Almira Larkin White, 1903), 1 (April 1903): 38–39.

108. Peabody, Letter, *CC*, 24 January 1903, 3.

109. Dr. Farnham, Letter, *CC*, 24 January 1903, 3.

110. "Dr. E. Edwin Spencer Dies Very Suddenly," 3.

111. Cambridge Board of Health, *Annual Report for 1902* (Cambridge, 1903), 641–63, 642. See 649 for rental cost.

112. Ibid., 644. The stations vaccinated 5,793 people in 1901 and 2,745 individuals in 1902.

113. Cambridge Board of Health, *Annual Report for 1902*, 641–63, 642–43.

114. Letter to Mayor McNamee, 25 June 1902, *CC*, 28 June 1902, 4.

115. Massachusetts State Board of Health, "Smallpox," in *Thirty-Third Annual Report* (for 1901), xi.

116. Cambridge Board of Health, "Report," in *Annual Reports Made to the City Council for the Year 1901* (Cambridge, 1902), 432. See also Massachusetts State Board of Health, "Health of Towns—Cambridge," *Thirty-Third Annual Report* (for 1901), 571.

117. Smallpox cases almost doubled from twelve for January to twenty-three cases by late February. Cambridge Board of Health, *Annual Report for 1902*, 657.

118. "Seventeen Physicians at Work," *BET*, 8 March 1902, 3.

119. "Compulsory Vaccination," *CC*, 8 March 1902, 5.

120. Cambridge Board of Health, *Annual Report for 1902*, 643–44; Cambridge population from Massachusetts State Board of Health, *Thirty-Fourth Annual Report* (1903), 553.

121. Cambridge Board of Health, *Annual Report for 1902*, 643–44. Total 1902 population was 96,334.

Chapter Four

1. "Vaccinators Often Deceived," *Boston Daily Advertiser*, 13 February 1902, 6.

2. C. S. Carr, "Good Common Sense," reporting on Dillingham in *Medical Talk for the Home*, 2 (July 1901): 311.

3. William R. Fisher, "School Vaccinations," *American Medicine* 4 (1902): 508.

4. McCollom, "Vaccinations," 206.

5. Ibid., 203.

6. Boston Board of Health, *Thirtieth Annual Report for 1901*, 53.

7. *Massachusetts Year Book and Business Directory* (Worcester: F. S. Blanchard & Company, 1901), 1242, gives the student population as 90,144 with 1,995 teachers.

8. Testimony before the Joint Committee on Public Health; see "Anti-Vaccination," *BET*, 19 February 1902, 3.

9. "Roxbury People Aroused," *BET*, 6 September 1901, 2.

10. Testimony before the Joint Committee on Public Health, in "Doctors in Protest," *Boston Herald*, 4 February 1902, 3. See also "More Protest against Repeal of Law," 4.

11. Boston Board of Health, *Thirtieth Annual Report for 1901*, 43.

12. Ibid., 45. Durgin did not provide the source for his assertion of three hundred thousand private vaccinations. He gave several estimates that varied to the newspapers in late 1901 but never explained where he got his information.

13. Table 1, "Population of Cities and Large Towns Estimated for 1901," and "Vaccinations Performed at Public Cost, 1901," Massachusetts State Board of Health, *Thirty-Third Annual Report* (1902), 544, 558.

14. Cambridge Board of Health, "Report," *Annual Reports for 1902*, 644. See discussion in chapter 3.

15. Theresa Bannan, MD, "The Vaccination Question," *New York Medical Journal* 76 (1902): 230. Paper given at the Syracuse Academy of Medicine, 20 May 1902.

16. Durgin interview, in "Under Grave Disadvantages," 3.

17. "Editorial Echoes," *American Medicine* 3 (4 January 1902): 6.

18. Durgin, "Vaccination and Smallpox," 115.

19. "'Major' Taylor Will Try for Bicycle Championship of World with Frank Kramer," *BP*, 21 July 1901, 7. See also "Cycle Whirlwind, Major Taylor," *BP*, 7 July 1901, 7.

20. "Langtry a Victim," *BG*, 1 December 1901, 24.

21. "The Vaccinated," *BP*, 1 December 1901, 18.

22. "A Vaccine Point," *BET*, 13 February 1902, 6.

23. "Small-Pox Cure and Preventative," advertisement, *Our Home Rights* 1 (November 1901): 45.

24. "For Vaccinated Arms," advertisement, *BP*, 16 December 1901, 2.

25. "Twenty New Cases," 2.

26. "May or May Not Be Vaccinated," *BET*, 19 November 1901, 1.

27. "Only Fourteen Cases," *BET*, 27 November 1901, 3.

28. "All Will Have Sore Arms," *BET*, 15 November 1901, 5.

29. Ibid.

30. Alex McAllister, "The Cause of Sore Arms during the Recent Vaccinations," Paper Read at the Medical Society of the State of New Jersey, reported in *American Medicine* 4 (1902): 88.

31. Bannan, "Vaccination Question," 230.

32. Russell, "A Case of Fatal Vaccination Infection," 35.

33. "American News and Notes," *American Medicine* 4 (1902): 997. See also "Victory over Vaccination," *The Liberator* 2 (January 1903): 100.

34. "Vaccination or Filth," Medical News, *JAMA* 38 (1902): 593. The item describes the case in detail, noting that physician accused the mother's "filthy hygiene" as the cause of the infection. See also "American News and Notes," *American Medicine* 3 (1902): 297; and J. M. Greene, "Legal Blood-Poisoning in Massachusetts," *The Animals' Defender* 7 (March 1902): 36, for another mention of the case.

35. "American News and Notes," *American Medicine* 4 (1902): 922. Sadly the physician erred in his judgment of the risks his patient's family ran. The mother died from smallpox and every member of her family who had washed their vaccinations contracted it.

36. Harvey P. Towle, "Vaccination Eruptions," *BMSJ* 147 (1902): 271.

37. Greene, "A Great Medical Scandal," 31.

38. Immanuel Pfeiffer, "The Fruit of Vaccination," *Our Home Rights* 1 (November 1901): 9–10.

39. Joseph M. Greene, "Eighty Victims," *The Liberator* 3 (April 1903): 212.

40. Joseph M. Greene, "Some Fruits of Vaccination," *The Animals' Defender* 6 (December 1901): 31. Greene, "Eighty Victims," 212, 213. Greene edited *The Animal's Defender*, a monthly publication of the New England Anti-vivisection Society. Greene took advantage of his position to comment on vaccination, the Boston Board of Health, and to report accounts of adverse vaccination effects in his journal.

41. R. Swinburne Clymer, *Vaccination Brought Home to You* (Terre Haute, IN: Press of G. H. Hebb, 1904), 54–55, for a detailed account of both children. Clymer probably learned about them from Pfeiffer when he joined Pfeiffer's practice as his assistant in early 1902.

42. The Infant's Hospital, 33 Blossom St., Boston. See Greene, "Eighty Victims," 212.

43. See Pfeiffer, "Fruit of Vaccination," 9; and Greene, "Eighty Victims," 213.

44. Greene, "Eighty Victims," 212.

45. All quotations except Hatch from "Vaccination Opposed," 1902, 3; see also "Last Arguments," *BG*, 4 February 1902, 9 (Eve.); Hatch quotation from "Hearing Over," *BG*, 5 February 1902, 4.

46. "Many Victims," *Our Home Rights* 1 (December 1901): 16.

47. Thomas P. Lohan, Letter dated 30 November 1901, *Our Home Rights* 1 (November 1901): 37.

48. Letter from an unidentified employee of the Boston Elevated Railway Company, quoted in *Our Home Rights* 1 (October 1901): 17–18.

49. Greene first advertised for affidavits in late 1901. See "A Request," *The Animals' Defender* 6 (December, 1901): 26.

50. Greene, "Notes on Vaccination," 16, for first mention of Hollis; quote from Greene, "Eighty Victims," 213.

51. Greene "Vaccination Scourge," 26; and Greene, "Eighty Victims," 212.

52. Greene, "Legal Blood-Poisoning in Massachusetts," 36; and Greene, "Eighty Victims," *The Liberator* 3 (May 1903): 241.

53. Ibid.

54. Greene, "Eighty Victims," 211.

55. Greene, "Legal Blood-Poisoning in Massachusetts," 36; and Greene, "Eighty Victims," 241.

56. J. M. Greene, "Law versus Order," *The Animals' Defender* 7 (August 1902): 21; and Greene, "Eighty Victims," *The Liberator* 3 (June 1903): 271.

57. "Compulsory Vaccination," Editorial, *Boston Courier*, 8 February 1902.

58. Greene, "Facts about Vaccination," 21.

59. "Experts Favor Vaccination," *BP*, 4 February 1902, 2.

60. Martin Friedrich, "How We Rid Cleveland of Smallpox," *Cleveland Medical Journal* 1 (February 1902): 77–89. See also "The Confession of a Vaccinator," *Medical Talk for the Home* 3 (June 1902): 295. Although Freidrich claimed that a formaldehyde disinfection campaign worked to control Cleveland's 1901 smallpox epidemic, he apparently began it when "the epidemic was already subsiding, in fact nearly extinct." See "How Cleveland Was Rid of Smallpox?," *Cleveland Medical Journal* 1 (September 1902): 472.

61. Joseph M. Greene briefly noted Friedrich's decision in "Vaccination Stopped," *The Animals' Defender* 6 (September, 1901): 10.

62. "Vaccination Pro and Con," Letter from Charles E. Page to the Editor, *BER*, 10 February 1902, 8.

63. Benjamin O. Flower, "How Cleveland Stamped Out Smallpox," Topics of the Times, *The Arena* 27 (1902): 426–27.

64. Joseph McFarland, "Tetanus and Vaccination—An Analytical Study of Ninety-Five Cases of This Rare Complication," *Medicine* 8 (June 1902): 442; paper read originally on 28 March 1902 at the annual meeting of the American Association of Pathologists and Bacteriologists.

65. "Tetanus after Vaccination," Editorial, *JAMA* 38 (1902): 769.

66. McFarland, "Tetanus and Vaccination," 443–44.

67. Friedrich, "How We Rid Cleveland of Smallpox," 79. Antivaccinationists quoted Friedrich extensively, making much of his disinfection campaign. See *Medical Talk for the* Home 3 (October 1901): xi; and Charles F. Nichols, *A Blunder in Poison* (Boston: Rockwell and Churchill Press, 1902), 22–28.

68. Friedrich interview with *The Medical Visitor* (n.d.), quoted in "the Trouble with Vaccination," *Our Home Rights* 1 (December 1901): 10.

69. McFarland, "Tetanus and Vaccination," 450.

70. Excerpt from an editorial in the *Cleveland Journal of Medicine*, reprinted in "Editorial Echoes," *American Medicine* 2 (28 September 1901): 474. The *Cleveland Journal of Medicine* became the *Cleveland Medical Journal* in 1902.

71. "Tetanus following Vaccination," American News and Notes, *American Medicine* 2 (1901): 51. Joseph M. Greene also commented on her death in "Some Vaccination Triumphs," *The Animals' Defender* 6 (September 1901): 14.

72. "Tetanus from Vaccination," *Medical Talk for the Home* 3 (December 1901): xv; from a news item originally placed in *American Medicine*.

73. "Tetanus from Diphtheria-Antitoxin," Editorial, *American Medicine* 2 (1901): 759; "The Coroner's Verdict in St. Louis," Editorial, *American Medicine* 2 (1901): 842. Several civil suits arose from these tragedies. In one case, a jury found the former city bacteriologist Dr. A. Ravold negligent, penalizing him $1,000. See "American News and Notes," *American Medicine* 4 (1902): 997.

74. "Army of Parents Fight School to Save Their 4,000 Children from Lockjaw," *New York Journal*, 16 November 1901, reprinted in *Our Home Rights* 1 (November 1901): 1–2.

75. "Investigation of Antitoxin and Vaccine Virus," News Item, *BMSJ* 146 (1902): 124.

76. Editorial Points, *BG*, 19 November 1901, 6. See also "Alarmed By Tetanus Cases," and "Tetanus in Philadelphia," *BG*, 19 November 1901, 3.

77. Robert N. Willson, "Tetanus Appearing in the Course of Vaccinia: Report of a Case," *American Medicine* 2 (1901): 904. Willis S. Cooke, "Report of a Case of Tetanus following Vaccination," *New York Medical Journal* 77 (1903): 62. On 61, Cooke cites medical authority that estimated the death rate "at about 80 per cent," although he noted that use of tetanus antitoxin recently seemed to be reducing that rate to about 40 percent.

78. "Tetanus and Vaccination," Editorial, *American Medicine* 2 (1901): 840.

79. Willson, "Tetanus Appearing," 903.

80. "Cases of Tetanus following Vaccination," Editorial, *American Medicine* 2 (1901): 801.

81. "Life History of the Tetanus Bacillus," Editorial, *American Medicine* 2 (1901): 840.

82. "Tetanus and Vaccination in Camden, N.J.," Medical Notes, *BMSJ* 145 (1901): 635.

83. Alex McAllister, "Cause of Tetanus following Vaccination," Paper read before the Medical Society of the State of New Jersey, reported in *American Medicine* 4 (1902): 89.

84. Clymer claimed to quote an editorial in *Pennsylvania Grit*, 1 December 1901, in *Our Home Rights* 1 (December 1901): 2. There is an editorial, "Vaccination vs. Lockjaw," *Pennsylvania Grit*, 1 December 1901, 3, which does not contain the language quoted by Clymer.

85. "Tetanus after Vaccination," 768.

86. "Tetanus following Vaccination," American News and Notes, *American Medicine* 2 (1901): 889.

87. Lyman Allen, "Two Cases of Tetanus following Vaccination," *BMSJ* 146 (1902): 545.

88. Cooke, "Report of a Case of Tetanus," 62.

89. Willson, "Tetanus Appearing," 905.

90. Willson, "An Analysis of Fifty-Two Cases of Tetanus following Vaccinia, with Reference to the Source of Infection: 1839–1902," Parts 1 and 2, JAMA 38 (1902): 1150, 1229–31.

91. I am indebted here to Jonathan Liebenau's discussion of Joseph McFarland and the involvement of H. K. Mulford, Parke-Davis, and H. M. Alexander vaccines in the Camden tetanus deaths, in Liebenau, *Medical Science and Medical Industry*, 80–90. Liebenau found the names of the vaccine producers in McFarland's unpublished papers archived at the College of Physicians in Philadelphia.

92. McFarland, "Tetanus and Vaccination," 441. Various medical journals commented on McFarland's article. See, for instance, "Tetanus and Vaccination," Editorial, *BMSJ* 146 (1902): 639–40.

93. Joseph McFarland, "The Relationship of Tetanus to Vaccination," Paper given at the 2nd Annual Meeting of the American Association of Pathologists and Bacteriologists, 28 March 1902, *BMSJ* 146 (1902): 442.

94. McFarland, "Tetanus and Vaccination," 449.

95. See Liebenau for detailed discussion, *Medical Science and Medical Industry*, 80–90. He asserts that H. K. Mulford, H. M. Alexander, and Parke-Davis ultimately joined together to lobby Congress to pass the Biologics Control Act in order to suppress smaller rival vaccine farms.

96. Rosenau, *Bacteriological Impurities of Vaccine Virus*, 50.

97. *Boston Journal*, 31 December 1901, quoted in Greene, "Eighty Victims," 211.

98. "Annie Caswell Dies as a Result of Vaccination," *Cambridge Democrat*, 4 January 1902, 7.

99. "Hearing Over," *BG*, 5 February 1902, 4.

100. Greene, "Eighty Victims," 211; and "Lockjaw from Vaccination," *BER*, 1 January 1902, 7.

101. "Lockjaw from Vaccination," 7; "Nantucket Lightship Captain's Ordeal," *BER*, 8 January 1902, 2; Untitled news item describing Capt. Jorgenson's return to his lightship, *Boston Daily Advertiser*, 12 February 1902, 4.

102. J. M. Greene, "Lockjaw and Vaccination," *The Animals' Defender* 6 (August 1901): 15–16, reporting on the lockjaw death of Charles Mara on 11 July 1901; and Greene, "Vaccination Stopped," 10.

103. Greene, "Some Vaccination Triumphs," 14, describing the death of Maria McGinley as well as that of Ellen Lamey of Chester, Pennsylvania.

104. Greene, "Facts about Vaccination"; Greene, "The Legitimate Result: Infant Slaughter in St. Louis," *The Animals' Defender* 6 (December 1901): 20–30; Greene, "Vaccination Scourge"; and Greene, "Notes on a Form of Animal and Human Vivisection Called Vaccination," *The Animals' Defender* 7 (February 1902): 11–17.

105. J. M. Greene, "Law versus Order," *The Animals' Defender* 7 (August 1902): 22; and Greene, "Eighty Victims," 272.

106. Greene, "Facts about Vaccination," 21.

107. "Pres. Eliot's Views," *BG*, 10 February 1902, 9.

108. "Dr. Galvin's Offer," *BP*, 21 November 1901, 4.

109. Bactil Chemical Company, "Vaccination: Some Important Facts," *BP*, 2 December 1901, 1.

110. See also Bactil, "Smallpox Spreading, Board of Health Alarmed," *BP*, 3 December 1901, 1; and "That Vaccinated Arm," *BP*, 5 December 1901, 1.

111. "State Should Make Virus," *BET*, 3 December 1901, 1.

112. "Tuberculous Cows as Sources of Vaccine Lymph," Editorial, *American Medicine* 3 (1902): 847.

113. Durgin believed more than two hundred thousand needed vaccinations, "Six New Smallpox Cases," 4. See also "Vaccination Stations Closed," Medical Notes, *BMSJ* 145 (1901): 690.

114. Several legislators noticed the convenient timing of the order and questioned Durgin rather harshly on the matter during hearings held in late January 1902. See chapter 7.

115. "Durgin Is Very Reassuring," *BER*, 2 January 1902, 1. The *Record* reports the cases as "the Cambridge case of tetanus after vaccination and the Brockton case." Christina Jorgenson lived in Braintree and Annie Caswell was a child living in Cambridge. Brockton might be an error, the reporter meaning instead Braintree, since the companion editorial refers to both cases correctly.

116. "Durgin Is Very Reassuring," 1.

117. Editorial, *BER*, 2 January 1902, 4.

118. Editorial, *BER*, 23 June 1902, 4. I do not know who the Belmont case is.

119. "Vaccination vs. Lockjaw," Editorial, *Pennsylvania Grit*, 1 December 1901, 3.

120. "Sore Arms on the Brookline Division," *BP*, 13 September 1901.

121. "Smallpox Record Grows," 14.

122. "Pres. Eliot's Views," 9.

123. "For Vaccination," *BG*, 7 February 1902, 4. See also "Vaccination Upheld By Homeopathists," *BMSJ* 146 (1902): 181.

124. For the archbishop's advisory, see "Eight New Cases," *BG*, 25 November 1901, 8; on Father Murphy, see "Churches and Schools Closed," *BG*, 16 February 1902, 6.

125. "Smallpox Record Grows," 14; and "Health Board Urges All to Be Vaccinated," 4.

126. Heaton & Co., "If Smallpox Is Epidemic in Boston, Have No Fear!" *BP*, 4 December 1901, 7.

127. "Smallpox G.G.," advertisement, *BP*, 26 November 1901, 2.

128. Coomb's Germicide Tablets, "Smallpox Prevented," *BP*, 16 December 1901, 2.

129. Lifebuoy, "Lifebuoy Soap," *CC*, 28 June 1902, 3.

Chapter Five

1. Shea, "Smallpox and Vaccination," 24–25.

2. Boston Board of Health, *Thirty-First Annual Report for 1902*, 36.

3. Matthew 16:18, 19. New English Bible.

4. Other medical professionals also relied on religious metaphors to describe opposition to vaccination. Azel Ames, a Wakefield, Massachusetts, physician who directed the Marine Hospital Service vaccination program in Puerto Rico, referred to antivaccination as an "absurd and unwanted heresy." See Azel Ames, Letter to the Editor, *American Medicine* 4 (1902): 531–32. Others also used the "hot-bed" metaphor. See "The Cambridge Smallpox Epidemic," Editorial, *Medical News* 80 (1902): 1230.

5. Massachusetts Revised Statues 1855, chapter 414.

6. Giles, *Iniquity of Compulsory Vaccination*, Prefatory. Vaccination Pamphlet files, Ebling Library, University of Wisconsin–Madison. Giles's pamphlet was a revised reprint of a long letter originally generated by an exchange of articles for and against compulsory vaccination between himself and Dr. W. S. Everett in the *Norfolk County Gazette* in October and November of 1881. Giles also published the same views more succinctly in a letter to the British antivaccination journal *The Vaccination Inquirer*. See Alfred E. Giles, "Vaccination a Violation of the Constitution of Massachusetts," Letter dated 10 February 1880, *The Vaccination Inquirer* 1 (1879–80): 185. Giles's full name is listed in the Opposition to Vaccination Pamphlets file, Countway Library, Harvard University.

7. Giles, *Iniquity of Compulsory Vaccination*, 6.

8. Commonwealth of Massachusetts, *Journal of the House of Representatives for the Year 1894* (Boston, 1894), 240 (Petition of James B. Bell and others for the abolition of compulsory vaccination), 290 (Petition of Edward A. Pierce and others to allow unvaccinated children to attend public schools), 306 (Petition of Solomon Schindler and others for the abolition of compulsory vaccination), 317 (Petition of William Lloyd Garrison and others for the abolition of compulsory vaccination).

9. Contemporary sources spell the doctor's name both as "Sanders" and "Saunders," but for consistency, I use the "Sanders" spelling. Joshua T. Small lauded Sanders's two-hour testimony as the impetus for the amendment; see "Anti-Vaccination Department," Our Home Rights 1 (December 1901): 25. Joseph M. Greene also remembered Sanders's key role in the amendment; see The Animals' Defender 7 (November 1902): 27.

10. Massachusetts Statutes 1894, chapter 515. The bill was first introduced as S. 37, but then redrafted as S. 195. The document packet in the Massachusetts State Archives indicates that the Senate and House batted it back and forth throughout the spring of 1894. They even considered raising the fine to ten dollars, but rejected it. See penciled-in text on the legislative documents in "Acts-1894, Chapter 515, Act relative to vaccination," Massachusetts State Archives. The Senate at first refused to concur, but after the Conference Committee recommended concurrence on the House amendment, it passed. Commonwealth of Massachusetts, *Journal of the House of Representatives for 1894*, 851. See also Commonwealth of Massachusetts, *Journal of the Senate for the Year 1894*, 125, 527, 782–83, 861, 1043–44. For a brief, bare mention of the law, see Peabody, "Historical Study of Legislation," 51.

11. C. W. Amerige, *Vaccination a Curse* (Springfield, MA: n.p., 1895). Vaccination Pamphlet files, Ebling Library, University of Wisconsin-Madison.

12. Amerige's family was fairly well known. One brother, George M. Amerige, was a judge, and another, William H. Amerige, was a spiritualist who conducted public healings and readings in the late 1890s. See "Spiritualistic Meetings," *BG*, 28 January 1899, 10; 4 February 1899, 10; 21 November 1897, 20. Both the death of his mother

and his sister-in-law were occasion for articles in the *Globe*. See "Mrs. Frances Amerige Dead," *BG*, 27 January 1898, 8; "Mrs. Amerige Dead," *BG*, 7 October 1909, 10. The *Globe* covered Amerige's arrest and trial extensively. See "Both Released on Bail," *BG*, 16 October 1893, 5; "Now Laugh!" *BG*, 25 October 1893, 1; "Doctors Now in Jail," *BG*, 26 October 1893, 7; "Amerige and Larkeque Out," *BG*, 27 October 1893, 1; "His Chum," *BG*, 17 October 1893, 1; "Acquits Both Doctors," *BG*, 11 November 1893, 5.

13. Amerige, *Vaccination a Curse*, preface, 31.

14. See "Books and Pamphlets on Vaccination," advertisement, *The Liberator* 3 (May 1903), back page of the issue.

15. See handwritten marginal note "Presented By A. F. Hill, Sept., 1908 Boston, Mass.," in Amerige, "Vaccination a Curse," top of preface page. The cover bears the stamp of the State Library of Massachusetts, State House, Boston. But this pamphlet now resides in the Vaccination Pamphlet file, Ebling Library, University of Wisconsin-Madison.

16. The prize was considerable, $250. Angell offered a total of $500 split between two essays, one against vivisection and one supporting it. See Joseph M. Greene, "In the Interests of Humanity, Should Vivisection Be Permitted, and If So, under What Restrictions and Limitations?" in *Vivisection: Five Hundred Dollar Prize Essays*, ed. George T. Angell (July 1891): 7–25. For information about the founding of the New England Anti-Vivisection Society, see the NEAVS website, www.neavs.org/about/history/1895-1920 (accessed 23 March 2013).

17. See, for instance, J. M. Greene, "The Hearing on Vivisection," *The Animals' Defender* 5 (April 1900): 6–26.

18. Every issue from February 1901 through 1904 advertised the law on the end page or back cover. Issues in 1905 present the text of the law as an item in the body of the journal. The journal began as the *New England Anti-Vivisection Quarterly* in 1895, was renamed the *Monthly* in 1898, and then *The Animals's Defender* in 1900. I have reviewed issues from 1900 to 1905 (when the journal probably ceased publication, according to its OCLC catalog entry).

19. "Vaccination in Rockland," *The Animals' Defender* 5 (September 1900): 7.

20. *Vaccination Is the Curse of Childhood*, No. 15 in Opposition to Vaccination Pamphlets, 1874–1901, Boston Medical Library in the Francis A. Countway Library of Medicine, Harvard University. The author of this pamphlet is not named, but the address given is Room 77, 1 Beacon Street—the same address as the office of NEAVS in 1901. Thus I surmise that Greene was its author. See any cover of *The Animals' Defender* for this address. No publication date appears on the pamphlet, but library catalogue sources indicate it as 1901.

21. Shea, "Smallpox and Vaccination," 20. A newspaper article tells of antivaccination circulars distributed by the secretary of the New England Anti-vivisection Society. See "Mayor Advises Vaccination," *BET*, 26 November 1901, 2.

22. J. M. Greene, *Vaccination Is the Curse of Childhood* (Boston, 1901). Capitals and italics in original.

23. "Pres. Eliot's Views," 9.

24. Sanders graduated from Cleveland Homeopathic Medical College, "considered one of the best in the country," in 1886. See William Harvey King, *History of Homeopathy and Its Institutions in America*, 4 vols. (New York: Lewis Publishing, 1905): 3:39 for Sanders graduation date; 3:56 for quote.

25. J. M. Greene, "Beating Vaccination," *The Animals' Defender* 5 (October 1900): 4. Sanders's office address in 1896 was 74 Boylston; see *Polk's Medical and Surgical Register* (Chicago: R. L. Polk & Co., 1896), 704. By 1901, he had moved his office: Sanders is listed as a homeopath, address at 355 Massachusetts Avenue, in *Massachusetts Year Book and Business Directory* (1901), 1471. Sanders became a member of MACVS, but died in October 1902. See J. M. Greene, "Mass. Anti-Compulsory Vaccination Society," *The Animals' Defender* 7 (November 1902): 26–27.

26. Joshua T. Small, "Anti-Vaccination Department," *Our Home Rights* 1 (December 1901), 25.

27. Durgin, "Vaccination and Smallpox," 115. See also his remarks in discussion, *JMABH* 12 (April 1902): 26.

28. Testimony of Samuel Durgin before the Joint Committee on Public Health, in "Anti-Vaccination," *BET*, 19 February 1902, 3.

29. Green recounted his meeting with Pfeiffer in "We Eat Too Much," *The Animals' Defender* 6 (August 1901), 15. The ads began July 1901 and lasted until July 1904. See inside front cover, *The Animals' Defender* 6 (July 1901) through 9 (May 1904). It was the only other magazine consistently advertised, except for occasional ads from antivivisection or anticruelty publications.

30. Immanuel Pfeiffer, "A Violent One of the Emma Goldman School," *Our Home Rights* 2 (January 1902): 32.

31. Immanuel Pfeiffer, "Justice! Justice! Justice!" *Our Home Rights* 2 (January 1902): 33.

32. Greene, "Notes on a Form of Animal and Human Vivisection," 11.

33. Greene, "Facts about Vaccination," 20–22.

34. Pfeiffer, "Justice! Justice! Justice!" 33; and "Second Jury Disagreement in Vaccination Cases," *BMSJ* 149 (1903): 635.

35. Letter from an employee of the Boston Elevated Railway Company, quoted in Pfeiffer, "Vaccination," *Our Home Rights* 1 (October 1901): 17–18.

36. Thomas P. Lohan to Immanuel Pfeiffer, letter dated 30 November 1901, *Our Home Rights* 1 (November 1901): 37, and Pfeiffer's comments, 37.

37. N. K. Noyes, question posed to Samuel Durgin in discussion, *JMABH* 12 (April 1902): 34.

38. Mr. Scott, comment in discussion, *JMABH* 12 (April 1902): 34–35.

39. Greene, "Facts about Vaccination," 21–22.

40. For a typical solicitation, see Greene, "A Request," 26.

41. Greene, "Eighty Victims," 212, 213.

42. Greene reported regularly on the progress of the appeals; see "Vaccination," *The Animals' Defender* 8 (March 1903): 6; "State vs. Pear and Jacobson," *The Animals' Defender* 8 (April 1903): 27; "The Supreme Court Decision" and "Important Notice," *The Animals' Defender* 8 (June 1903): 26; "Important Notice," *The Animals' Defender* 8 (July 1903): 26; "Important Notice," *The Animals' Defender* 8 (November 1903): 31; "The Test Case," *The Animals' Defender* 9 (January 1904): 13; and "A Progressive Body," *The Animals' Defender* 9 (April 1904): 11. Greene also reported on it to other antivaccination journals; see "An Adverse Decision," *The Liberator* 3 (April 1903): 208.

43. The 1901 annual meeting of the New England Anti-vivisection Society reported that "50,000 pamphlets and leaflets have been circulated," and that "the

monthly magazine of the Society is sent throughout the country to many editors and physicians." "Our Annual Meeting," *The Animals' Defender* 6 (February 1901): 17.

44. See "Against Vivisection," *BG*, 5 March 1902, 1, for a partial list of petitions for a bill to prevent cruelty to animals and prohibit cruel vivisection. The list included two former Massachusetts governors, the Surgeon General of the United States, several congressmen, as well as Julia Ward Howe and Elizabeth Stuart Phelps Ward. The Massachusetts Federation of Women Clubs, comprised of twenty-three thousand members, also "gave their moral support to the bill."

45. Joseph M. Greene, "Hearing on Vivisection," *The Animals' Defender* 6 (April 1901): 5–30, 8 for Bell's 1901 testimony and quotation. For the 1894 abolition bill, see "By Mr. Blanchard, Petition of James B. Bell and Others for the Abolition of Compulsory Vaccination," Commonwealth of Massachusetts, *Journal of the Senate for 1894*, 190 (Thursday, 8 February 1894), "Leave to Withdraw," 529. James Batchelder Bell was born in 1838, graduated from the Hahnemann Medical College of Philadelphia in 1859, studied in Vienna, and practiced in Augusta, Maine, until he moved to Boston in 1880 to join William P. Wesselhoeft's practice. See King, *History of Homeopathy*, 1:311. Bell is listed as a surgeon at the Massachusetts Homeopathic Hospital, a member of the International Hahnemannian Society, American Institute of Homeopathy, Massachusetts Homeopathic Society, Massachusetts Surgical and Gynecological Society, and Boston Homeopathic Medical Society in the *Medical Directory of Greater Boston* (Boston: Boston Medical Publishing Co., 1906), 22, 59.

46. Greene, "Hearing on Vivisection," 9 for Hastings's testimony, 11 for Merrick letter.

47. Ibid. Greene gives the initial date (10 January 1902) and lists the officers, but unfortunately provides no membership list. See also "Preparing for Work," *BET*, 13 January 1902 for Bassett's occupation.

48. "Compulsory Vaccination," *Boston Courier*, 8 February 1902. See also Greene, "Notes on a Form of Animal and Human Vivisection," 11–17.

49. In March 1903, Joseph Greene reported that the Society had gained twenty-nine new members in February. See "Vaccination," 6.

50. Hill spoke at a 23 March 1903 hearing on vaccination. See J. M. Greene, "Legislative Hearings on Vaccination," *The Animals' Defender* 8 (May 1903): 20. For his correspondence, see Aurin F. Hill, "To the Editor of the Liberator," *The Liberator* 4 (December 1903): 91. In 1909, he petitioned the state legislature for the abolition of compulsory vaccination. See Massachusetts General Court, *Journal of the House of Representatives of the Commonwealth of Massachusetts* (1909), 96. In 1913, *The Vaccination Inquirer* described him as "one of the most untiring supporters of our cause in the States." See "American Notes," *The Vaccination Inquirer* 35 (1913): 79. Hill was quite a character, a "free thinker, a carpenter and labor activist, a building inspector, unemployed worker, a Spiritualist, and self-styled 'insane architect' of Boston." He "waged his reformist campaigns largely through a series of letters to the editors of both liberal and mainstream press." See "Background of Aurin F. Hill," in Aurin F. Hill Papers, 1887–1930 (MS 579), Special Collections and University Archives, University of Massachusetts Amherst Libraries.

51. For Simpson's education and profession, see "Register of Former Students of MIT," *Bulletin of the Massachusetts Institute of Technology* 44 (1909): 283. For his patent,

see "Patent 1,203,919: Bottle Stopper and Pipette, Filed 1 November 1915, Granted 7 November 1916," *Official Gazette of the United States Patent Office* 232 (1917).

52. Small edited the "Anti-Vaccination Department." See, for example, *Our Home Rights* 1 (December 1901): 25.

53. Immanuel Pfeiffer, "The Anti-Compulsory Vaccination Society of Massachusetts and the U.S. Supreme Court," *Our Home Rights* (June–July 1903): 10–11.

54. "Preparing for Work," *BET*, 13 January 1902.

55. "Anti-Vaccination," *Cambridge Courier*, 29 March 1902, 5.

56. Johnston, *Radical Middle Class*, xi, 178.

57. Starr, *Social Transformation of American Medicine*, 144. See also Barbara Gutmann Rosenkrantz, "The Search for Professional Order in Nineteenth-Century American Medicine," in Leavitt and Numbers, *Sickness and Health in America*, 219–32; and Ronald L. Numbers, "The Fall and Rise of the American Medical Profession," in Leavitt and Numbers, *Sickness and Health in America*, 185–96.

58. Benjamin O. Flower, *Progressive Men, Women, and Movements of the Past Twenty-Five Years* (Boston: The New Arena, 1914), 300, 316.

59. "On Compulsion," editorial, *The Animals' Defender* 10 (January 1905): 19. The German researcher Robert Koch isolated the bacillus that caused tuberculosis in 1882. In 1890, to great global excitement, he announced that he had developed "tuberculin," which he believed could both prevent and cure tuberculosis. "It soon became obvious that tuberculin killed many more patients than it helped, and the treatment fell into discredit almost everywhere." See René and Jean Dubos, *The White Plague: Tuberculosis, Man, and Society* (New Brunswick, NJ: Rutgers University Press, 1996 [1952]), 106.

60. Cyrus Edson, "The Present and Future of Medical Science," *North American Review* 154 (1892): 118. Edson (1857–1903) was a New York City health department officer and prolific author on "medical and sanitary subjects." See "Dr. Cyrus Edson Dead," *New York Times*, 3 December 1903.

61. Louis Pasteur honored Jenner in 1881 by proposing to term all immunizations "vaccination." See Derrick Baxby, "Author's Note," in Baxby, *Jenner's Smallpox Vaccine*, xiii. The *British Medical Journal* devoted an entire issue to celebrating Jenner. See Jenner Centenary articles, *British Medical Journal* (1896): 1246–1312. Edward J. Edwardes quoted by C.-E. A. Winslow in his review of Edwardes, *A Concise History of Smallpox and Vaccination in Europe*, in "The Case for Vaccination," *Science* 18 (July 1903): 102.

62. See, for instance, N. S. Davis, "Dr. Edward Jenner and the History of His Discovery of the Protective Value of Vaccination," *The Sanitarian* 36 (June 1896): 514–22, an abstract of an address given at the Centennial Anniversary, Atlanta, Georgia, May 1896; Dock, "Works of Edward Jenner"; and William M. Welch, "The Work of Jenner and His most Faithful Disciple, Waterhouse," annual address before the Associated Health Authorities and Sanitarians of Pennsylvania, 7 May 1902, *American Medicine* 3 (1902): 959–65.

63. Dr. Pepper, remarks at the Kings County Medical Society, Brooklyn, New York, celebration of Jenner's centennial, in *The Sanitarian* 36 (June 1896): 523.

64. Henry Bergh, "The Lancet and the Law," *North American Review* 134 (February 1882): 169. Bergh was referring to the views of a physician friend. Bergh was the president and founder of the New York Humane Society.

65. "Smallpox and Vaccination," editorial, *New York Medical Journal* 76 (1902): 112.

66. "The Proven Proved Again," editorial, *New York Times*, 2 October 1896, 4.

67. Ernest Wende, "The Smallpox Problem," *Medical News* 80 (1902): 1026.

68. Martin Kaufman, "Homeopathy in America: The Rise and Fall and Persistence of a Medical Heresy," in Gevitz, *Other Healers*, 109. See also Anne Taylor Kirschmann, *A Vital Force: Women in American Homeopathy* (New Brunswick, NJ: Rutgers University Press, 2004), 113–31.

69. For instance the Boston Homeopathic Medical Society passed a resolution supporting compulsory vaccination on 6 February 1902. See "For Vaccination," *BG*, 7 February 1902, 4. See also "Vaccination Upheld By Homeopaths," editorial, *BMSJ* 146 (1902): 181. The president of the Massachusetts Homeopathic Society, George S. Adams, also expressed support for compulsory vaccination in his presidential address that year. See George S. Adams, "Presidential Address," *The New England Medical Gazette* 10 (October 1902): 435. The *Hahnemannian Monthly* editorialized in support of vaccination, as reported in *American Medicine* 2 (1901): 977.

70. Several historians have noted that homeopaths generally supported vaccination. See Eberhard Wolff, "Sectarian Identity and the Aim of Integration," *British Homeopathic Journal* 85 (April 1996): 95–114 (my thanks to Ron Numbers for providing this source); and Davidovitch, "Negotiating Dissent," 11–28.

71. "More Protest against Repeal of Law," 4.

72. Below are some of the physicians who testified or wrote against vaccination that I have found by correlating mention of their names in various newspapers, antivaccination journals, and petitions with the *Massachusetts Yearbook and Business Directory* for 1901. James B. Bell (hom), George C. Hale, Caroline E. Hastings (hom), William B. Hidden, Noble Hind Hill (hom), J. D. Judge, Sara Newcomb Merrick (hom), Charles F. Nichols (hom), R. K. Noyes, Charles E. Page, Immanuel Pfeiffer, Julia M. Plummer (Hastings's lifelong housemate and thus probably also an antivaccinationist), William B. Sanders (hom), Conrad Wesselhoeft (hom), Morris P. Wheeler (hom).

73. Wesselhoeft was the nephew of William Wesselhoeft, a pioneer in establishing homeopathy in the United States. The American Institute of Homeopathy was established as national professional organization in 1844, three years before the founding of the American Medical Association in 1847. He was also a member of the Massachusetts Homeopathic Medical Society and the Boston Homeopathic Medical Society. See King, *History of Homeopathy*, 3:180–81, 187–88, and 4:403. Louisa May Alcott dedicated *Jo's Boys* to "her friend and physician" Conrad Wesselhoeft. Quoted in Kirschmann, *Vital Force*, 32.

74. This success proved illusory, however, as male medical elites who derided their competence and questioned their innate abilities succeeded in raising barriers once again to their entrance into the field. Women's medical colleges closed and coeducational schools severely limited the numbers of female students they accepted. By 1910, only 13.7 percent of Boston's physicians were women, and that percentage kept on declining for the next seventy years. See Walsh, *"Doctors Wanted,"* 186. Also see Kirschmann, *Vital Force*, appendix B, 176, for numbers of female homeopaths versus regulars. See Rothstein, *American Physicians in the Nineteenth Century*, appendix 4, "Enumerations of Physicians, 1850–1900," 344–45, for percentage of homeopaths.

75. Kirschmann, *Vital Force*, 73.

76. Boston University, *Historical Register of Boston University* (Boston: University Offices, 1911), 47, 48, and 49 lists Hastings as assistant demonstrator and lecturer in anatomy from 1873 to 1874, demonstrator and lecturer in embryology from 1874 to 1879, and assistant demonstrator and lecturer in anatomy from 1879 to 1881. See also "Hastings, Caroline Eliza," in *The Biographical Cyclopedia of American Women*, ed. Mabel Ward Cameron (New York: The Halvord Publishing Company, 1924): 239 for quoted material.

77. King, *History of Homeopathy*, 3:172.

78. "Hastings, Caroline Eliza," in *Biographical Cyclopedia of American Women*, 240.

79. "Hastings, Caroline," in *Daughters of America; or Women of the Century*, ed. Phebe A. Hanaford (Augusta, ME: True & Co., 1882), 323. See Caroline E. Hastings, "Lecture II," in *Dress Reform: A Series of Lectures Delivered in Boston on Dress as It Affects the Health of Women*, ed. Abba Goold Woolson (Boston: Roberts, 1874): 42–67.

80. "Hastings, Caroline Eliza," in *Cleave's Biographical Cyclopedia of Homeopathic Physicians and Surgeons*, ed. Egbert Cleave (Philadelphia: Galaxy Publishing Company, 1873), 498. My thanks to Eve Fine for pointing out this source. Hastings was born on 21 April 1841. She died on 10 July 1922. Hastings is listed as a homeopath at 160 Huntington Ave. in the *Massachusetts Year Book and Business Directory* (1901), 1467.

81. Julia Morton Plummer graduated from Boston University School of Medicine in 1887. See King, *History of Homeopathy*, 3:206. They lived together from at least 1894 until Hastings's death in 1922. An 1894 letter from Plummer to a colleague gives the same address as that of Hastings, 160 Huntington Ave. See Julia Morton Plummer to Howard Crutcher, 16 June 1894, in *Proceedings of the Fifteenth Annual Session of the International Hahnemannian Association Meeting of 1894* 15 (1894): 4–5. United States Census data shows them living together in 1900 through 1920. See entry for Caroline E. Hastings, *Twelfth Census of the United States* (1900), Suffolk County, Ward 10, Boston, Massachusetts, Series T623, Roll 680, 250; *Thirteenth Census of the United States* (1910), Norfolk County, Sharon, Massachusetts, Series T624, Roll 610, 54; and *Fourteenth Census of the United States* (1920), Norfolk County, Sharon, Massachusetts. Plummer was a homeopath but she did not list herself as one. See *Massachusetts Year Book and Business Directory* (1901), 1470. Plummer worked also as a consulting physician for the Women's Educational and Industrial Union in 1889. See Kirschmann, *Vital Force*, 49.

82. "Hastings, Caroline Eliza," in *Biographical Cyclopedia of American Women*, 239. Hastings served as medical director for seven years but was involved with the home for over fifty years. Hastings's companion, Julia Morton Plummer, took over the job as director after Hastings retired and also worked as corresponding secretary for the New England Female Moral Reform Society, writing the annual reports for the Talitha Cumi Home for a number of years.

83. For the New England Female Moral Reform Society, 1836–60, see Barbara Meil Hobson, *Uneasy Virtue: The Politics of Prostitution and the American Reform Tradition* (Chicago: University of Chicago Press, 1987), 53–56.

84. New England Female Moral Reform Society, *Annual Report of the New England Moral Reform Society for 1917* (Boston: The Fort Hill Press, 1917), 5. The *Annual Reports* for 1893, 1907, 1913, 1916, and 1917 list Hastings as president. The phrase "Talitha Cumi" refers to a biblical passage meaning "girl, rise up." It was later renamed Hastings House in honor of Caroline E. Hastings's lifelong devotion. It continues

today as a system of shelters named the Crittenton Hastings houses and shelters throughout New England. Hastings apparently served as president of the society until her death on 10 July 1922. See *Journal of the American Institute of Homeopathy* 15 (1922): 460, for notice of her passing.

85. "Hastings, Caroline Eliza," in *Biographical Cyclopaedia of American Women*, 239.

86. Caroline E. Hastings, "The Indicated Remedy vs. the Knife," *Proceedings of the Massachusetts Homeopathic Medical Society* 14 (1900): 204–12.

87. "Caroline E. Hastings Report of Talitha Cumi Home," *Transactions of the American Institute of Homeopathy* 55 (1900): 141.

88. See chapter 7 for a detailed description of the Durgin-Hastings controversy.

89. "Compulsory Vaccination," *Boston Courier*, 8 February 1902.

90. She is listed in the *Medical Directory of Boston* for 1906 as having her office at 359 Massachusetts Avenue; the same address is given for the office of MACVS in all of its notices. See, for instance, Aurin F. Hill, "To the Editor of the Liberator," *The Liberator* 4 (December 1903): 91, which uses the same address for MACVS.

91. See "Important Notice," *The Liberator* 3 (September 1903): 356; and Sara Newcomb Merrick, "Review of the U.S. Supreme Court Decision in the Massachusetts Vaccination Case," *The Liberator* 7 (August 1905): 113–15.

92. Albert E. Moyer, *The Scientist's Voice in American Culture: Simon Newcomb and the Rhetoric of Scientific Method* (Berkeley: University of California Press, 1992), xi. See also "Sara Newcomb Merrick, M.D.," *The Liberator* 7 (August 1905): 112.

93. Simon Newcomb (1835–1909) was nine years older than his sister, and he spent most of his professional career in at the Naval Observatory in Washington, DC. Sara might have taken the teaching job in Manassas, Virginia, because it is but 32 miles outside of that city. She might also have gotten it through her brother's influence in the federal government, since it was funded by the Freedmen's Bureau.

94. Bureau of the Census, "Sarah J. Merrick," "Morgan W. Merrick," and "Julia Merrick," in *1880 United States Federal Census Record*, Bexar, Texas, Roll T9-1291, Page 298.1000, Enumeration District 22. See also "Morgan Wolfe Merrick," www.cemetery. state.tx.us/pub/user_form.asp?pers_id=1267, accessed 21 March 2013, for biographical details of their marriage and Morgan Merrick's life. Morgan W. Merrick is now known for the journal he kept during the Civil War. See *From Desert to Bayou: The Civil War Journal and Sketches of Morgan Wolfe Merrick*, ed. Jerry D. Thompson (El Paso: Texas Western Press, 1991). The spelling of Merrick's name varied in her lifetime. Both "Sarah" and "Sara" appear as the appropriate spelling in various places.

95. "Sarah Newcomb Merrick," in *A Woman of the Century: Fourteen Hundred-Seventy Biographical Sketches Accompanied By Portraits of Leading American Women in All Walks of Life*, ed. Frances E. Willard and Mary A. Livermore (New York: Charles Wells Moulton, 1893), 500.

96. Patent No. 361,535, granted 19 April 1887, in US Government, *Women Inventors to Whom Patents Have Been Granted By the United States* (Washington, DC: Government Printing Office, 1888), 39.

97. A news item in the *San Antonio Daily Light*, 11 February 1892, notes her work as chair of the decoration committee for that year's State Press Association meeting.

98. She may have been inspired to try medicine by her niece Anita Newcomb McGee, who graduated in 1892 from Columbian University Medical School (now George Washington School of Medicine) in Washington, DC. Merrick probably also brought her

daughter, Julia, to Boston. The 1900 federal census records her as head of the household. Bureau of the Census, "Sarah Merrick," in *1900 United States Census Record*, Boston Ward 10, Suffolk, Massachusetts, Roll T623-680, Page 2B, Enumeration District 1307. This record gives her immigration year as 1858, two years earlier than her biographical article in *Woman of the Century*. A biographical note on www.cemetery.state.tx.us/pub/user_form.asp?pers_id=1267 characterizes Morgan W. Merrick as a "free spirit" who was gone a great deal on his surveying work. He enjoyed living outside to the extent that he would sleep on a tree platform rather than in a bed. Money was not very important to him—he was reputed to prefer payment for his services in whiskey rather than cash. He and Sara may have had some religious differences. Whereas he proclaimed his lack of religious belief, she taught Sunday school. They may also have had differing views about African Americans. He joined the Knights of the Golden Order in the 1850s, a group of adventurers who attempted to create a slave empire in Mexico, and he had fought for the Confederacy whereas she was a northerner who made her living teaching the children of former slaves. Love may have played a role too: his first marriage in 1865 was to a woman from a prominent Spanish family. She died in 1871, and he was said to have never quite recovered from the tragedy. By 1909 he was penniless, and he was admitted to the Confederate Home in Austin, Texas, in 1911. He died at age eighty in 1919. Although he listed his marital status as single, there is no mention or record of a divorce. One indication of an alteration in their marital status is a change in Sara's name. San Antonio papers refer to her as Sarah J. Merrick, and the 1892 biographical dictionary entry refers to her as "Mrs. Sarah Newcomb Merrick," but the Boston University School of Medicine lists her as "Sara Newcomb Merrick." In later years she used the title "Dr." but was referred to as a "widow" in 1912 even though Morgan did not die until 1919. See "Doctor, a Widow, on How to Be Happy If Married," *Rockingham Daily Record* (Harrisonburg, Virginia), 26 December 1912.

99. For Merrick's graduation, see King, *History of Homeopathy*, 3:204.

100. See ibid., 3:186–90.

101. "Roxbury Dispensary," *Medical Directory of Greater Boston* (Boston Medical Publishing Company, 1906), 27. See King, *History of Homeopathy*, 3:190, for the Roxbury Dispensary affiliation.

102. Greene, "Hearing on Vivisection" (April 1901): 11.

103. Sara Newcomb Merrick, "Consumption, What Causes It and What Prevents It—Its Health Treatment at Home," review and notice, *The Liberator* 4 (March 1904): 179; and advertisement for "S. N. Merrick, M.D." on the back page of *The Liberator* 8 (December 1905).

104. "Women's Clubs," *BET*, 1 April 1905; and "Keep Your Nose Clean," *BG*, 7 April 1905.

105. "Criminals Made in the Cradle," *BG*, 24 April 1912, 13.

106. "Government Aid to Marriage," *Fort Wayne Sentinel* (Indiana), 22 June 1912. See also "Good Advice to Husbands," *Fort Wayne Sentinel*, 13 June 1914.

107. "Sara Newcomb Merrick, M.D.," *The Liberator* 7 (August 1905): 112.

108. Simon Newcomb, *Reminiscences of an Astronomer* (Boston: Houghton Mifflin, 1903). Sara Newcomb Merrick, "John and Simon Newcomb: The Story of a Father and Son," *McClure's Magazine* 35 (1910): 677–87.

109. Charles Edward Page is listed in the 1902 medical registry as a "Form B" physician, which meant that he had applied for registration before 1 January 1895

and could show that he had practiced medicine for three years continuously in Massachusetts up to 7 June 1894. He did not have to prove that he had attended a legally chartered school, nor did he have to pass an exam to be registered to practice medicine. See *Ninth Annual Report of the Board of Registration in Medicine: January 1903* (Boston, 1903), 55. He was a regular physician: see his business listing, *Massachusetts Year Book* (1901), 1470. His listing in the 1906 *Medical Directory of Greater Boston*, 147, does not mention which medical school he attended.

110. See "Vaccination, Pro and Con," *Boston Evening Record*, 10 February 1902, 8, for the exchange with Eliot; "The Anti-Vaccinationist 'Explanation' of Dr. Pfeiffer's Case," *Boston Evening Record*, 15 February 1902, 8; "Favors Sanitation," *Cambridge Tribune*, 5 July 1902, 8; and Charles E. Page, "Are Bacilli the Cause of Disease, or a Natural Aid to Its Cure?" Paper read at the American Social Science Association, Washington, DC, 8 May 1900, reprinted in *The Liberator* 2 (December 1902): 67–69.

111. See, for instance, Charles E. Page, "Vaccination," *The Animals' Defender* 6 (July 1901): 14. Greene mentions that Page had authored "Natural Cure of Consumption," "How to Treat the Baby," and "Pneumonia and Typhoid Fever."

112. Charles E. Page, letter to the editor, *Boston Transcript*, 6 November 1902, quoted in J. M. Greene, "Compulsory Vaccination," *The Animals' Defender* 8 (February 1903): 19. See also "Contagion Theories Evidently Wrong," editorial citing a letter by Page to the *Boston Record*, *The Liberator* 2 (October 1902): 13; Charles E. Page, letter originally printed in *Physical Culture*, reprinted in *The Liberator* 2 (December 1902): 88; Charles E. Page, "Sanitation, Not Vaccination," letter printed in the *Boston Record*, reprinted in *The Liberator* 2 (January 1903): 117; and "Boston, Mass.," under "American Notes," *The Vaccination Inquirer* 38 (1916): 121.

113. Charles E. Page, *Vaccination: The Whole Truth about It*, pamphlet dated 27 March 1916, in Vaccination Pamphlet files, Ebling Library, University of Wisconsin-Madison.

114. Nichols was born 20 February 1846 to Charles Saunders Nichols and Amelia Ann Ainsworth Nichols. He died on 5 April 1915 at the age of sixty-nine. There are several sources for biographical information on Nichols. See "Nichols, Charles Fessenden," in King, *History of Homeopathy*, 4:282; "Nichols, Charles Fessenden," *The Cyclopedia of American Biography* (New York: James T. White & Co., 1917), 14:133–34; and "Charles Fessenden Nichols," *In Memorium* Index, Archives of the Hawaiian Medical Society, Mamiya Medical Heritage Center website, http://hml.org/mmhc/mdindex/nicholsc.html.

115. Quotation in Kirschmann, *Vital Force*, 31. There is a discrepancy in these dates. The *Cyclopedia of American Biography* places Nichols in Hawaii 1872–74, but a Hawaiian source claims this is incorrect, locating him in Hawaii from 1870 to 1872, and thus theorizes that he must have studied with Wesselhoeft between 1866 and 1868, before his admission to Harvard. The Hawaiian source is more persuasive because it notes the ships and exact dates on which he traveled to and from Hawaii. See "Charles Fessenden Nichols," *In Memorium* Index.

116. "Charles Fessenden Nichols," *In Memorium* Index.

117. This bit of information courtesy of the *In Memorium* Index. Other biographic essays mention his tenure on *Science*, but not the exact nature of his writing for the journal.

118. "Nichols, Charles Fessenden," *Cyclopedia of American Biography*, 133–34.

119. "Homemade Treatment," *Hahnemannian Monthly* 15 (1879): 762; *Multum in Parvo* (1879), *Quantum Sufficit: A Summary of Cases Chiefly Treated By the Higher Homeopathic Attentuations, with Comments* (1881), *Homeopathy, Its Reason* (1881), and *Homeopathy and Modern Serum Therapy, and Homeopathy's Claim as a Science in Medicine* (1905). See Francesco Cordasco, *Homeopathy in the United States: A Bibliography of Homeopathic Medical Imprints, 1825–1925* (London: Junius-Vaughan Press, 1991), 119, 183 for Nichols entries.

120. Cordasco lists *Blunder* as being published simultaneously in New York and Boston in 1902, and then published in a second edition in Boston in 1903. See Cordasco, *Homeopathy in the United States*, 183. The *Index Catalogue*, 2nd Series, lists Charles Fessenden Nichols, *The Outrage Vaccination: The Arraignment of Vaccination By Eminent Men and By Medical Specialists* (Boston, 1908). I found the other work, *Syphilis and Vaccination*, 4th ed. (Boston, 1911), in a WorldCat search.

121. Greene, "Legislative Hearings on Vaccination," 22.

122. See "Nichols, Charles F., Hotel Pelham," in 1901 *Massachusetts Year Book*, 1470. The Hotel Pelham, located at 74 Boylston and the oldest residential hotel in Boston, also provided medical offices for a number of physicians. Nichols kept his office there for years. See 1906 *Medical Directory of Greater Boston*, 144. In 1912, his office is listed at the same address. See the *American Medical Directory* (Chicago: AMA, 1912), 553.

123. Nichols, *Blunder*, 64, in Vaccination Pamphlet files, Ebling Library, University of Wisconsin-Madison. Internal references to the tuberculous cow scandal in Boston lead me to believe that Nichols did not publish the book until after April 1902.

124. Nichols, *Blunder*, 39 (cow), 51 (Pfeiffer), and 55–57 (*Courier* editorial).

125. Wallace, *Wonderful Century*, viii, quoted in Nichols, *Blunder*, 3.

126. Nichols, quoting the June 1901 *Report of the Surgeon General of the United States Army*, in *Blunder*, 4. He did not explain to his readers why these vaccinations might have failed—some argued, for instance, that hot weather over 80° Fahrenheit (like the tropical heat of the Philippines) could "speedily injure vaccine" and even "enormously increase the number of germs in fluid lymph." See Elgin, "Influence of Temperature on Vaccine Virus," 80–83.

127. Nichols, *Blunder*, 28, 37.

128. Ibid., 46.

129. Ibid., 22–23. Antivaccinationist sentiment was so strong in Leicester, England, that its health authorities famously dispensed with compulsory vaccination in favor of isolation and disinfection in the 1870s. British and American anti-vaccinationists claimed that the city successfully controlled smallpox for many years using these methods. See, for instance, J. W. Hodge, MD, *How Small-Pox Was Banished from Leicester*, pamphlet reprinted from *Medical Century* (January 1911); and J. T. Biggs, *The Leicester Experience: Sanitation vs. Vaccination* (1910), both in Vaccination Pamphlet files, Ebling Library, University of Wisconsin-Madison. C. Killick Millard, however, who served as medical health officer for Leicester, argued in *The Vaccination Question in Light of Modern Experience* (London: H. K. Lewis, 1914) that Leicester demonstrated the success of strict surveillance and containment of smallpox cases rather than sanitary measures. For a historical analysis of Leicester, see Stuart M. F. Fraser, "Leicester and Smallpox: The Leicester Method," *Medical History* 24 (1980): 315–32. See also Durbach, "'They Might as Well Brand Us,'" 45–62.

130. Nichols, *Blunder*, 27.

131. Ibid., 46, 17, 16–17.

132. Iibid., 65–66.

133. Ibid., 69.

134. Clymer was twenty-four years old in 1902; he was born 25 November 1878 and died in June 1966.

135. R. Swinburne Clymer, Letter to Pfeiffer, 5 December 1901, in "Lockjaw in the Air," *Our Home Rights* 1 (December 1901): 4.

136. Ibid. Clymer first appeared in Boston on 8 February 1902, explaining that Pfeiffer had met with him in Philadelphia and hired him. See "Dr. Pfeiffer is Missing," *Boston Herald*, 8 February 1902, 1, 2; and "Pfeiffer Not at His Office—Is He Ill?" *Boston Evening Record*, 8 February 1902, 8, for a transcription of a conversation with Clymer about Pfeiffer's whereabouts.

137. R. S. Clymer, "Smallpox and Vaccination," *The Medical Brief* 30 (1902): 1330–31.

138. Clymer's biography is confusing as to the timing and extent of his studies. A 1906 letter claims Clymer graduated from Illinois State, "a born physician, chemist and philosopher." See T. M. Woodhouse, "A Fight for Freedom," *Medical Talk for the Home* 7 (January 1906): 304. In 1901, Clymer claimed to hold a PhD and MS as well as an MD degree. See *Our Home Rights* 1 (December 1901): 1–4. Yet his medical school diploma shows that he graduated from the College of Medicine and Surgery at Chicago, Illinois, months later in April 1902. Founded as an eclectic institution in 1901, this college probably counted Clymer as one of its first graduates. Abraham Flexner inspected the College of Medicine and Surgery in 1909, and he reported that it accepted students with "a high school education or equivalent," and that it accorded advanced status to transfer students "of even the worst night schools." If Clymer applied credits from another medical school toward advanced status, that would explain how he managed to work as a physician at a Philadelphia hospital in December 1901 and then as Pfeiffer's assistant in February and March 1902, yet graduate with a medical degree dated April 1902. It appeared that as long as the students paid the tuition and fees, this college was happy to accept them regardless of their previous academic background. See Abraham Flexner, *Medical Education in the United States and Canada* (1910; reprint, New York: Arno Press, 1972), 209–10. Clymer also studied osteopathy in New York City at the Health League Sanitarium in 1902. Possibly he had finished his courses at the Chicago school before fall semester of 1901, but did not receive the diploma until April 1902.

The website for The Fraternitas Rosae Crucis: The Authentic Rosicrucian Fraternity in the Americas and the Isles of the Sea, www.soul.org, reproduces copies of his diploma, among other documents. For osteopathy, see Norman Gevitz, "Osteopathic Medicine: From Deviance to Difference," in Gevitz, *Other Healers*, 124–56. Arthur Allen documents the lasting influence Clymer has had on contemporary opposition to immunization in the career of one of his disciples, Dr. Harold Buttram, an expert witness in child abuse cases who argues that immunizations and vitamin deficiencies are the real culprits. See Allen, *Vaccine*, 87 (for Clymer), 337–42 (for Buttram).

139. The Health Sanitarium, Inc. was "a Sanitarium and College duly Incorporated under and by the virtue of the Laws of the State of New York." Clymer studied and

worked there as its superintendent for at least two terms in 1902. See an affidavit sworn by Leopold H. R. Hibbe, MD, 23 January 1919, reproduced at www.soul.org.

140. T. M. Woodhouse, "Medical Laws Not Constitutional," *Medical Talk for the Home* 7 (January 1906): 304–5. Woodhouse was Clymer's assistant in November 1903. The article describes Clymer's legal troubles.

141. Dr. I. L. Keperling, "The Rights of the People," *Medical Talk for the Home* 7 (January 1906): 305–6.

142. The title page declares Clymer "licensed by the Territorial Board of Health to practice Medicine and Surgery in Oklahoma." In "Author's Acknowledgment," Clymer gives his location as Guthrie, Oklahoma, at the time of writing. See Clymer, *Vaccination Brought Home*, title page and 10.

143. See Clymer, *Vaccination Brought Home*, 36–38, and "Appendix: Smallpox in Cleveland," 89–92.

144. Clymer, *Vaccination Brought Home*, 53–54. Clymer got the dates wrong, declaring that the Shore girl was vaccinated in August 1902 when in fact she was vaccinated in August 1901. The original story is in Pfeiffer, "Fruit of Vaccination," 9–10.

145. Guillaume Desmoulins, "The Charge of the Hundred and Fifty," in Clymer, *Vaccination Brought Home*, 88.

146. Clymer, *Vaccination Brought Home*, 82–83. By "Russian coercion," he meant that of tsarist Russia, not the Soviet Union, although he became intensely nationalistic and anticommunist in the 1950s and 1960s, authoring books like *America's Betrayal: Is America, the Home of a Once Proud, Cultured and Highly Successful People, Doomed, as So Many Fear?* (Quakertown, PA: Humanitarian Society, 1961).

Clymer eventually returned to Pennsylvania to practice as a registered osteopath in Allentown, Pennsylvania, and established a medical center in 1904. He was registered to practice medicine in Michigan, Oklahoma, and Arkansas. He joined the Rosicrucian Fraternity of the Americas order in 1897, attained the office of Grand Master in 1905, and was selected as the Supreme Grand Master in 1907, an office he held until his death in 1966. This Rosicrucian organization regards him with reverence. His medical institute and treatment center, the Clymer Healing Center, brought wealth to this Rosicrucian sect, creating a campus for it, Beverly Hall, in Quakertown, Pennsylvania. Most of his works focus on Rosicrucian spirituality, running to over fifty titles. He also wrote medical advice books that reflect his early training as an eclectic physician: see, for instance, *Nature's Healing Agents; the Medicines of Nature (or the Natura System)* (Quakertown, PA: Humanitarian Society, 1906); and *The Medicines of Nature: The Thomsonian System: A Course of Medical Treatment as Taught By Dr. Samuel Thomson* (Quakertown, PA: Humanitarian Society, 1926).

The Rosicrucians apparently connected a few early twentieth-century antivaccination leaders on an interstate level. The eclectic physician and journalist Alexander Wilder, who founded the first antivaccination society in the United States, led the Rosicrucian Order as a member of its Council of Three until his death in 1908, and he undoubtedly knew Clymer. Another Rosicrucian connection surfaces when L. H. Piehn, the president of the Anti-vaccination Society of America, invited Clymer in June 1902 to serve as its vice president, apparently on Frank D. Blue's recommendation. Frank D. Blue edited the Indiana antivaccination journal *Vaccination*. In *Blue v. Beach* (1900) he unsuccessfully appealed the Terre Haute, Indiana, board of health decision to exclude his unvaccinated son from school. Piehn referred to Blue as

"Brother Blue" and also addressed Clymer as "My Dear Bro.," appellations that might refer to their common membership in the Order. Piehn hoped that his society would serve to unify all the scattered forces of antivaccination in the United States: "we all must concentrate our forces into one grand national society: In union is strength." See L. H. Piehn to Dr. R. S. Clymer, New York, 21 June 1902, in Clymer, *Vaccination Brought Home*, 5. Clymer accepted the "honored appointment," but Piehn's society never attained the truly national scope that he had intended for it. See www.soul.org.

Chapter Six

1. William T. Sedgwick, "Remarks on 'Opposition to Vaccination,'" *JMABH* 12 (April 1902), 5–19; Durgin's comments, 17–18. The *Journal* printed transcriptions of informal discussions as well as papers presented during quarterly meetings of the Association. The meeting in question took place on 30 January 1902.

2. "In spite of the measures taken, cases increased to 12 in August, to 30 in September, to 49 in October, to 195 in November, to 201 in December, and 177 in January [1902]." See Boston Board of Health, "Smallpox," *Thirtieth Annual Report for 1901*, 44.

3. "Dr. Durgin on the Case," *BG*, 10 February 1902, 4.

4. Steven J. Ross, "Single-Tax Movement," in *Oxford Companion to American History*, ed. Paul Boyer (Oxford: Oxford University Press, 2000), 709. Henry George (1839–97) inspired the single-tax movement in his 1879 work *Progress and Poverty*. Ross claims that the single tax was "a great panacea" for all social and economic ills that supposedly would "generate funds sufficient to eliminate all other taxes." Robert D. Johnston argues that "the single tax movement represented a genuine class struggle" in which "single taxers articulated a utopian vision of a modern small-enterprise economy where the relationship between wage labor and self-employment remained fluid—and where, therefore, wage slavery would be eliminated." See *Radical Middle Class*, 159–76, quote on 159.

5. Immanuel Pfeiffer, "Anti-Compulsory Vaccination vs. Anti-Vaccination," *Our Home Rights* 2 (February–April, 1902): 45.

6. "Official List of Practitioners of Medicine," in the *Eighth Annual Report of the Board of Registration in Medicine* (Boston, 1902), 55, in *Public Documents of the State of Massachusetts*, vol. 4, document no. 56. He never specified the institution or whether he actually obtained a diploma. Obituaries for Pfeiffer are vague about his education, noting his Danish origin and commenting only that he was educated "abroad." Pfeiffer was born on 29 March 1841. He died on 2 May 1918 at the age of seventy-seven. See "Passed Away Friday, Dr. Immanuel Pfeiffer of Bedford Dies at Age 77," *Bedford Enterprise*, 3 May 1918, 1; and "A Former Boston Specialist," *BET*, 4 May 1918, 3. Pfeiffer did not always identify himself as a physician. The 1880 United States Federal Census Record for Pfeiffer locates him in Franklin, New Jersey, working as "a dealer in real estate," but by 1890, a New Bedford directory lists him as a physician. This information from Ancestry.com.

7. See Pfeiffer, "Dr. Pfeiffer's Statement, 34, for information about his family. Although the newspapers claimed that his wife, Olive, was his second marriage, he refuted them and declared that he had married only once. See also "He Is Better,"

BG, 10 February 1902, 1, which declared that four children still lived at home: Immanuel Jr., a veterinary surgeon, managed the farm; Louis worked as a clerk in a wool house in Boston; daughters Hannah, a high school student, and Alice, a grammar school student, were the youngest. According to his obituary notices, another son, William, lived in New York City, and a daughter, Mrs. Oline Blaaberg, lived in London. (This may have been a typo: her first name was Olive, according to the 1880 United States Census.) Pfeiffer's fourth son, Albert, became a physician who served as a major in the Medical Reserve Corps in 1918. See "Passed Away Friday," *Bedford Enterprise*, 3 May 1918, 1; and "A Former Boston Specialist," *BET*, 4 May 1918, 3.

8. Pfeiffer refers to the farm as Orchard Farm in "Dr. Pfeiffer's Statement," 44. Bedford is located about 15 miles from Boston and in 1901 had a population of 1,208, according to the *Massachusetts Year Book and Business Directory* (1901), 334. Description of his house in "Dr. Durgin on the Case," 4. The address was 413 Hotel Pelham. See 1901 *Massachusetts Year Book*, 1470. Pfeiffer probably commuted to Boston from his farm in Bedford and stayed in town during the business week, so the hotel may have been his home away from home. In 1902, however, one newspaper listed his office address as 247 Washington St. See "He Is Better," *BG* 19 February 1902, 1.

9. See "A Most Remarkable Cure of a Well-Known Citizen," *North Adams Transcript*, 23 August 1899, in which the milk dealer Harry Crews describes "the great healing power of the natural physician, Dr. Immanuel Pfeiffer." For his speciality, see "A Former Boston Specialist," *BET*, 4 May 1918, 3. For his approach, see "Dr. Durgin on the Case," 4.

10. "Healer Fails to Cure," *Chicago Daily Tribune*, 27 April 1896, 8. Pfeiffer practiced in North Adams in 1899, according to a testimonial published in a local paper. See "A Most Remarkable Cure of a Well-Known Citizen." The *Boston Medical and Surgical Journal* noted that he had practiced in New Bedford, Pittsfield, and North Adams before coming to Boston sometime between late 1900 and early 1901. See "The Case of Dr. Pfeiffer," Editorial, *BMSJ* 146 (1902): 210–11.

11. "Case of Dr. Pfeiffer," 211. From 1895, the Massachusetts medical registration law required physicians to graduate from medical school and pass an examination. It allowed established physicians to continue their practices if they met certain conditions. Pfeiffer registered under "Form B," which allowed physicians with three years of continuous practice in the state before 7 June 1894 to register. "Form B" physicians did not have to take the test or produce a diploma. See *Eighth Annual Report of the Board of Registration in Medicine*, 6.

12. House Bill no. 936, in Commonwealth of Massachusetts, *The Journal of the Senate for the Year 1901* (Boston, 1901), 230, 486, 505. The *North Adams Transcript* reported on Pfeiffer's 1901 bill. See "Dr. Pfeiffer Takes Action," *North Adams Transcript*, 24 January 1901. See also "Local Intelligence," *North Adams Transcript*, 7 March 1901.

13. "Pending Legislation," *The New England Medical Gazette* 36 (March 1901): 147. See "Legislation," *The New England Medical Gazette* 36 (April 1901): 207, for a short discussion of the Pfeiffer bill's failure to pass through the Committee.

14. "By-Laws of the Medical Rights League of Massachusetts," *Our Home Rights* 1 (October 1901): 34–36. "Proclamation to the Liberty Loving People of Massachusetts and Elsewhere," *Our Home Rights* 2 (January 1902): 31. Senate No. 225, *Documents Printed By Order of the Senate of the Commonwealth of Massachusetts during the Session of the General Court, 1903* (Boston, 1903).

15. See "Will Fast 21 Days," *North Adams Transcript*, 2 March 1900; and "Dr. Pfeiffer Fasting," *North Adams Transcript*, 6 March 1900. The *Boston Journal* also noted his 1900 fast: "Account of his Long Fast and Portraits Before and After," *Boston Journal*, 25 March 1900, 1; and "Ends His Fast of 21 Days with a Loss of Only 20 lbs of Weight and with Little If Any Loss of Strength," *Boston Journal*, 27 March 1900, 2. The *Boston Post* reported on a 1901 fast: "Begins His Thirty-Day Fast," *BP*, 1 July 1901, 2; "New 'Fasting' Race," *BP*, 4 July 1901, 2; "Pfeiffer Has Fasted a Week," *BP*, 7 July 1901, 12; "Carnegie's Chance to Recover Health: Dr. Pfeiffer, the Faster, Says He Can Cure the Millionaire's Ills," *BP*, 11 July 1901, 2; "First Meal in 30 Days," *BP*, 31 July 1901, 3; "Why Dr. Pfeiffer Fasted," *BP*, 4 August 1901, 3. See also "Case of Dr. Pfeiffer," 210–11, for reference that he "had achieved considerable notoriety" for the fasts.

16. "Pfeiffer Dying of Smallpox [Dr. Pfeiffer's Fast]," *BP*, 9 February 1902, 1, 9.

17. "First Meal in 30 Days," 3.

18. "Dr. Durgin on the Case," 4. Pfeiffer gave "practical demonstrations" of hypnosis at spiritualist meetings in the 1890s. See "Spiritualist meetings," *BG*, 10 March 1894, 8.

19. Pfeiffer probably exaggerated. He could claim ten thousand subscribers only because he had taken over the subscription list of J. M. Peebles's *Temple of Health* for a brief period. See "The 10,000 Mark," *Our Home Rights* 1 (October 1901): 11.

20. "Our Home Rights," advertisement, *Medical Talk for the Home* 4 (October 1902): 67.

21. "The Journal of Universal Antiism," *American Medicine* 3 (1902): 293.

22. John Allen Wyeth, "The President's Address," *BMSJ* 146 (1902): 618. Delivered at the 53rd annual meeting of the AMA, 10–13 June 1902.

23. See Starr, *Social Transformation of American Medicine*, 108–12, for a brief discussion of how the AMA effected a transition in outlook among physicians, "the replacement of a competitive orientation with a corporate consciousness" (111), at this time.

24. Samuel Hopkins Adams, *The Great American Fraud* (n.p.: Collier & Son, 1905 and 1906), 84; quoted in Starr, *Social Transformation of American Medicine*, 131. See also Starr's discussion of advertising, 127–34.

25. He charged an initial five-dollar fee with subsequent advice discounted to two dollars. See "Consultation By Letter," *Our Home Rights* 1 (October 1901): 29.

26. "System=Energy," advertisement, *Our Home Rights* 3 (June–July 1903), 47.

27. Immanuel Pfeiffer, "For Postal Reform," letter to the editor, *New York Times*, 14 February 1905, 8. In this letter, Pfeiffer signed himself, "Vice President and General Manager Postal Reform League." He also mentions other "liberal healers" and their problems with the Postal Service in *Our Home Rights* 2 (February–April 1902): 45. Pfeiffer was still carrying on his campaign as late as 1910, identifying himself as president and founder of the Postal Reform League and issuing an open letter to President Taft on postal reform. See "Takes Taft to Task on the Postal Situation," editorial, *Indiana Democrat*, 2 February 1910.

28. Howard Health Company Advertisement, *Our Home Rights* 1 (November 1901): 45. The company's address was 246 Washington St.; Pfeiffer's office was located at 247 Washington St.

29. Samuel Durgin responding to a question about a remedy based on cream of tartar and other smallpox cures. "Cream of Tartar Cannot Cure," *BET*, 3 December 1901, 9.

30. Wyeth, "President's Address," 618.

31. The New England Eclectic Medical Association's 1901 resolution against compulsory vaccination was one exception. See Pfeiffer, "Vaccination," 14.

32. "Dr. Durgin on the Case," 4.

33. "The Organization of the Medical Profession," *JAMA* 38 (1902): 113.

34. Pfeiffer, "Vaccination," 13, 14. The Board of Health member was probably Samuel Durgin, since he usually gave the interviews to the newspapers.

35. "Dr. Durgin Warns as to Spread of Smallpox," *BP*, 30 October 1901, 8. Pfeiffer reprinted the interview in *Our Home Rights* 1 (November 1901): 36–37.

36. Immanuel Pfeiffer, "Dr. Durgin as Prosecutor," *Our Home Rights* 1 (November 1901): 11–12.

37. "Its Big Benefits: John H. McCollum Talks about Vaccination." *BG*, 20 December 1901, 5. Joseph M. Greene also attended this lecture, noting that Pfeiffer "put some pointed questions to the speaker." See Greene, "Vaccination Scourge," 21.

38. Founded in 1848, it still exists as "one of the oldest continuous women's organizations . . . in America." By the 1890s "it became a public platform among women for whom health ranked high on a long agenda of social needs." See Martha H. Verbrugge, *Able-Bodied Womanhood: Personal Health and Social Change in Nineteenth-Century Boston* (New York: Oxford University Press, 1988): 49–96; 51, 81 for quoted material.

39. Immanuel Pfeiffer, "Make Up Your Mind," *Our Home Rights* 1 (December 1901): 16.

40. Editorial, *Our Home Rights* 1 (December 1901): 22.

41. "Durgin Issues a Challenge," *Our Home Rights* 2 (January 1902): 30. The quoted material is taken from an interview that Durgin gave to *The Traveler* before Christmas 1901, because the article leads with the Board of Health notice that there is no smallpox in the big stores. Durgin corroborated that he made the offer in discussion following Sedgwick, "Remarks on 'Opposition to Vaccination,'" 18. "Some weeks ago, I made an offer to these people that, if I could get a few adult leaders of the anti-vaccination faith who had never been vaccinated, I would give them the privilege of seeing some cases of small-pox, studying the disease personally, and exhibiting the sincerity which they professed before the community." In an interview on 2 December for the *Boston Post*, Durgin also had deliberately provoked the antivaccinationists, stating that the epidemic provided a "golden opportunity . . . to put their theories to the test" even though he believed "they all die while there is a chance for those who have been vaccinated." See "12 New Smallpox Cases," *BP*, 2 December 1901, 5.

42. Pfeiffer to Samuel H. Durgin, 18 January 1902, reprinted in *Our Home Rights* 2 (January 1902): 30. Local papers also reprinted the letters. See "Pfeiffer Has Smallpox," *Boston Herald*, 8 February 1902, 1.

43. Durgin to Immanuel Pfeiffer, 20 January 1902, reprinted in *Our Home Rights* 2 (January 1902): 30; also "Pfeiffer Has Smallpox," *Boston Herald*, 8 February 1902, 1.

44. Immanuel Pfeiffer, "Proclamation," *Our Home Rights* 2 (January 1902): 33; and "Dr. Pfeiffer Has Smallpox," *BG*, 9 February 1902, 1.

45. Pfeiffer, "Dr. Pfeiffer's Statement," 33, 34. Pfeiffer and Durgin disagreed as to when the visit took place. Pfeiffer claimed 21 January and Durgin put it at 23 January. I am taking Pfeiffer at his word, since he, after all, was the person who visited the hospital.

46. "Pfeiffer Attacks Durgin," *BP*, 27 January 1902, 6. Possibly it was the Massachusetts Anti-compulsory Vaccination Society, which held its monthly meetings there.

47. Ibid. The *Boston Globe* also received a letter; see "His Opinion of Pfeiffer's Action," *BG*, 27 January 1902, 11. Pfeiffer also published the letter in full in his magazine; see "Proclamation," *Our Home Rights* 2 (January 1902): 33.

48. Pfeiffer, "Dr. Pfeiffer's Statement," 41–42.

49. Pfeiffer, "Proclamation," 33. Pfeiffer uses nearly identical language about Durgin in his *Post* interview.

50. "His Opinion of Pfeiffer's Action," 11.

51. Samuel Durgin, discussion following Sedgwick paper, "Remarks on 'Opposition to Vaccination,'" 19.

52. "Case of Dr. Pfeiffer," 211.

53. First quotation: "Is Dr. Pfeiffer Ill?" *Boston Globe*, 8 February 1902, 4. Second quotation: "Dr. Pfeiffer Is Missing," *Boston Herald*, 8 February 1902, 1, 2.

54. "Is Dr. Pfeiffer Ill?" 4.

55. "Pfeiffer Exposed Many to Disease," *BP*, 10 February 1902, 2.

56. "The Case of Dr. Pfeiffer," Editorial, *BP*, 10 February 1902, 6.

57. Editorial, *Boston Evening Record*, 8 February 1902, 4.

58. "Dr. Pfeiffer's Illness," *Boston Herald*, 10 February 1902, 9.

59. "Complied with Regulations," *BER*, 10 February 1902, 8. See Pfeiffer, "Dr. Pfeiffer's Statement," 34, for his account.

60. "Is Dr. Pfeiffer Ill?" 4.

61. Pfeiffer, "Dr. Pfeiffer's Statement," 37–38.

62. "Complied with Regulations," 8.

63. "Dr. Pfeiffer Is Missing," 1, 2. See also "Pfeiffer Not at His Office—Is He Ill?" *BER*, 8 February 1902, 8, for a transcription of short conversation with Clymer about Pfeiffer's whereabouts.

64. "Dr. Pfeiffer Has Smallpox," *BG*, 9 February 1902, 1. See "Pfeiffer Has Smallpox," *Boston Herald*, 9 February 1902, 1, for identification of Mrs. Bordman [Boardman] as his chief clerk.

65. "Dr. Pfeiffer Is Missing," 1, 2. See also "Dr. Pfeiffer Has Smallpox," 1.

66. "Pfeiffer Dying of Smallpox," *BP*, 9 February 1902, 1.

67. "Dr. Pfeiffer Is Missing," 1, 2. See also "Dr. Pfeiffer Has Smallpox," 1.

68. "Dr. Pfeiffer Has Smallpox," 1.

69. Ibid.

70. Untitled editorial item, *Boston Herald*, 10 February 1902, 2.

71. See "Exposed to Smallpox," *New York Times*, 8 February 1902, 2; Dr. Pfeiffer Has Smallpox," 1; "Pfeiffer May Recover," *BET*, 10 February 1902, 6; "Pfeiffer Has Smallpox," *Boston Herald*, 9 February 1902, 1; "Pfeiffer Dying of Smallpox," 1; "Pfeiffer Home Strictly Quarantined," *BER*, 10 February 1902, 8; "Patrols Guarding House," *Boston Daily Advertiser*, 10 February 1902, 1; "Two Bad Methods of Fighting the Antivaccination Craze," *American Medicine* 3 (1902): 294; "Case of Dr. Pfeiffer," 210–11; "Immanuel Pfeiffer," *Cleveland Medical Journal* 1 (July 1902): 392; "The Smallpox versus Dr. Pfeiffer," *Medical News* 80 (1902): 363–64.

72. "He May Not Recover," *BG*, 9 February 1902, 3.

73. "Dr. Pfeiffer Has Smallpox," 1.

74. "Pfeiffer Dying of Smallpox," 1.

75. "He May Not Recover," 3.

76. "Pfeiffer Has Smallpox," 1.

77. "Pfeiffer Yet Alive," *BG*, 10 February 1902, 1, 4.

78. "Pfeiffer Exposed Many to Disease," *BP*, 10 February 1902, 2.

79. "He May Not Recover," *BG*, 9 February 1902, 3.

80. "Dr. Pfeiffer Has Smallpox," 1.

81. "Pfeiffer Exposed Many to Disease," 2.

82. "Dr. Pfeiffer Holding His Own," *BP*, 11 February 1902, 10.

83. Ibid.

84. "Pfeiffer Exposed Many to Disease," 2.

85. "Dr. Pfeiffer Has Smallpox," *BG*, 10 February 1902, 1, 3.

86. Pfeiffer, "Dr. Pfeiffer's Statement," 39, 43.

87. Ibid., 38–39.

88. Ibid., 39–40.

89. "Pfeiffer Case Excites Bedford," *BER*, 17 February 1902, 8.

90. Pfeiffer, "Dr. Pfeiffer's Statement," 42–43.

91. "Pfeiffer Has Not Decided to Sue," *BER*, 16 May 1902, 1.

92. Pfeiffer, "Dr. Pfeiffer's Statement," 43.

93. Ibid.

94. Ibid.

95. Ibid., 35, 41.

96. "The Anti-Vaccinationist 'Explanation' of Dr. Pfeiffer's Case," *BER*, 15 February 1902, 8.

97. Pfeiffer, "Dr. Pfeiffer's Statement," 42.

98. "Ten Thousand Vaccinated," *BP*, 12 February 1902, 2; and "Vaccinators Invade North and West Ends," *BP*, 11 February 1902, 10. See also "Smallpox Decreasing Here," Editorial Suggestions, *Boston Daily Advertiser*, 12 February 1902, 4; and "The Smallpox versus Dr. Pfeiffer," 364.

99. See, for instance, "Pfeiffer Case Nearing Crisis," *BP*, 12 February 1902, 2; "Dr. Pfeiffer May Recover," *BP*, 14 February 1902, 8; "Dr. Pfeiffer Very Feverish," *BP*, 15 February 1902, 1; "Pfeiffer Past Crisis," *BP*, 17 February 1902, 6; "He Is Better," *BG*, 10 February 1902, 1; "Pfeiffer May Recover," 6; "No Change in Condition," *BET*, 12 February 1902, 10; "He Is a Very Sick Man," *BET*, 13 February 1902, 3; and "Dr. Pfeiffer's Illness," *Boston Herald*, 10 February 1902, 9.

100. "Two Bad Methods of Fighting the Antivaccination Craze," and "A Further Object Lesson in Vaccination," *BMSJ* 146 (1902): 239, 611.

101. "The Smallpox versus Dr. Pfeiffer," 364.

102. "An Object Lesson in Anti-Vaccination," *JAMA* 38 (1902): 518–19.

103. "Case of Dr. Pfeiffer," 211.

104. "Two Bad Methods of Fighting the Antivaccination Craze," 294.

105. "Dr. Pfeiffer Remains an Antivaccinationist," Editorial Echoes, *American Medicine* 3 (1902): 415.

106. See "An Antivaccination Insurance Company," Editorial Comment, *American Medicine* 3 (1902): 454; "Secret and Ignored Vaccination," Editorial Comment, *American Medicine* 3 (1902): 759; and "Smallpox Is Due to Overwork," Editorial Comment, *American Medicine* 3 (1902): 893.

107. "Case of Dr. Pfeiffer," 6.

108. Nichols, *Blunder*, 51.

109. "Compulsory Vaccination," *BG*, 10 February 1902, 9.

110. "Vaccination Bills In," *BET*, 19 February 1902, 3.

111. "A Further Object Lesson in Vaccination," 611.

112. "Pfeiffer Exposed Many to Disease," 2.

113. Untitled editorial item, *Boston Herald*, 10 February 1902, 2.

Chapter Seven

1. Newspapers vary in their estimates of attendance. The *Transcript* put it at "about seventy-five," whereas the *Globe* declared "upward of 80 person [*sic*] were present," and the *Herald* asserted "nearly a hundred members . . . attended." See "Discussed Vaccination," *BET*, 30 January 1902, 2; "Smallpox Talk," *BG*, 31 January 1902, 2; and "To Avoid Smallpox," *Boston Herald*, 31 January 1902, 8. According to its *Journal*, the Association had 248 members as of January 1902, and they were adding new members at every meeting. See "Members of the Massachusetts Association of Boards of Health," *JMABH* 12 (April 1902): 49–50.

2. Shea, "Smallpox and Vaccination," 20.

3. Massachusetts Revised Statues 1855, chapter 414.

4. Peabody, "Historical Study of Legislation," 50.

5. Abbott, "Legislation with Reference to Smallpox and Vaccination," 266, 267.

6. Massachusetts Statutes 1894, chapter 515.

7. Sedgwick, "Remarks on 'Opposition to Vaccination,'" 6–10.

8. Alfred Russel Wallace, the codiscoverer of the theory evolution, also wrote books for the general audience. In one "appreciation" of the nineteenth century, he discussed the history of some of its great scientific and technological innovations and failures, devoting an entire chapter to vaccination under the category of "failure." See Wallace, "Vaccination a Delusion," 213–315.

9. Sedgwick, "Remarks on Opposition to Vaccination," 16–17.

10. Ibid., 6–7.

11. Samuel Durgin, discussion following Sedgwick's talk, *JMABH* 12 (April 1902): 26–27.

12. Edwin L. Pilsbury, discussion following Sedgwick's talk, *JMABH* 12 (April 1902): 27.

13. Discussion following Sedgwick's talk, 31–32. A list of the twenty-eight members on the committee appears on 31.

14. "Compulsory Vaccination," *Boston Courier*, 8 February 1902.

15. "More Protest against Repeal of Law," 4.

16. "Doctors in Protest," *Boston Herald*, 4 February 1902, 3.

17. Commonwealth of Massachusetts, "Rules of the Senate" and "Rules of the House of Representatives," in *Manual for the Use of the General Court: Containing the Rules of the Two Branches* (Boston, 1902): 455, 485.

18. Representative Issac M. Small (Republican of Truro, Barnstable County) presented his bill (based on the petition of Reuben F. Brown and others) "at the request of the people of Provincetown," on 22 January 1901. Joshua T. Small,

"Anti-Vaccination Department," *Our Home Rights* 2 (January 1902): 8. Representative Issac M. Small, who proposed the first abolition bill, apparently supported the anti-vaccinationists. By 1902, Issac Small was no longer in the House: he had moved on, and Immanuel Pfeiffer identified him as working as a correspondent for the Provincetown *Advocate.* Quite possibly he was related to the Provincetown resident Joshua T. Small, editor of the antivaccination column in *Our Home Rights* and vice president of MACVS in 1903. See "A Most Worthy Representative," *Our Home Rights* 2 (January 1902): 25–26. The 1901 bill was later joined by petitions of Everett D. Hatch (6 February 1901), George A. Smith (7 February 1901), and House No. 226. See Commonwealth of Massachusetts, *Journal of the House of Representatives* (Boston, 1901): 104, 276, 295, 478, 495, 526. The bill may have been held over because the legislature had allowed a huge backlog of bills to accumulate, forcing it to extend the session until 10 June 1901. See Michael E. Hennessy, *Twenty-Five Years of Massachusetts Politics* (Boston: Practical Politics, 1917), 96. On 14 January 1902, Rep. John F. Foster of Somerville, a Republican, revived Small's bill by moving that the House take the petition of Reuben F. Brown and others from the 1901 files. Foster is listed as a Republican in the *Massachusetts Yearbook and Business Directory* (1901): 114. See also Commonwealth of Massachusetts, *Manual for the Use of the General Court for 1901*, 402.

19. House No. 128 Relative to Compulsory Vaccination, Unenacted Legislation, Massachusetts State Archives. See also Commonwealth of Massachusetts, *Journal of the House of Representatives* (Boston, 1902), 65.

20. "Mr. Small presents the petition of Reuben F. Brown and others for the abolition of compulsory vaccination, Jan. 22, 1901," and "Mr. Small of Truro presents the remonstrance of John W. Small and others against the passage of legislation for the abolition of compulsory vaccination, Feb. 7, 1901," in Document Packet for H. 128, Unenacted Legislation for 1902, Massachusetts State Archives.

21. "Mr. Small of Truro presents the petition of George M. Smith and others in aid of the petition for abolition of compulsory vaccination, Feb. 7, 1901," and "Mr. Small of Truro presents the petition of Everett D. Hatch and others in aid of the petition for the abolition of compulsory vaccination, Feb. 6, 1901," in H. 128, Unenacted Legislation for 1902, Massachusetts State Archives.

22. Rep. John F. Foster of Somerville presented House No. 636 on 31 January 1902. This bill sought to create a medical exemption for adults from the vaccination law. See Commonwealth of Massachusetts, *Journal of the House of Representatives* (1902), 190. The petition lists eight names, none known antivaccinationists, although three give East Boston for their district. For petition and text of proposed bill, see Document Packet for H. 636, Unenacted Legislation for 1902, Massachusetts State Archives. Foster also presented a second bill with a similar objective, House No. 980, which he presented at the conclusion of vaccination hearings on 5 February 1902. See Massachusetts, *Journal of the House* (1902), 248. The petition lists just four names, one of whom signed H. 636 petition too. Text of bill and petition in Document Packet for H. 980, Unenacted Legislation for 1902, Massachusetts State Archives.

23. Presented 4 February 1902, H. 847 was based on a petition of Charles J. Belknap and three others. The accompanying bill proposed amendments that would abolish the five-dollar fine, the vaccination requirement for school attendance, and prohibit health officials from assaulting, injuring, imprisoning citizens or destroying their property. See petition and accompanying bill in Document Packet for

H. 847, Unenacted Legislation for 1902, Massachusetts State Archives. See also Massachusetts, *Journal of the House* (1902), 225; and "Vaccination Bills In," *BET*, 20 February 1902, 3, for a description of the bill.

24. "Vaccination Bills In," 3.

25. Immanuel Pfeiffer probably wrote the bill himself. It is handwritten, not typed, and Pfeiffer is the sole signatory. For text of the bill, see Document Packet for H. 982, Unenacted Legislation for 1902, Massachusetts State Archives. Representative Fred A. Bearse, a Republican from Springfield, presented it. See also Massachusetts, *Journal of the House* (1902), 248. Bearse may have been connected in some way to Pfeiffer's fight against medical registration laws.

26. They started on 29 January 1902 and continued for three more sessions—31 January, 3 February, and 4 February. Librarians at the State Library of Massachusetts and the Massachusetts State Archives assure me that there are no transcripts for these hearings or floor debates at this time. Newspapers reported comprehensively, though, and even occasionally transcribed testimony; Joseph M. Greene also provides detailed reports on these hearings in *The Animals' Defender*.

27. "Compulsory Vaccination," *BET*, 31 January 1902, 6.

28. "Vaccination Opposed," 3.

29. "Vaccination," *BG*, 1 February 1902, 4.

30. "Compulsory Vaccination," *BET*, 31 January 1902, 6.

31. "Compulsory Vaccination," *BG*, 10 February 1902, 9. Although Nichols was sympathetic to antivaccination and shared the same surname with Charles Fessenden Nichols, I have not found any genealogical evidence to support close kinship between them. I also do not know whether or not Nichols was a homeopathic druggist. The *Massachsetts Year Book and Business Directory* (1901), 1323, just lists him as a druggist.

32. "Compulsory Vaccination," *BG*, 10 February 1902, 9.

33. From the Senate: J. Frank Porter (Republican), Justice of Peace from Danvers; Chester B. Williams (Republican), [I could not find him listed in the *Business Directory*] from Wayland (Cochituate); Cornelius R. Day (Republican), coal dealer from Blackstone (Millville). From the House: William J. Bullock (Republican), possibly a druggist from New Bedford [the *Business Directory* lists Bullock & Waldron under New Bedford druggists, 840]; William F. Craig, Republican from Lynn; Jeremiah J. Desmond, Democrat, druggist from Lawrence; John G. Hagberg, Republican from Worcester; Francis D. Newton, Republican insurance agent from Fayville, residing in Southborough; Walter E. Nichols, Republican druggist from Boston; J. William Williams, Republican from Medford; George A. Hall, Republican from Haverhill. The occupations are listed in the *Massachusetts Year Book and Business Directory* (1901); party affiliation and residence in *Manual of the Court*. See entries in *Massachusetts Yearbook and Business Directory*, 1323 for Nichols; 672 for Desmond; 840 for Bullock ("Bullock & Waldron"). None of the committee members was a physician.

34. William Bassett, president of the Massachusetts Anti-compulsory Vaccination Society, "conducted the case of the petitioners." George W. Allen, a "traveling man," J. M. Greene, editor of the antivivisectionist *Animal Defender*, and Hulda M. Loud, editor of a Rockland newspaper, also testified. See "Vaccination Opposed," *BET*, 4 February 1902, 3; and "Repeal Wanted," *BG*, 30 January 1902, 2. Hulda Loud also signed the 1901 Rockland petition for abolition of the law. See "Petition of George M. Smith, Feb. 7, 1901," H. 128, Unenacted Legislation for 1902, Massachusetts State Archives.

35. "Repeal Wanted," 2.

36. The *Globe* article refers to the letter as coming from "Dr. Frederick Martin, chairman of the Cleveland board of health," but this is an error. The correct name is Martin Friedrich.

37. Quotation from "Repeal Wanted," 2. The *Globe* describes J. D. Judge as "an allopathic physician and a graduate of the American medical school of Pennsylvania." He is listed at 358 Columbus Ave. in the *Massachusetts Year Book*, 1468. Joseph M. Greene identifies him also as working as superintendent and physician of the House of the Angel Guardian, Vernon St., Roxbury, in 1871, in "Notes on Vaccination," 13. Greene describes Judge's 1872 experience in "Legal Blood-Poisoning in Massachusetts," 19–20.

38. "Repeal Wanted," 2.

39. See chapter 4, note 9.

40. "Vaccination Opposed," 3.

41. "State Should Make the Virus," *BET*, 3 December 1901, 9; Durgin's remarks following Sedgwick, "Remarks on 'Opposition to Vaccination,'" 19. See also "Smallpox Talk," *BG*, 31 January 1902, 2; and "To Avoid Smallpox," *Boston Herald*, 31 January 1902, 8.

42. "Vaccination," *BG*, 1 February 1902, 4.

43. "Dr. Hastings Calls Durgin's Story False," *BP*, 5 February 1902, 1. Durgin also had told his fellow health officers about his encounter with Hastings at the Massachusetts Association of Boards of Health meeting just a few days before. There Durgin first mentioned that Hastings had asked him for a job and also asked about his opinion on the best lymph. See Durgin, remarks in discussion, *JMABH* 12 (April 1902): 18.

44. Hastings may have gotten wind of Durgin's story before he mentioned it at the vaccination hearings. The *Boston Herald*, *Globe*, and *Evening Transcript* had reported on Durgin's remarks at the Association meeting in some detail. The *Herald* and *Globe* offered detailed articles that paraphrased the talks and discussion. See "Smallpox Talk," *BG*, 31 January 1902, 2; "To Avoid Smallpox," *Boston Herald*, 31 January 1902, 8; and "Discussed Vaccination," *BET*, 30 January 1902, 2.

45. "Vaccination Opposed," 3.

46. "Dr. Hastings Calls Durgin's Story False," 1.

47. "Vaccination Opposed," 3. The same quote and confirmation is given in "Dr. Hastings Calls Durgin's Story False," 1.

48. Both quotations from Hastings in "Compulsory Vaccination," *Boston Courier*, 8 February 1902. For her gentility, see "Vaccination Bills In," 3.

49. "Last Arguments," *BG*, 4 February 1902, 9.

50. Ibid. See "Vaccination Opposed, 3.

51. "Compulsory Vaccination," *Boston Courier*, 8 February 1902.

52. "Compulsory Vaccination," *BET*, 31 January 1902, 6. McCollom was the lecturer who had argued with Pfeiffer about vaccination at the Ladies Physiological Institute in December 1901. See chapter 6, note 38. He began work as the city physician in 1881. See Boston Board of Health, "City Physician's Report," in *Tenth Annual Report of the Board of Health of the City of Boston, for the Financial Year 1881–1882* (Boston, 1882), 72–75.

53. "Vaccination," 4.

54. "Compulsory Vaccination," *BET*, 31 January 1902, 6.

55. Ibid.

56. "Vaccination," 4.

57. The *Globe* reported that Durgin "desired to present representatives of the great educational institutions, physicians and heads of mercantile establishments," which I interpret to mean that he orchestrated their appearance. The medical experts testifying represented the spectrum of medical disciplines and practice: Dr. Francis Draper, president of the Massachusetts Medical Society; William T. Councilman, Harvard professor of pathology and pathologist for Boston City Hospital; Dr. Horace Packard, professor of surgery, Boston University School of Medicine, according to *The New England Medical Gazette* 37 (June 1902); Dr. Mann, superintendent of the Massachusetts Homeopathic Hospital; Dr. Howard of Massachusetts General Hospital; Dr. Sherman, homeopath and smallpox specialist; Dr. Bancroft, resident physician at Boston City Hospital; Dr. Miles, president of the Massachusetts Eclectic Medical Society; and Dr. Azel Ames, medical inspector of Puerto Rico. See "More Protest against Repeal of Law," 4.

58. They included Horace D. Williams of Jordan Marsh Company, Wallace W. Chilson for Houghton & Dutton, B. F. Pitman for L. P. Hollander & Co., John Shepard for Shepard, Norwell Co., Mr. McGavin for Plant Shoe Co., and C. P. Jameson for Dominion SS Co. See "Doctors in Protest," *Boston Herald*, 4 February 1902, 3.

59. "Doctors in Protest," 3. The letters were from Harvard president Charles W. Eliot, MIT president Henry F. Pritchett, Archbishop Williams, and Bishop Beavan.

60. See Eliot letter in "More Protest against Repeal of Law," 4.

61. Ibid., 4.

62. All of these petitions failed to pass through committee: Pfeiffer petition (H 982) withdrawn 26 February 1902; Rueben Brown petition (H 128) withdrawn 4 March 1902; Foster petition (H 980) withdrawn 7 March 1902; Brooks petition (H 636) withdrawn 11 March 1902; Belknap petition (H 847) withdrawn 4 April 1902. See Commonwealth of Massachusetts, *Journal of the Senate* (1902).

63. "State Should Make the Virus," *BET*, 3 December 1901, 9. Senator Edward Seaver introduced Sen. 179. See Commonwealth of Massachusetts, *Journal of the Senate* (1902), 172. The bill, Sen. 179, was then sent to the House on 4 February 1902. See Commonwealth of Massachusetts, *Journal of the House of Representatives* (1902), 236. See chapter 2 for a discussion of S. 179.

64. Commonwealth of Massachusetts, *Journal of the Senate* (1902), 172. Senator Seaver also presented Durgin's vaccination bill, Sen. 178, in the Senate on 3 February 1902, which sent it to the House on 5 February 1902. See Commonwealth of Massachusetts, *Journal of the House of Representatives* (1902), 254.

65. Petition of Samuel Durgin, S. 178, S. 179, Unenacted Legislation, Massachusetts State Archives.

66. "Vaccination Bills In," 3.

67. "Anti-Vaccination," *BT*, 19 February 1902, 1, 3. The *Boston Globe* also reported on the hearing in "Make It Clear," *BG*, 19 February 1902, 4. E. M. Greene was the inspector for Bowdoin, Somerset, Sharp, Phillips, Grant, and Baldwin on Chardon Street schools in 1902. W. F. Temple was the medical inspector for Rice, Boys' Latin, Boys' High, Girls' Latin, and Girls' High schools in 1902. The *Transcript* identifies

286 ᜶ NOTES TO PP. 158–161

him as "Dr. Granger," but the Boston Health Department lists only a "William H. Grainger" as a medical inspector for Chapman, Tappan, and Parochial schools. See Boston Board of Health, *Thirty-First Annual Report for 1902*, 46, 47. Both their full names and addresses are listed in the *Massachusetts Year Book and Business Directory* (1901), 1467 and 1472.

68. "Anti-Vaccination," 1, 3.

69. Ibid.

70. "Vaccination Bills In," 3.

71. "Anti-Vaccination," 1, 3. The *Boston Globe* identifies him as "Dr. Cowles of Wakefield"; see "Make It Clear," 4.

72. "Anti-Vaccination," 1, 3.

73. "Make It Clear," 4, description of Hale as an allopath. See "Anti-Vaccination," 1, 3 for Hale quotations. George Carleton Hale was a registered physician under "Form B," which meant that he had practiced in Massachusetts for three years prior to the passage of the medical registration law of 7 June 1894. Physicians who registered under "Form B" did not have to pass a state exam or graduate from a legally chartered medical school. The "Form B" exception was a compromise designed to elicit support for the 1894 medical registration law from practicing physicians. See Massachusetts State Board of Registration, *Ninth Annual Report of the Board of Registration in Medicine* (Boston, 1903), 38. Hale's full name and address are listed in the *Massachusetts Year Book*, 1467.

74. "Make It Clear," 4, for description of Wheeler's education. The *Massachusetts Year Book*, 1473, has five Wheelers, one of which, Morris P., is listed as a homeopath. For quotations, see "Anti-Vaccination," 1, 3.

75. "Make It Clear, 4.

76. "Anti-Vaccination," 1, 3.

77. Senator Williams quoted in "Antis Gain Point," *BG*, 11 March 1902, 11. For the amendment to H. 1113, see Commonwealth of Massachusetts, *Journal of the Senate* (1902), 390.

78. Quotatation from "Antis Gain Point," 11. Out of a total of 39 voting state senators (Senator Rufus Soule, the president of the Senate, did not cast a vote), 17 voted for the amended version, 15 against it, and 6 either abstained or were absent.

79. Commonwealth of Massachusetts, "Senate, By Districts," in *Manual for the Use of the General Court* (1902), 373–76.

80. "Antis' Triumph Brief," *Boston Daily Advertiser*, 12 March 1902, 6; "Anti-Vaccinationists Lose," *Boston Evening Record*, 12 March 1902, 7; and "Antis Gain Point," 11.

81. Seventeen to thirteen, with eight abstentions. He picked up votes from four senators who had abstained, although two senators who had previously voted with him then abstained, holding his majority down to four votes. See Commonwealth of Massachusetts, *Journal of the Senate* (1902), 401–2.

82. See Commonwealth of Massachusetts, "Rules of the Senate—Voting," Rules 55–57, in Manual for the Use of the General Court (1902), 466.

83. See Commonwealth of Massachusetts, *Journal of the Senate* (1902), 390–91.

84. As of January 1902, Boston had by far the most smallpox cases in the state, 514. New Bedford was the next highest at 38, Fall River at 22, Cambridge at 15, Loeminster at 13, Lowell at 12, and Worcester at 11. Most of the other towns had

only one or two cases. Massachusetts State Board of Health, *Thirty-Third Annual Report* (1902), xi.

85. Williams lived in Wayland and represented Lexington, Lincoln, Marlborough, Medford, Sudbury, Waltham, Wayland, and Winchester. For Mrs. Henderson's testimony, see "Legal Blood-Poisoning in Massachusetts," 31. Also "About Smallpox," BG, 21 February 1902, 5. Mrs. Henderson became the president of MACVS in 1903. See Pfeiffer, "Anti-Compulsory Vaccination Society of Massachusetts and U.S. Supreme Court," 10. The mother of six children, she attended the Supreme Court hearing of Jacobson's appeal with "an eight-month-old babe" in her arms. See "The Brief and Argument of the Hon. George Fred Williams," The Liberator 6 (February 1905): 142.

86. Willard Howland represented Ward 1 (East Boston, noted for its cool reception of the vaccination sweep); John K. Berry represented Wards 16, 20, and 24 (all Dorchester wards also unhappy with the sweeps); Perlie Dyar represented Wards 11 (Back Bay), 19 (West Roxbury), and 25 (Roxbury Heights), which were among some of the wealthiest and noted for their patronage of physicians who advised against vaccination. Albert S. Aspey represented Cambridge Wards 1, 2, 4, and 5. John T. Sparks represented Lowell Wards 1–8. See appendix b for a more detailed breakdown of each senator's district and votes.

87. Joshua T. Small, "Anti-Vaccination Department," *Our Home Rights* 2 (January 1902): 8.

88. "Indignation: No Compulsory Vaccination for Rockland," *BG*, 8 August 1900, 2; and "In the Public Eye," *Boston Daily Advertiser*, 17 February 1902, 4. For Harvell, see Commonwealth of Massachusetts, "Senate, By Districts," *Manual for the Use of the General Court* (1902), 375.

89. Senator Williams quoted in "Antis Gain Point," 11.

90. It certainly does not surface in historical accounts of the development of Massachusetts health laws. In a thesis published just seven years later, Susan Wade Peabody does not even mention the 1902 amendment controversy in her discussion of the Massachusetts vaccination laws. Although her intent was to account for legislation that passed rather than dwell on reasons bills failed, she curiously also omitted any mention of the successful Durgin amendment to require physicians to personally examine candidates for unfitness certification. See Peabody, "Historical Study of Legislation," 50–51. Indeed it seems that others who witnessed this controversy also quickly forgot it had ever occurred. Just a little over fifteen years later, a former *Boston Globe* reporter's history of noteworthy 1902 legislation announced simply that "vaccination was made compulsory." Hennessy, *Twenty-Five Years of Massachusetts Politics*, 100.

Chapter Eight

1. Boston Board of Health, "Vaccination," Thirtieth Annual Report for 1901, 45.

2. In 1902, county authorities criminally prosecuted thirty-eight cases for violation of the Massachusetts vaccination statutes in Middlesex (nineteen from Cambridge) and Suffolk (nineteen from Boston) Counties. See Massachusetts Board of Prison Commissioners, *Second Annual Report of the Board of Prison Commissioners of Massachusetts . . . for the Year Ending September 30, 1902* (Boston, 1902), 104.

3. "Dr. Durgin Warns as to Spread of Smallpox," 8. Dr. Immanuel Pfeiffer also reprinted the interview. See "Dr. Durgin as Prosecutor," 37.

4. "Vaccination Opposed," 3.

5. Abbott, "Legislation with Reference to Smallpox and Vaccination," 267.

6. Massachusetts State Board of Health, "Smallpox," *Thirty-Third Annual Report* (1902), xi–xii. The year covered by the report is 1901.

7. Massachusetts State Board of Health, "Vaccination," *Thirty-Second Annual Report* (1901), xx–xxiii, xxi.

8. Medford population in the *Massachusetts Year Book and Business Directory* (1901), 785. Quotations from Massachusetts State Board of Health, "Smallpox" and "Health of Towns—Medford," *Annual Report* [for 1901], xi and 579.

9. Brookline population in *Massachusetts Year Book*, 381. Quotations from Massachusetts State Board of Health, "Health of Towns—Brookline," *Annual Report* [for 1901], 568–70, 569. The report for 1902 does not even mention smallpox. Massachusetts State Board of Health, "Health of Towns—Brookline," *Thirty-Fourth Annual Report* (1903), 570–73.

10. Massachusetts State Board of Health, "Health of Towns—Somerville," *Report* [for 1901], 586, 544 for Somerville population total.

11. Massachusetts State Board of Health, "Health of Towns—Newton," *Report* [for 1901], 581, population on 544.

12. Massachusetts State Board of Health, "Health of Towns—Newton," *Report* [for 1902], 580, cases on 545.

13. Massachusetts State Board of Health, Table 1, *Report* [for 1901], 544.

14. Massachusetts State Board of Health, "Smallpox" and "Health of Towns—Quincy," *Report* [for 1901], xi–xii (for locations of smallpox cases), 584 (Quincy report). Despite its stated emphasis on smallpox as a "principal point of interest," the State Board of Health did not feature any extract from the Hyde Park report and it omitted any mention of vaccination or smallpox in its extract from the Quincy report for 1901. Perhaps these towns undertook a vaccination campaign that the State Board of Health omitted from its extracts, but I think it unlikely given the board's concern about vaccination that year.

15. Massachusetts State Board of Health, "Health of Towns—Watertown," *Report* [for 1901], 589.

16. Massachusetts State Board of Health, "Cases of Infectious Diseases Reported to the State Board of Health from Two Hundred and Sixty-One Cities and Towns during 1902," *Report* [for 1902], 545. The Somerville extract for 1902 (582) does not mention vaccination, but newspapers reported the order. See "Stands By Albert M. Pear," *BG*, 2 December 1902, 4 for the forty-one refusals. See also J. M. Greene, citing the *Boston Post*, 26 October 1902, and the *Boston Record*, 27 October 1902, for the Somerville vaccination order, in "A Medical Crime," *The Animals' Defender* 7 (December 1902): 23.

17. Massachusetts State Board of Health, "Health of Towns—Southbridge," *Report* [for 1902], 583.

18. Massachusetts State Board of Health, "Health of Towns—North Adams," *Report* [for 1901], 582.

19. Dr. James C. Coffey, secretary of the Association and member of the Worcester Board of Health, comments following Dr. Thomas B. Shea, "Small-pox and Vaccination," *JMABH* 12 (April 1902): 42–43.

20. Massachusetts, *An Act Relative to Vaccination, Acts* (1894), chapter 515, section 5, 667–68.

21. "Smallpox Record Grows," 14.

22. Greene, "Vaccination Scourge," 23.

23. "No Small Pox in Department Stores," Boston Board of Health notice, *BET*, 23 November 1901, 1; "No Smallpox in Big Stores," *BP*, 22 November 1901, 8; "Stores Are Clean," *BP*, 24 November 1901, 1; and "No Smallpox in Large Stores," Boston Board of Health notice, *BP*, 14 December 1901, 1, and 15 December 1901, 1.

24. Advertisement for Manhattan Market, *CC*, 28 June 1902, 16.

25. Edward M. Greene, "On Giving Certificates of Vaccination," letter dated 11 December 1902, *BMSJ* 147 (1902): 687.

26. "No Smallpox in Big Stores," 8.

27. "Wholesale Vaccination," *Cambridge Democrat*, 30 November 1901, 8.

28. "Osgood's Employees Vaccinated," *Boston Post*, December 2, 1901, 5.

29. "American News and Notes," *American Medicine* 2 (1901): 434; and "Two More Cases," *BET*, 31 August 1901, 3.

30. "This Evening's News," *BET*, 2 November 1901, 1; and "All Will Have Sore Arms," *BET*, 15 November 1901, 5.

31. "One Death in Cambridge," *BET*, 27 November 1901, 3; and "Mayor Advises Vaccination," *BET*, 26 November 1901, 2.

32. "Twenty-Seven More Cases," *BET*, 29 November 1901, 3.

33. "American News and Notes," *American Medicine* 2 (1901): 889.

34. "Vaccination at Bostock's," *BP*, 2 December 1901, 5.

35. Dr. James B. Bell, testimony before the Joint Committee on Public Health, quoted in "Vaccination Opposed," 3.

36. Unnamed correspondent, Letter, quoted in *Our Home Rights* 1 (October 1901): 17–18.

37. Greene, "Eighty Victims," *The Liberator* 4 (October 1903): 27–28.

38. Ibid., 271.

39. "More Protest against Repeal of Law," 4.

40. "Damage Suit in Massachusetts," *The Liberator* 4 (January 1904): 109.

41. "Smallpox Now Epidemic in Philadelphia," News Items, *New York Medical Journal and Philadelphia Medical Journal* 78 (1903): 1050. The church, known as the Church of God and Saints in Christ, had attracted the attention of the authorities because its founder, Bishop Crowdy, preached that prayer alone could heal the sick. With three smallpox deaths in the neighborhood, and church members known to have visited the sick "indiscriminately," the health department deemed them "a threatening menace to the community of Philadelphia." See also "Faith Curists Again" and "Negro Faith Curist Escapes the Philadelphia Authorities," News Items, *New York Medical Journal and Philadelphia Medical Journal* 78 (1903): 1000, 1001; and "Bigotry and Persecution Rampant in Philadelphia," *The Liberator* 4 (December 1903): 79–81.

42. "Held Up the Train," *BG*, 8 February 1902, 2.

43. J. M. Greene, quoting a story on the traders' vaccinations on 18 January 1902, from the *New York Herald*, 19 January 1902, in "Notes on Vaccination," 12.

44. The *Philadelphia Evening Bulletin*, quoted in Clymer, *Vaccination Brought Home*, 81.

45. Clymer set his account of the Italian laborers in a section titled "The Despotism of Darkest Russia in America." Lora Little titled her account of the Philadelphia congregation "Bigotry and Persecution Rampant in Philadelphia," *The Liberator* 4 (December 1903): 79–81.

46. The *Philadelphia Evening Bulletin*, quoted in Clymer, *Vaccination Brought Home*, 80.

47. "Held Up the Train," 2.

48. "Factory Girls' Resistance," *BG*, 12 April 1901, 3.

49. Editorial Item, *CC*, 19 July 1902, 2.

50. "Tramp, Stopped By Doctor, Had Small-Pox," *BER*, 6 February 1902, 1. Sadly Roche died a few days later. See "Disinfect Their Office," *BG*, 8 February 1902, 2.

51. "Another Tramp Found Ill with Smallpox," *BER*, 7 February 1902, 1; and "One More Tramp with Smallpox in Court Sq.," *BER*, 12 February 1902, 1.

52. "Homeless Man with Smallpox," *BER*, 13 February 1902, 2.

53. Quotation in "Smallpox Record Grows," 14; see also "Health Board Urges All to Be Vaccinated," 4.

54. "Health Board Vigilant," *BG*, 8 February 1902, 3.

55. "Tramps Object to Vaccination," *BP*, 26 January 1902, 8.

56. "Virus Squad Out," *BG*, 18 November 1901, 7.

57. Greene, "Facts about Vaccination," 23. Italics in original.

58. Greene, "Notes on Vaccination," 12.

59. "Tramps Object to Vaccination," 8.

60. "He Had Smallpox," *BG*, 3 February 1902, 1.

61. Boston Board of Health, "Vaccination," *Thirtieth Annual Report for 1901*, 45.

62. "Eight Smallpox Cases," *BP*, 8 February 1902, 12.

63. Warner, *Streetcar Suburbs*.

64. Boston Board of Health, "Tenement Houses," *Report for 1901*, 40.

65. Warner, *Streetcar Suburbs*, 86.

66. Woods and Kennedy, *Zone of Emergence*, 136. The original manuscripts were composed between 1907 and 1914 but not published until 1962.

67. "To East Boston," *BG*, 27 January 1902, 1.

68. The East Boston subway tunnel was constructed in 1905.

69. Woods and Kennedy, *Zone of Emergence*, 151–83, describing East Boston; quotations on 180, 152, and 176.

70. Schoolmaster Prince, testimony before the Joint Committee on Public Health, in "Anti-Vaccination," 3. See chapter 4 for discussion of various vaccination rates among schoolchildren.

71. "To East Boston," 1.

72. Frank M. Davis, "Defendant's Exceptions," 3, in *Commonwealth v. John H. Mugford*, in vol. 183, *Massachusetts Reports: Papers and Briefs* (1903).

73. Mugford's neighbors were a marine engineer, ironworker, printer, cigar maker, salesman, expressman, drummer, cabinetmaker, and two teamsters, according to the Bureau of the Census, *Twelfth Census of the United States, Suffolk County, Massachusetts, June 4, 1900*. Many thanks to Judy Bates for supplying this information through ancestry.com. Bessie is listed under "milk and cheese dealers," *Massachusetts Year Book and Business Directory* (1901), 1281. For Mugford's grocery store, see Greene, "Prosecution or Persecution?" 5.

74. Woods and Kennedy, *Zone of Emergence*, South Boston information on 128–50; quotations on 138, 136, 134.

75. "About 10,000 Vaccinated in South Boston," *BG*, 28 January 1902, 14.

76. Greene, "Legal Blood-Poisoning in Massachusetts," 17.

77. "About 10,000 Vaccinated in South Boston," 14.

78. Emmons full name given in the *Massachusetts Year Book*, 180.

79. "Board of Health Wins," *BG*, 7 February 1902, 4.

80. "Eight Smallpox Cases," 12; "Board of Health Wins," 4 for quotations. See also "Board of Health Wins," *BG*, 8 February 1902, 3.

81. "Vaccination Cases," *BG*, 1 March 1902, 12; and "Refused to Be Vaccinated," *BP*, 2 March 1902, 12. The court did not explain why it fined Mugford fifteen dollars for failure to vaccinate his daughter.

82. The formal complaint was filed 1 April and entered 7 April 1902. See "Complaint" and "Record of Superior Court," in Davis, "Defendant's Exceptions," *Commonwealth v. John H. Mugford*.

83. There are two "Defendant's Exceptions" in Mugford's appeal. One concerns John Mugford's refusal for his own vaccination, the other his refusal to vaccinate his daughter, Eva.

84. Frank M. Davis had practiced law since 1883. See William T. Davis, *Bench and Bar of the Commonwealth of Massachusetts* (1895; reprint, New York: DeCapo Press, 1974), 467.

85. Cross examination of Charles E. Davis, Jr., secretary to the Boston Board of Health, and cross examination of the health department physician John L. Ames, in M. J. Sughrue, "Brief for the Commonwealth," 2 and 3, in *Commonwealth v. John H. Mugford*, in vol. 183, *Massachusetts Reports: Papers and Briefs* (1903).

86. Davis, "Defendant's Exceptions," *Commonwealth v. John H. Mugford*.

87. Editorial, *BER*, 26 April 1902, 4. See also Greene, "Legal Blood-Poisoning in Massachusetts," 17.

88. "Record of the Superior Court," *Commonwealth v. John H. Mugford*, in vol. 183, *Massachusetts Reports: Papers and Briefs* (1903). Why Sheldon stalled on accepting Mugford's exceptions is a mystery; he gave no reason for the delay.

89. See "Cate Will Not Pay Fine," *BER*, 20 February 1902, 1, for "lumper"; and "Would Not Be Vaccinated," *BG* [Evening], 20 February 1902, 1, for furniture moving detail. A "lumper" is a person who unloads fishing vessels.

90. "Would Not Be Vaccinated," 1, for first quotation. The article gives the address of the lodging house where Cate and his wife occupied "one room" as "281 Shawmut av." Second quotation in "Cate Will Not Pay Fine," 1.

91. See "Cate's Costly Obstinacy," *BDA*, 21 February 1902, 8, for reference to his vaccination status. For quotation, see "Would Not Be Vaccinated," 1.

92. "Would Not Be Vaccinated," 1.

93. "Fifteen Days In Jail," *BG*, 21 February 1902, 5. A first *Globe* article mentions a ten-day sentence and then later a fifteen-day sentence. See "Would Not Be Vaccinated," 1. Police told another newspaper that it would take Cate thirty days to serve out his five-dollar fine, but that "he may be held only eight days." See item in "In the Public Eye" section, *BDA*, 21 February 1902, 4.

94. An act of 1701–2 empowered "selectmen of towns to remove, isolate, and provide for persons sick or infected with contagious disease, intended particularly to prevent the spread of smallpox." See Peabody, "Historical Survey of Legislation," 44.

95. Durgin quoted in a news item from "In the Public Eye" section, *BDA*, 21 February 1902, 4.

96. "Would Not Be Vaccinated," 1.

97. "More Arrests Next Monday," *BET*, 21 February 1902, 12, puts the vaccination in the evening, but the *Boston Evening Record* declared it happened the next morning; see "Cate Says He Has Had Smallpox Once," *BER*, 24 February 1902, 5. See also "Fifteen Days in Jail," 5.

98. "Cate Says He Has Had Smallpox Once," *BER*, 5.

99. "Costs Him Dear," *BG*, 7 November 1903, 11.

100. "More Arrests Next Monday," 12.

101. Editorial Note, *BER*, 21 February 1902, 4.

102. "Cate Will Know Better Next Time. Perhaps," Letter from Charles E. Page, Boston, dated 25 February 1902, *BER*, 26 February 1902.

103. "Pretty Mary Would Go to Jail Rather Than Be Vaccinated," *BG*, 26 February 1902, 5.

104. Sarah Deutsch, *Women and the City: Gender, Space, and Power in Boston, 1870–1940* (Oxford: Oxford University Press, 2000), 101.

105. Ibid.

106. Boston Board of Health, *Report for 1901*, 39. Italics added for emphasis.

107. J. M. Greene, citing the story about Mrs. Clifford Sykes in the *Boston Record*, 17 October 1902, in "A Great Medical Scandal," 26.

108. "Made a Test Case," Medical News, *JAMA* 44 (1905): 135.

109. Greene, "A Great Medical Scandal," 25; and "A Medical Crime," 22–23.

110. Greene, "Legal Blood-Poisoning in Massachusetts," 18.

111. "Pres. Eliot's Views," 9.

112. "Vaccination at Harvard," *BET*, 3 December 1902, 9.

113. Cambridge Board of Health, "Report," in *Annual Reports Made to the City Council for the Year 1902* (Cambridge, 1903), 643. See also "Compulsory Vaccination," *CC*, 8 March 1902, 5; and "Seventeen Physicians at Work," *BET*, 8 March 1902, for Harvard coverage.

114. Cambridge Board of Health, "Report" (1902), 643.

115. J. M. Greene, "Crime in Massachusetts," *The Animals' Defender* 7 (May 1902): 21–22.

116. J. M. Greene states that the letter was sent 25 March 1902 in "Crime in Massachusetts," 22. The sweep began on 8 March 1902 and continued through at least 15 March 1902. See J. W. Pickering, "Defendant's Exceptions," in *Henning Jacobson, Plaintiff in Error, v. The Commowealth of Massachusetts*, in *Supreme Court Records and Briefs* (Washington DC: Judd & Detweiler, July 13, 1903), 5; and "Compulsory Vaccination," *CC*, 8 March 1902, 5.

117. Cambridge Board of Health, "Report" (1902), 658.

118. "Small Pox Scourge," *CC*, 21 June 1902, 4.

119. "Small Pox Epidemic Closes the Schools," *CC*, 21 June 1902, 5.

120. "Small Pox Scourge," 4.

121. Ibid. See also "Prosecution!" Official notice placed in *Cambridge Democrat*, 28 June 1902, 1. The board met on 20 June 1902.

122. Cambridge Board of Health, "Report" (1902), 643.

123. "Small Pox Scourge," 4.

124. "Smallpox Fully under Control," *CC*, 28 June 1902, 4.

125. "The Chronicler," editorial, *CC*, 28 June 1902, 2.

126. "The Cambridge Smallpox Epidemic," *Medical News* 80 (1902): 1230.

127. "News Items," *New York Medical Journal* 76 (1902): 27.

128. "The Chronicler," editorial, *CC*, 28 June 1902, 2; and "Small Pox Fully under Control," 4.

129. Letter to Mayor McNamee dated 25 June 1902, *CC*, 28 June 1902, 4.

130. "More Smallpox Cases in North Cambridge," *CC*, 12 July 1902, 2.

131. "Mayor McNamee Scores a Point," *CC*, 12 July 1902, 4.

132. "The Revival of Smallpox," Editorial, *CC*, 12 July 1902, 4.

133. Greene, citing the *Boston Post*, 13 July 1902, in "Law versus Order," 17.

134. J. W. Pickering, "Criminal Complaint" attached to "Defendant's Exceptions," 4–5, in *Commonwealth v. Albert M. Pear*, vol. 183, *Massachusetts Reports: Papers and Briefs* (1903); and J. W. Pickering, "Criminal Complaint," attached to "Defendant's Exceptions," 7, in *Commonwealth v. Jacobson*, vol. 183, *Massachusetts Reports: Papers and Briefs* (1903).

135. "Not Vaccinated," *Cambridge Tribune*, 19 July 1902. The *Boston Medical and Surgical Journal* described them as "several citizens of more or less prominence." See "In Court for Refusing to Be Vaccinated," *BMSJ* 147 (1902): 141. The other defendants were Ephraim Gould, his wife, Maggie Gould, and Paul Morse, a brickmaker. See "Anti-Vaccinationists Must Go into Court, Board of Health Has Proceeded against Six Recalcitrants—Assistant City Clerk Pear One of the Number," *CC*, 19 July 1902, 1.

136. S. G. Häggland, "Henning Jacobson," *My Church: An Illustrated Manual* 17 (1931): 160–63.

137. "Cambridge's Electric Plant," *BG*, 20 November 1895, 7.

138. For Pear's salary, see *Massachusetts Year Book*, 390. "Bancroft Said No," *BG*, 5 February 1896, 4, mentions Pear's first reelection. "Won't Submit, Albert M. Pear an Antivaccinationist," *BG*, 18 July 1902, 12, notes that Pear "has held the position of assistant city clerk for the past eight years."

139. "Won't Submit," 12.

140. See Massachusetts State Board of Health, "List of Salaries," vol. 3, *Records of the State Board of Health of Massachusetts*, beginning May 1886, unnumbered page inserted between pages 308 and 309, Massachusetts State Archives. Salaries of clerks, salespeople, and bookkeepers ranged from $480 to $960 in 1902. See Stephan Thernstrom, *The Other Bostonians: Poverty and Progress in the American Metropolis, 1880–1970* (Cambridge, MA: Harvard University Press, 1973), 301.

141. "Won't Submit," 12.

142. "Anti-Vaccinationists Must Go into Court," 1.

143. "Anti-Vaccination," *CC*, 29 March 1902, 5. Caroline Hanks Hitchcock served as chairman.

144. "Anti-Vaccinationists Must Go into Court," 1.

145. See, for instance, "Won't Submit," 12 (with photograph); "Anti-Vaccinationists Must Go into Court," 1 (with photograph); "Vaccination Test Case," *BG*, 13 November 1902, 4 (with photograph).

146. "Won't Submit," 12.

147. The hearing was postponed from 19 July to 23 July 1902 because the health department failed to send a representative; see "Cambridge," News Item, *BG*, 19 July

1902, 7. Pickering signed a legislative petition in 1903 as a member of a committee authorized by the Massachusetts Anti-compulsory Vaccination Society. See his
signature in "H 698: Petition of John F. Foster and others for legislation to prevent
persons being vaccinated against their will," in Unpassed Legislation Files (1903),
Massachusetts State Archives.

148. "Three Cases Appealed," *Cambridge Tribune*, 26 July 1902, 1; and "Four
Prosecutions By Board of Health," *CC*, 26 July 1902, 4.

149. "Four Prosecutions By Board of Health," 4.

150. "Vaccination Cases in Court," *BET*, 23 July 1902, 11.

151. "Four Prosecutions By Board of Health," 4.

152. "Three Cases Appealed," 1.

153. "Four Prosecutions By Board of Health," 4.

154. "Vaccination Cases in Court," 11; "Three Cases Appealed," 1; "Four
Prosecutions By Board of Health," 4; and "Fined Them $5 Each," *BG*, 23 July 1902, 7.
The insurance agent George A. Giles posted Jacobson's $200 bond. Giles represented
several insurance companies, according to the *Cambridge Directory of the Inhabitants,
Institutions, Manufacturing Establishments, Societies, Business, Business Firms, Map, State
Census, etc.* (Boston: W. A. Greenough & Co., 1902), 223. For Giles as bondsman, see
"Memorandum" attached to "Plea of Not Guilty," in "Record in the Third District
Court," *Henning Jacobson v. The Commonwealth of Massachusetts*, in *United States Supreme
Court Records and Briefs*, 4 [6 in the original].

155. "Not Vaccinated," *Cambridge Tribune*, 19 July 1902, no page number available.

156. Pickering, "Defendant's Exceptions," 4, *Commonwealth v. Henning Jacobson*.

157. "Vaccination Case in the U.S. Supreme Court," *The Liberator* 6 (December
1904): 78. The incident with Jacobson's daughter must have occurred between 1892,
when Jacobson moved to Cambridge, and before the 1894 amendment permitting
unfitness certificates for vaccination, which would explain Jacobson seeking a special
exemption from Abbott. Henning Jacobson married Hattie C. Anderson in 1882.
They had five children, Julia, Ruth, Joseph, David, and Marcus. The *Twelfth Census of
the United States* lists just the three sons living at home in 1900, but Hattie as having
had five children altogether, meaning that Julia and Ruth had died or left home by
1900. Hattie attended Gustavus Adolphus College. Two of the sons became attorneys.
For Jacobson's family, see Häggland, "Henning Jacobson," 160; and "Mrs. Hattie C.
Jacobson," *Lutheran Companion* 45 (1931): 151.

158. Henning Jacobson, "Sermon Notes for Marriages, 1894–1910" Folder, Box 2,
Faith/Augustana Lutheran Church of Cambridge (209 Chestnut Street, Cambridge,
MA), Lutheran Archives Center, Northeast Region Archives, Evangelical Lutheran
Church of America, Germantown, PA.

159. This characterization is based on a translation from Swedish: "Han sjöng ut
utan omsvep och var if rädd att saga: 'Du är den mannen!'" in "Henning Jacobson,"
Korsbaneret: Kristlig Kalendar för Året 1932 (Rock Island, IL: Augustana Book Concern,
1932). Dr. Kim Eric Williams of the Lutheran Archives Center translated this quotation for me in a 1999 personal communication: "he was without hostility and not
afraid to say 'You are the man!'" Dr. Williams observed that this saying referred to
the Old Testament in the Bible when the Prophet Nathan counseled David to stand
up for himself and meant that Jacobson "was not afraid to speak out in the face of
extreme opposition and pressure not to."

160. Jacobson made $672 per year, placing him in the low white-collar earnings range, according to Thernstrom's *Other Bostonians*, 300. Skilled manual laborers made more, ranging from fifteen to twenty dollars per week. For Jacobson's salary, see Augustana Lutheran Church, *After Fifty Years, 1892–1942* (Cambridge, MA: Augustana Lutheran Church, 1942), 13, in Archives of the Evangelical Lutheran Church in America, Chicago, Illinois.

161. Augustana Lutheran Church, *After Fifty Years*, 13–14.

162. He served as a student pastor in Wataga, Illinois, Davenport, Iowa, and New Haven and South Manchester, Connecticut, and one mentor called him "an uncommonly gifted speaker." He also attended Yale Divinity School while living in New Haven. His brother Fritz Jacobson was pastor to a congregation of several thousand in Brooklyn, New York. For detailed biographical information see Häggland, "Henning Jacobson," 160–62. Jacobson was born on 15 September 1856 in Yllestad, Sweden, and died on 14 October 1930 in Belmont, Massachusetts. For obituaries, see New York Times, 15 October 1930, Cambridge Chronicle, 17 October 1930, and Belmont Citizen, 18 October 1930. None of them mention his United States Supreme Court case.

163. See *Historik: Öfver Förberedel och Organizeringen af Svenska Ev. Luth. Augustana Församlingen i Cambridge Massachusetts, Jemte Dess Tio-åriga Versamhet, Räknadt Från den 21 August 1892 till och med Nyårssämman 1902.* (Svenska Tryckeriet, 1902). Held by Archives of the Evangelical Lutheran Church in America, Elk Grove, IL.

164. See *Missionären* (Mars, Maj, June, Juli, 1902), Archives of the Evangelical Lutheran Church in America, Elk Grove, IL.

165. J. M. Greene notes that Jacobson spoke at a MACVS meeting on 3 November 1902, in "A Medical Crime," 22.

166. "Goes to Supreme Court," *Cambridge Tribune*, 15 November 1902, 10. Jacobson's trial came up on 27 February 1903. See "Record in the Third District Court," 5 [8 in the original].

167. "Test Vaccination Case," *CC*, 15 November 1902, 12; "Goes to Supreme Court," *Cambridge Tribune*, 15 November 1902, 10; and "Vaccination Test Case," *BG*, 13 November 1902, 4.

168. "Test Vaccination Case," 12.

169. "Goes to Supreme Court," 10.

170. "The Vaccination Question," *CC*, 15 November 1902, 2.

171. "Goes to Supreme Court," 10.

172. John Mugford's case came to trial 25 April 1902. Although he filed exceptions immediately, the Supreme Judicial Court did not accept them until 29 October 1902. See "Record of the Superior Court," *Commonwealth v. John H. Mugford* (1903).

173. The society gave up funding Mugford "because of complications testing too severely its finances," and his attorney may have been too ill to prepare an adequate brief, for he died in the summer of 1903, according to Greene, in "Prosecution or Persecution?" 5. It voted instead "to sustain" Pear "in his contest with the board of health." See "Stands By Albert M. Pear," 4. Pear went to trial 12 November 1902, according to "Goes to Supreme Court," *Cambridge Tribune*, 15 November 1902, 10. Jacobson's trial came up on 27 February 1903. See "Record in the Third District Court," *Henning Jacobson v. The Commonwealth of Massachusetts*, 5 [8 in original].

174. "Good Work," Letter from C. Asbury Simpson, secretary-treasurer, MACVS, *The Liberator* (December 1902): 75.

175. The vaccination law was changed to require that a physician personally examine a child before granting him or her a certificate of unfitness for vaccination. See chapter 190, "An Act Relative to Vaccination," *Acts and Resolves Passed By the General Court of Massachusetts in the Year 1902* (Boston, 1902), 138–39. The Act took effect 19 March 1902.

176. "Mistake as to Facts," *BG*, 20 January 1903, 5.

177. "Defendant's Exceptions," 2, *Commonwealth v. Henning Jacobson*, vol. 183, *Massachusetts Reports: Papers and Briefs* (1903).

178. Jacobson's trial took place on 27 February 1903. Pickering filed exceptions on 2 March 1903. See "Record in Third District court," 5 [8 in the original].

179. "On Adverse Decision in Massachusetts: Case to be Appealed, Aid Needed," Letter from C. Asbury Simpson, secretary-treasurer, MACVS, *The Liberator* 3 (June 1903): 265.

180. Pickering, "Defendant's Exceptions," 2–4, in *Commonwealth v. Henning Jacobson*, vol. 183, *Massachusetts Reports: Papers and Briefs* (1903).

Chapter Nine

1. Marcus Dubber, *The Police Power: Patriarchy and the Foundations of American Government* (New York: Columbia University Press, 2005).

2. See Novak, *People's Welfare*, for a compelling and thorough discussion of how states and localities used police power to regulate nearly every aspect of their citizens' lives, property, and business. I base much of my discussion below on Novak's history.

3. Novak, *People's Welfare*, 1, 14. That does not mean that Americans did not resist government regulation of their businesses and lives. After all, Novak's study looks at appellate court decisions that grew out of objections to police power regulations. His point was that "the well-regulated society" was an idea that the courts tended to back up when they upheld state authority to make such laws. That said, we must remember it might not have been so easy to enforce regulations in cities and states lacking the necessary administrative apparatus to do so. My thanks to Tom Broman for reminding me of this important qualification.

4. U.S. Const. amend. XIV, §1.

5. Novak, *People's Welfare*, 323.

6. *Slaughterhouse Cases*, 83 U.S. 36 (1872), 62.

7. *Munn v. Illinois*, 94 U.S. 113 (1877), 126.

8. Loren P. Beth, *John Marshall Harlan: The Last Whig Justice* (Lexington: University Press of Kentucky, 1992), 208.

9. Novak, *People's Welfare*, 233.

10. Rodney L. Mott, *Due Process of Law: A Historical and Analytical Treatise of the Principles and Methods Followed By the Courts in the Application of the Concept of the "Law of the Land"* (Indianapolis, IN: The Bobbs-Merrill Company, 1926), 338.

11. Novak, *People's Welfare*, 247. The cases were: *Mugler v. Kansas*, 123 U.S. 623 (1887); *Powell v. Pennsylvania*, 127 U.S. 678 (1888); *Budd v. New York*, 143 U.S. 517 (1892); and *Lawton v. Steele*, 152 U.S. 133 (1894).

12. Beth, *John Marshall Harlan*, 210. See also his concise discussion of substantive due process on 208–15.

13. The Court upheld the constitutionality of a medical licensing law, for instance, because it concerned public health in 1889, but decided in 1897 that a state statute fining purchasers of insurance from businesses outside the state violated "liberty of contract" and thus due process because it interfered with private business and did not affect the public interest. See *Dent v. West Virginia*, 129 U.S. 114 (1889), and *Allgeyer v. Louisiana*, 165 U.S. 578 (1897). Justice Rufus Wheeler Peckham wrote *Allgeyer* and connected liberty of contract to substantive due process in many opinions. As Bernard Schwartz put it, *Allgeyer* "made due process dominant as the doctrine virtually immunizing economic activity from regulation deemed contrary to the laissez-faire philosophy of the day." Bernard Schwartz, A History of the Supreme Court (New York: Oxford University Press, 1993), 180. According to the legal scholar Wendy Parmet, this scrutiny ended in 1937 when the Court decided "it would no longer review whether state regulations truly protected the public health. The case was *West Coast Hotel v. Parish*, 300 U.S. 379 (1937). See Parmet, "From Slaughter-House to Lochner," 476 n. 5.

14. *Wong Wai v. Williamson*, 103 U.S. (1900), and *Jew Ho v. Williamson*, 103 U.S. (1900).

15. See "Doctors Accompanied By Policeman," Letter from H. A. Libbey, Boston, MA, 20 February 1903, *The Liberator* 2 (March 1903), 181; and Simpson, "On Adverse Decision in Massachusetts," 265.

16. Quotations from "Henry Ballard Dead," *BG*, 24 September 1906, 9. For his effectiveness as a public speaker, see "The Campaign in Malone," *New York Times*, 9 September 1876, 1.

17. Henry Ballard and J. W. Pickering, "Brief for Defendant," 3, 4, in *Commonwealth v. Albert M. Pear*, in vol. 183, *Massachusetts Reports: Papers and Briefs* (1903); and Ballard and Pickering, "Brief for Defendant," 3, 4, in *Commonwealth v. Henning Jacobson*, in vol. 183, *Massachusetts Reports: Papers and Briefs* (1903).

18. Ballard and Pickering quoting Justice Dunbar, Supreme Court of Washington, in *State v. Buchanan*, 55 Cent. L. J. 428 (1902), in Ballard and Pickering, "Brief for Defendant," 4, in *Commonwealth v. Albert M. Pear*, and "Brief for Defendant," 4, in *Commonwealth v. Henning Jacobson*. Italics in original.

19. Ballard and Pickering, "Brief for Defendant," 5–7, 18, in *Commonwealth v. Albert M. Pear*, and "Brief for Defendant," 5–7, 18, in *Commonwealth v. Henning Jacobson*.

20. Henry Ballard and J. W. Pickering, "Medical Authorities," in "Brief for Defendant," 20–24, in *Commonwealth v. Albert M. Pear*, and "Medical Authorities" in "Brief for Defendant," 20–24, in *Commonwealth v. Henning Jacobson*. Ballard and Pickering provided the following citation: Joseph McFarland, "Tetanus and Vaccination: An Analytical Study of Ninety-Five Cases of This Rare Complication," *Boston Journal of Medical Research* (May 1902). He read the paper at a meeting of the American Association of Pathologists and Bacteriologists on 28 March 1902, and it was also published in *Medicine* 8 (June 1902): 441–56.

21. J. M. Green, quoting Pickering in "State vs. Pear and Jacobson," *The Animals' Defender* 8 (April 1903): 27; and Greene, "An Adverse Decision," *The Liberator* 3 (April 1903): 208.

22. Henry Ballard, "Additional Points and Considerations," in "Brief for Defendant," 25–39, 25, 28, 29, 30, in *Commonwealth vs. Henning Jacobson*. Italics in original.

23. Greene, "State vs. Pear and Jacobson," 27; and Greene, "An Adverse Decision," 208.

24. Information on Bancroft from various articles. See "Hugh Bancroft, 53, Publisher, Is Dead," *New York Times*, 18 October 1933, 21; "Hugh Bancroft, at 32, in $15,000 Position," *BG*, 10 December 1911, 35; "Hugh Bancroft Has Resigned," *BG*, 4 January 1906, 14; "Sleeps in Holyhood," *BG*, 2 November 1903, 4; and "County Officials Organize," *BG*, 2 January 1902, 12. After the tragic death of his first wife in childbirth in late 1903, he married the daughter of Clarence W. Barron, publisher of financial papers like the *Wall Street Journal* and *Barron's Weekly*. From 1911 to 1914, Bancroft served as chairman of the Port of Boston, a very lucrative position. Later he entered the publishing business, eventually rising to take over as president of his father-in-law's businesses.

25. Hugh Bancroft, "Brief for the Commonwealth," 4, in *Commonwealth v. Henning Jacobson*, vol. 183, *Massachusetts Reports: Papers and Briefs* (1903); and Bancroft, "Brief for the Commonwealth," 2, in *Commonwealth v. Albert M. Pear*, vol. 183, *Massachusetts Reports: Papers and Briefs* (1903) for identical language.

26. Bancroft, "Brief for the Commonwealth," 4, 7, in *Commonwealth v. Henning Jacobson*.

27. Massachusetts Constitution, art. 14, forbids unreasonable seizure of the person. Bancroft, "Brief for the Commonwealth," 5, 7, in *Commonwealth v. Henning Jacobson*, and "Brief for the Commonwealth," 5, in *Commonwealth v. Albert M. Pear*.

28. The Supreme Judicial Court considered the case important enough to warrant a hearing before the full bench of justices. Justices present were Knowlton, Barker, Hammond, Loring, and Braley. See "Judge Dewey Resigns," *BET*, 10 December 1902, 12.

29. Holmes resigned to accept a position as associate justice on the United States Supreme Court. "Judge Dewey Resigns," 12. "Knowlton Reunion," *BG*, 18 June 1896, 6.

30. "Ex-Chief Justice Knowlton Dead," *BG*, 8 May 1918, 9.

31. Joseph Hollister, "Letter to the Editor," *New York Times*, 12 January 1935, 14.

32. Marcus P. Knowlton, "Legislation and Judicial Decision: In Their Relations to Each Other and to the Law," *Yale Law Journal* 11 (December 1901): 107.

33. *Commonwealth v. Pear. Same v. Jacobson*, 183 Mass. 242, 66 Northeastern Reporter (Massachusetts), 720.

34. *Commonwealth v. Pear. Same v. Jacobson*, 721.

35. Bancroft, "Brief for the Commonwealth," 2, in *Commonwealth v. Henning Jacobson*.

36. *Commonwealth v. Pear. Same v. Jacobson*, 721.

37. Ballard and Pickering first posed the issue in "Defendant's Exceptions," 6, in *Commonwealth v. Jacobson*, and then explored the issue at length in "Additional Points and Considerations," attached to the "Brief for Defendant," 25–39, in *Commonwealth v. Jacobson*.

38. *Commonwealth v. Pear. Same v. Jacobson*, 722, 721.

39. Greene, "Supreme Court Decision," 21.

40. *Commonwealth v. Pear. Same v. Jacobson*, 722.

41. Ibid.

42. "Supreme Court Decides," *Cambridge Tribune*, 4 April 1903, 1.

43. Simpson, "On Adverse Decision in Massachusetts," 267. Italics in the original.

44. Ibid., 266. Italics in the original.

45. Greene, "Supreme Court Decision," 22, 23.

46. Immanuel Pfeiffer, "Anti-Vaccination and the Supreme Court," *Our Home Rights* 3 (June–July 1903): 8.

47. The Supreme Judicial Court overruled Mugford's exceptions, stating "this case is governed by Com. vs. Jacobson. Ante." See "Certificate of the Decision," in *Commonwealth v. John H. Mugford*, vol. 183, *Massachusetts Reports: Papers and Briefs* (1903).

48. "Costs Him Dear," *BG*, 7 November 1903, 11. See also "Recreant Massachusetts," *The Liberator* 4 (December 1903): 81.

49. Greene, "Prosecution or Persecution?" 5.

50. Lora Little, citing a story on Mugford in the *Boston Record*, 12 December 1903, in "More Persecution in Boston," *The Liberator* 4 (January 1904): 109.

51. Massachusetts Board of Prison Commissioners, "Criminal Prosecutions," *Fourth Annual Report of the Board of Prison Commissioners of Massachusetts for the Year Ending September 30, 1904* (Boston: Wright & Potter, 1905), 113; "Criminal Prosecutions," *Fifth Annual Report of the Board of Prison Commissioners of Massachusetts for the Year Ending September 30, 1905* (Boston: Wright & Potter, 1906), 116.

52. The disposition of Cone's case remains a mystery. Pickering may have gotten his case continued pending the Pear and Jacobson appeal.

53. "Important Notice," *The Animals' Defender* 8 (June 1903): 26. The society voted on 1 June 1903 to hire Williams. Joshua T. Small, vice president of the society, later wrote, "I have no confidence that we shall win our case before the U.S. Supreme Court." Letter dated 9 November 1904, *The Liberator* 6 (December 1904): 89.

54. George Fred Williams deposited his papers in two archives, the Massachusetts Historical Society and Duke University. Unfortunately none of the documents in these archives cover the years surrounding the Jacobson case, nor do they address the subject of vaccination, antivaccination, or contain correspondence with any of the individuals involved in MACVS.

55. "Williams Forms New Party," *New York Times*, 11 January 1903, 1. Williams favored "first, direct legislation; second, public ownership of all public utilities; third, a restriction upon the power of judges in equity to take the liberty of the citizen without trial by jury."

56. Williams's hiatus was short. In May 1903, his name circulated as a potential presidential or vice presidential candidate. See untitled editorial item, *New York Times*, 17 May 1903, 6. By 1904, he sat once again on the Democratic Party National Committee and supported William Randolph Hearst at the 1904 convention. See "Hearst against Olney," *New York Times*, 7 February 1904, 1. By late 1904, he pledged to work with William Jennings Bryan "in building up democracy." See "Geo. Fred Williams Election Statement," *BP*, 11 November 1904, 7.

57. Henry Ballard probably was too sick to continue his work for Jacobson and MACVS. He died of "consumption and complications" in 1906. See "Henry Ballard Dead," 9. J. W. Pickering also probably was not qualified to argue before the United

States Supreme Court. Quotation from Pfeiffer, "Anti-Compulsory Vaccination Society of Massachusetts and the U.S. Supreme Court," 11. See also "Petition for Writ of Error," 12, in *Henning Jacobson v. The Commonwealth of Massachusetts* in *United States Supreme Court Records and Briefs, October Term, 1903* (Washington, DC: Judd & Detweiler, 1903).

58. Compare "Defendant's Exceptions," in *Commonwealth v. Henning Jacobson* with "Defendant's Exceptions," in *Commonweath v. Albert M. Pear.*

59. His father, George William Wenigmann, was born in Prussia but ran away to sea as a boy, eventually ending up in the United States to be adopted and brought up on Cape Cod by his ship's captain. Changing his last name to Williams, he married Henrietta Whitney, who belonged to "an old Massachusetts family." In 1861, George William Williams went down with his ship, the *Maritana*, after making sure that his passengers and crew had reached safety. His son, George Fred Williams, had socially and commercially prominent relatives in Hamburg, Germany, with whom he stayed while attending university there.

60. "Running for Governor," *New York Times*, 20 October 1895, 21. An editor for the *American Law Review* observed that "an eminent lawyer of our acquaintance remarked the other day, that it was one of the best books he knew, and that he carried it around everywhere under his arm." See "Book Notices," *American Law Review* 13 (1879): 359.

61. Quotation from "Running for Governor," *New York Times*, 20 October 1895, 21; biographical information from the article and partly from the "Williams, George Fred," entry in *The National Cyclopedia of American Biography* (New York: James White & Company, 1943), 30:297–98.

62. "Running for Governor," 21.

63. "Leiber Ted," *New York Times*, 13 July 1932, 16.

64. For a detailed account of Williams's life up to 1895, see "Running for Governor," *New York Times*, 20 October 1895, 21. For a history of the Mugwumps with some reference to George Fred Williams, see Gerald W. McFarland, *Mugwumps, Morals and Politics, 1884–1920* (Amherst: University of Massachusetts Press, 1975). Also David M. Tucker, *Mugwumps: Public Moralists of the Gilded Age* (Columbia: University of Missouri Press, 1998).

65. First quotation from "A Small Piece of Spleen," *New York Times*, 9 July 1886, 3; second quotation from "William E. Russell's Candidacy," *New York Times*, 24 April 1896, 5.

66. He "menaced the plutocracy by boldly demanding an investigation of the ugly charges of corruption" made against Boston's West End Railway Company. See Flower, *Progressive Men, Women, and Movements*, 105.

67. "A Great Wave of Reform," *New York Times*, 2 November 1890, 1.

68. "Williams for Governor," *New York Times*, 2 October 1895, 16.

69. "Charles Ransom Miller," *New York Times*, 19 July 1922, 8, referred to Williams as "Mr. Miller's lifelong friend." Williams was the executor for Miller's estate; one obituary on Williams referred to him as "the oldest and closest friend" of Miller. See "Lieber Ted," 16.

70. "Running for Governor," 21.

71. Quoted phrase from "Lieber Ted," 16. See also "A Bay State Silverite," *New York Times*, 3 July 1896, 2; and "A Split in the Bay State," *New York Times*, 27 September 1896, 4.

72. "A Bay State Silverite," 2.

73. Michael E. Hennessy, political reporter for the *Boston Globe*, recalled that "practically every prominent and influential Democrat in this State was against free silver" in 1896. He claimed that Williams's sudden conversion created a division in the state party leadership that spoiled Williams's chances of receiving the nomination for vice president at the 1896 Democratic convention. See Hennessy, *Twenty-Five Years of Massachusetts Politics*, 63–69; quoted word on 64; quoted passage above in note on 63.

74. Quotation in "Split in the Bay State," *New York Times*, 27 September 1896, 4 (article on his second gubernatorial nomination); see also "Hot Politics in Boston," *New York Times*, 26 September 1896, 1; and the "The Bay State Democracy," *New York Times*, 29 September 1897, 3, for accounts of his machinations to obtain his third gubernatorial nomination.

75. "The National Committee," *New York Times*, 5 July 1900, 1.

76. "Williams for Vice-President," *New York Times*, 13 April 1900, 2; "Bryan and Williams in 1900," *New York Times*, 22 April 1900, 3; "Enthusiasm for Williams," *New York Times*, 22 April 1900, 1; and "George Fred Williams Talks," *New York Times*, 30 June 1900, 3.

77. Flower, *Progressive Men, Women, and Movements*, 106. Williams would go on to argue successfully before the United States Supreme Court for the constitutionality of the initiative and referendum provisions of the Oregon state constitution. See *Pacific States Telephone and Telegraph Company v. Oregon*, 223 U.S. 118 (1911).

78. "Geo. Fred Williams' Election Statement," *BP*, 11 November 1904, 7.

79. See Johnston, *Radical Middle Class*, for an exploration of the connection between middle-class radical populism and antivaccination.

80. Flower, *Progressive Men, Women, and Movements*, 106. Williams, as United States ambassador to Greece, learned that rival religious and ethnic groups engaged in systematic genocide in Albania. Outraged when President Woodrow Wilson told him to keep out of it, he resigned in order to advocate for victims of the violence.

81. "Held at Quarantine: Cabin Passengers on Steamships Detained By the Health Officers," *New York Times*, 13 September 1892, 9. See Howard Markel, *Quarantine! East European Immigrants and the New York City Epidemics of 1892* (Baltimore, MD: The Johns Hopkins University Press, 1997), 101–34, for a description of conditions aboard the detained ships.

82. "Williams, George Fred," *National Cyclopedia of American Biography*, 30:297.

83. George Fred Williams quoting J. Peckham in *The American School of Magnetic Healing v. McAnnulty*, 187 U.S. 94, "Brief and Argument for Plaintiff in Error," 6, in *Henning Jacobson, Plaintiff in Error v. The Commonwealth of Massachusetts, Defendant in Error*, reprinted in *Supreme Court Records and Briefs, October Term, 1904* (Washington, DC: Judd & Detweiler, 1904). My notes to follow refer to the original pagination of the briefs.

84. Williams, "Brief for Plaintiff in Error," 6–7. The thirty-four states lacking a compulsory vaccination law were: Alabama, Arkansas, California, Colorado, Delaware, Florida, Idaho, Illinois, Indiana, Iowa, Kansas, Louisiana, Maine, Michigan, Minnesota, Missouri, Montana, Nebraska, Nevada, New Hampshire, New Jersey, New York, North Dakota, Ohio, Oregon, Rhode Island, South Dakota, Tennessee, Texas, Utah, Vermont, Washington, West Virginia, and Wisconsin. The eleven states

that had a compulsory vaccination statute were: Connecticut, Georgia, Kentucky, Maryland (of children), Massachusetts, Mississippi, North Carolina, Pennsylvania (in second-class cities), South Carolina, Virginia, and Wyoming. Thirteen states excluded unvaccinated children from school: California, Georgia, Iowa, Maine, Massachusetts, New Hampshire, New Jersey, New York, Oregon, Pennsylvania, Rhode Island, South Dakota, and Virginia.

85. Williams quoting La Follette's 1901 veto of a compulsory vaccination bill, "Brief for Plaintiff in Error," 8.

86. It amended the law "to obviate" a court decision, *Blue v. Beach*, that had upheld the exclusion of unvaccinated pupils from public schools. Williams incorrectly cited this case as *Beech v. Blue*, 155, Ind. State, 121. It should be *Blue v. Beach*, 155 Ind. 121, 56 N.E. 89 (1900). Williams, "Brief for Plaintiff in Error," 8.

87. Williams, "Brief for Plaintiff in Error," 9.

88. Williams explicitly distinguished these three cases from those concerning school vaccinations, asserting that they simply did not apply since they involved exclusion from a "privilege" that "the state may regulate at its own discretion. It may exclude any one it chooses." See Williams, "Brief for Plaintiff in Error," 11.

89. *Re William H. Smith*, 146 N.Y. 68 (1895). The Brooklyn Health Commissioner's quarantine order was declared invalid because the law did not grant specific authority to quarantine unexposed and uninfected persons.

90. Williams, "Brief for Plaintiff in Error," 9, quoting *State v. Hay*, 126 N.C. 999 (1900).

91. Williams, "Brief for Plaintiff in Error," 10, referring to *Morris v. City of Columbus*, 102 Ga. 792 (1897), 11.

92. Williams, "Brief for Plaintiff in Error," 13, quoting *Lawton v. Steele*, 152 U.S. 133 (1894), which upheld a state's power to protect its fish stock by prohibiting "exhaustive methods of fishing."

93. Williams, "Brief for Plaintiff in Error," 15, 19–20, 23.

94. Ibid., 15, 14, 20, 29, 23.

95. Ibid., 15, 16, 17, 18.

96. Ibid., 18–19, 19, 27, 30, 26.

97. Ibid., 24.

98. Ibid., 25.

99. Ibid., 30–31, 31.

100. Herbert Parker, "Brief for the Defendant in Error," 8, 3, 6, 7 (paraphrasing *Powell v. Pennsylvania*, 127 U.S. 678 (1888)), in *Henning Jacobson, Plaintiff in Error v. The Commonwealth of Massachusetts, Defendant in Error*, in *United States Supreme Court Records and Briefs, October Term, 1904*. My notes to follow refer to the original pagination of the briefs.

101. Parker, "Brief for Defendant in Error, 15, citing *Morris v. City of Columbus*, 102 Ga. 792 (1897), and *State v. Hay*, 126 N.C. 999 (1900), 16.

102. "Brief for Defendant in Error," 16. Pear could have presented a compelling case for a medical excuse, but he did not raise the issue at his trial. Jacobson raised the issue but only in general terms—he did not claim ill health prevented him for getting vaccinated.

103. "Brief for Defendant in Error," 9, 8.

104. "Brief for Defendant in Error," 10, 15. Quote from *State v. Hay*, 126 N.C. 999 (1900).

105. The justices of United States Supreme Court in 1904–5 were: Chief Justice Fuller, Justices Edward D. White, Oliver Wendell Holmes, Henry B. Brown, William R. Day, John Marshall Harlan, Joseph McKenna, Rufus W. Peckham, and David J. Brewer.

106. Schwartz, A History of the Supreme Court, 180.

107. Arnold M. Paul, "David J. Brewer," in The Justices of the United States Supreme Court 1789–1969: Their Lives and Major Opinions, ed. Leon Friedman and Fred L. Israel (New York: Chelsea House Publishers, 1969), 2:1515.

108. Budd v. New York, 143 U.S. 517 (1892).

109. That said, he was swayed later by Louis Brandeis's argument that women's physiology and role as mothers placed them in a special protected category that allowed for state regulation of their work conditions. Muller v. Oregon, 208 U.S. 412 (1908). The "Brandeis brief" consisted of medical, social, economic, and legal documents supporting the necessity of limiting the maximum working hours of women.

110. Richard Skolink, "Rufus Peckham," in Friedman and Israel, Justices of the United States Supreme Court, 3:1686. The opinion was The American School of Magnetic Healing v. McAnnulty, 187 U.S. 94 (1902).

111. Skolnik, "Rufus Peckham," 1693, quoting Peckham's dissent in People v. Budd, 117 N.Y. 1 (1889).

112. Skolnik, "Rufus Peckham," 1695.

113. Schwartz, A History of the Supreme Court, 180.

114. Peckham in Allgeyer v. Louisiana, 165 U.S. 578 (1897), 165.

115. The American School of Magnetic Healing v. McAnnulty, 187 U.S. 94 (1902), 106.

116. Skolnik, "Rufus Peckham," 1696, quoting Harlan in Jacobson v. Massachusetts, 197 U.S. 11 (1905), 26.

117. The Chief Justice assigns opinions in secret conference with the other justices. No one takes notes and "strict secrecy, with no legal assistants or staff present," prevails. See Joan Biskupic, Congressional Quarterly's Guide to the United States Supreme Court, 2nd ed. (Washington DC: Congressional Quarterly, 1997), 731, 734. Henry J. Abraham, "John Marshall Harlan: A Justice Neglected," Virginia Law Review 41 (November 1955): 879.

118. Abraham, "John Marshall Harlan," 872; see also Frank B. Latham, The Great Dissenter: John Marshall Harlan, 1833–1911 (New York: Cowles Book Company, 1970); and Alan Westin, "John Marshall Harlan and the Constitutional Rights of Negroes: The Transformation of a Southerner," The Yale Law Journal 66 (April 1957): 637, quoting a 1954 New York Times editorial.

119. Civil Rights Cases, 109 U.S. 3 (1883).

120. Plessy v. Ferguson, 163 U.S. 537 (1896).

121. Brown v. Board of Education, 347 U.S. 483 (1954); Abraham, "John Marshall Harlan," 871; and Westin, "John Marshall Harlan and the Constitutional Rights of Negroes."

122. Linda Przybyszewski, The Republic according to John Marshall Harlan (Chapel Hill: University of North Carolina Press, 1999), 2. Harlan sided with discriminatory laws in two opinions: once in 1882 to support a state law that provided a harsher punishment for interracial adultery than that between persons of the same race, and then in an 1899 ruling where he supported the closure of a black public high school

for financial reasons whereas the white public high school remained open. Justice Felix Frankfurter famously described Harlan as "an eccentric exception" in 1947: see G. Edward White, "John Marshall Harlan I: The Precursor," *The American Journal of Legal History* 19 (January 1975): 1.

123. Tinsley Yarborough, *Judicial Enigma: The First Justice Harlan* (New York: Oxford University Press, 1995).

124. No biographical work on Harlan discusses *Jacobson* beyond the barest mention. Quotation from Abraham, "John Marshall Harlan," 878.

125. *Mugler v. Kansas*, 123 U.S. 623 (1887). Quoted word in Paul, "David J. Brewer," 1518.

126. *Jacobson v. Massachusetts*, 197 U.S. 11, 25, Supreme Court Reporter, 361, 362.

127. William J. Novak, "Intellectual Origins of the State Police Power: The Common Law Vision of a Well-Regulated Society," *Legal History Program Working Papers*, Series 3 (Madison: University of Wisconsin-Madison Law School, 1989), 90, 93.

128. Justice John Marshall Harlan, "James Wilson and the Formation of the Constitution," *The American Law Review* (July–August 1900): quotations on 502, 499, 500.

129. *Jacobson v. Massachusetts*, 361, 362.

130. Ibid., 363.

131. Ibid., 363.

132. Ibid., footnote, 363–64. Harlan quoted from entries on vaccination from the 1894 *Encyclopedia Britannica*, Johnson's *Universal Cyclopedia* (1897), and *American Cyclopedia* (1883). He quoted from two treatises on vaccination: Hardway, *Essentials of Vaccination* (1882), and Edwards, *Vaccination* (1882). He misspelled both authors' names and gave the wrong publication date for one. They should be William A. Hardaway, *Essentials of Vaccination* (Chicago: Jansen, McClurg, 1882); and Edward J. Edwardes, *A Concise History of Small-Pox and Vaccination in Europe* (London: H. K. Lewis, 1902). He also quoted the 1898 British Royal Commission on Vaccination.

133. *Viemester v. White*, 179 N.Y. 235, 72 N.E. 97 (1904).

134. William T. Councilman's article in the *Universal Cyclopaedia* ignores any possibility of lymph contamination and instead singles out "dirty instruments" for "extensive inflammations, etc." after vaccination. See Councilman, "Vaccination," in Johnson's *Universal Cyclopaedia*, vol. 8 (New York: D. Appleton and Company, 1895): 418. (The publication date is different from Harlan's citation, but the text matches his quotation.) The article on vaccination in *American Cyclopaedia* does not even mention the possibility of any complications after vaccination. See "Vaccination," in *The American Cyclopaedia*, vol. 16, ed. George Ripley and Charles A. Dana (New York: D. Appleton and Company, 1876): 240. (I could not obtain the 1883 edition, but the text matches Harlan's quotation.)

135. The *Britannica* article, though supportive of vaccination, acknowledges its many complications. See "Vaccination," in *Encyclopedia Britannica*, vol. 24 (New York: The Werner Company, 1898): 23–30. (The publication differs from Harlan's citation, but the text matches his quotation.)

136. *Jacobson v. Massachusetts*, 365, 366.

137. Charles Warren, "The Progressiveness of the United States Supreme Court," *Columbia Law Review* 13 (1913): 300; James Tobey, "Vaccination and the Courts,"

JAMA 83 (1924): 462–64; Tobey, *Public Health Law: A Manual for Sanitarians*, 90–92; Tobey, *Public Health Law*, 230–31; Benjamin Spector, "The Growth of Medicine and the Letter of the Law," *Bulletin of the History of Medicine* 26 (November–December 1952): 509; and Wing, *Law and the Public's Health*, 24–28. Lawrence Gostin is one exception in *Public Health Law*, 66–69, especially his discussion of "harm avoidance," 69. Michael Willrich also gave overdue recognition to this aspect of the opinion; see Willrich, *Pox*, 329.

138. *Griswold v. Connecticut*, 381 U.S. 479 (1965).

139. *Jacobson v. Massachusetts*, 366–67.

140. E.F., "Notes of Recent Cases," *The Green Bag* 17 (1905): 670. See also "Compulsory Vaccination," *The American Lawyer* 13 (1905): 227, for a similar analysis.

141. Merrick, "Review of the U.S. Supreme Court Decision in the Massachusetts Vaccination Case," 115, 114.

142. George Dock, "Compulsory Vaccination, Antivaccination, and Organized Vaccination," *The American Journal of Medical Sciences* (February 1907): 231.

143. Gostin, *Public Health Law*, 69 and 347 n. 43.

144. Boston Board of Health, "Report of the Medical Inspector," *Thirty-Third Annual Report of the Health Department of the City of Boston for the Year 1904* (Boston, 1905), 62.

145. Massachusetts Board of Prison Commissioners, "Cases Pending and Begun in Superior Courts," *Fourth Annual Report for the Year Ending September 30, 1904*, 108; "Cases Pending and Begun in Superior Courts," *Fifth Annual Report for the Year Ending September 30, 1905*, 116; and "Cases Pending and Begun in Superior Courts," *Sixth Annual Report for the Year 1906* (Boston, 1907), 99.

146. "The Memorial Hymnal," *Augustana Messenger* 2 (January 1931): 5.

147. "Rev. Henning Jacobson," *Augustana Messenger* 1 (October 1930): 1.

Conclusion

1. "Vaccination," *BMSJ* 161 (1909): 595.

2. Lora Little, "The Only Way: Educate," *The Liberator* 6 (March 1905): 158.

3. Merrick, "Review of the U.S. Supreme Court Decision," 114.

4. "Compulsory Vaccination and a Step Beyond," *Bench and Bar* 2 (1905): 86.

5. Editorial, *New York Times*, 22 February 1905, 6.

6. See Colgrove, *State of Immunity*, 45–80, for a discussion of antivaccinationism after *Jacobson*.

7. See Johnston, *Radical Middle Class*.

8. Colgrove, *State of Immunity*, 65.

9. "Is Vaccination Un-American?" Editorial Item, *BMSJ* 156 (1907): 279.

10. "Bills Before the Legislature," Editorial Item, *BMSJ* 156 (1907): 309. Where the language "regular practicing physicians" came from I do not know. It is not in the text of the last amended vaccination act in 1902, which provides that any "registered physician" may provide the exemption certificate. The editors may have simply made a mistake. See chapter 190, section 2 in *Acts and Resolves Passed By the General Court of Massachusetts for the Year 1902* (Boston, 1902), 138.

11. "Vaccination in Rockland, Mass.," *BMSJ* 157 (1907): 408.

12. For H. No. 351, see Commonwealth of Massachusetts, *Journal of the House of Representatives of the Commonwealth of Massachusetts, 1908* (Boston, 1908), 97. For the vote, see "To Third Reading," *Boston Daily Globe*, 3 March 1908, 8.

13. "Bills Before the Massachusetts Legislature," *BMSJ* 160 (1909): 318–19.

14. For the Senate vote, see "Vote on Vaccination," *Boston Daily Globe*, 10 April 1914, 4. For the House, see "Will Not Relax on Vaccination," *Boston Daily Globe*, 15 May 1914, 20.

15. "Vaccination Bill Pushed," *Boston Daily Globe*, 24 March 1916, 8.

16. "Ford Hall Town Meeting Lively," *Boston Daily Globe*, 23 March 1917, 16. The story also mentions the attendance of Miss Margaret Foley of the Massachusetts Noncompulsory Vaccination Society—probably a renaming of MACVS.

17. "Senate Advances Soldiers' Pay Bill," *Boston Daily Globe*, 13 March 1918, 10. The article also mentions that the "existing vaccination statute" did not "compel a physician to state that he has examined the child for whom he offers the exemption certificate." This is a bit of a mystery because the 1902 Act clearly contains language to that effect. I do not know when the legislature amended the law to revert back to the older 1894 text that allowed physicians to provide exemption certificates without personal examinations. But if it did so, that amendment represents quite a concession to the antivaccinationists.

18. *Massachusetts General Laws Annotated*, vol. 17, 452. The statute was upheld by the Supreme Judicial Court of Massachusetts in 1921. See *Spofford v. Carlton*, 131 N.E. 314, 238 Mass. 528 (1921).

19. "House Will Not Consider Vaccination Law Repeal," *Boston Daily Globe*, 2 April 1919, 10; and "State Senate Kills Vaccination Bill," *Boston Daily Globe*, 28 May 1919, 13.

20. Op.Atty.Gen. 1920, 463, cited in *Massachusetts General Laws Annotated*, vol. 17, 451.

21. George A. Sargent, "Report of George A. Sargent, M.D.," *Thirty-Second Annual Report of the Health Department of the City of Boston for the Year 1903* (Boston, 1904), 84.

22. "Anti-Vaccination Victory in Senate," *Boston Daily Globe*, 1 April 1921, 6.

23. "Vaccination Bill Beaten," *Boston Daily Globe*, 29 March 1922, 4.

24. "For Vaccination in Private Schools," *New York Times*, 21 March 1930, 31.

25. Charles Chapin, "Justifiable Measures for the Prevention of the Spread of Infectious Diseases," in *Papers of Charles V. Chapin, M.D.*, ed. Clarence L. Scammon (New York: Commonwealth Fund, 1934), 79, 82.

26. Biggs quoted in Colgrove, *State of Immunity*, 67.

27. "Vaccination of Newsboys," *BMSJ* 158 (1908): 28.

28. "The Constitutionality of the Compulsory Asexualization of Criminals and Insane Persons," *Harvard Law Review* 26 (1912–13): 163.

29. *Buck v. Bell*, 274 U.S. 200 (1927), 207.

30. *Griswold v. Connecticut*, 381 U.S. 479 (1965). *Griswold* "struck down laws prohibiting the distribution of birth control, information, and devices," and "introduced the idea of a fundamental right to privacy." See Paul A. Lombardo, "Medicine, Eugenics, and the Supreme Court: From Coercive Sterilization to Reproductive Freedom," *Journal of Contemporary Health Law and Policy Issues* 13 (1996–97): 1–25, 23.

31. *Buck v. Bell*, 274 U.S. 200.

32. William Fowler, *Smallpox Vaccination Laws, Regulations, and Court Decisions* (Washington, DC: Treasury Department, United States Public Health Service, 1927),

2–3. The states with laws authorizing compulsion were: Alabama, Connecticut, Georgia, Kansas, Kentucky, Massachusetts, Mississippi, North Carolina, Pennsylvania, South Carolina, Tennessee, Virginia, and Wyoming. Four states forbade it: Arizona, Minnesota, North Dakota, and Utah.

33. Fowler, *Smallpox Vaccination Laws*, 3. The states requiring vaccination for schoolchildren were: Arkansas, Kentucky, Maryland, Massachusetts, New Hampshire, New Mexico, New York, Pennsylvania, Rhode Island, South Carolina, and West Virginia. Puerto Rico and Washington, DC, also required it.

34. See note 84, chapter 9 for an enumeration of state vaccination laws in 1904. A 1945 United States Public Health Service study also tabulated similar data. See Selwyn D. Collins and Clara Councell, "Extent of Immunization and Case Histories for Diphtheria, Smallpox, Scarlet Fever, and Typhoid Fever in 200,000 Surveyed Families in 28 Large Cities," in *Illness and Medical Care among 2,500,000 Persons in 83 Cities, with Special Reference to Socio-Economic Factors* (Washington, DC: Federal Security Agency, United States Public Health Service, 1945), 2–32. Arkansas, District of Columbia, Kentucky, Maryland, Massachusetts, New Hampshire, New Mexico, New York, Pennsylvania, Rhode Island, South Carolina, Virginia, and West Virginia had laws requiring vaccination for school admission in 1939–40; Connecticut, Georgia, Maine, New Jersey, Ohio, and Oregon permitted local authorities to require it if they needed to. Although the study's authors did not distinguish whether the cities they surveyed had compulsory vaccination laws, at least one pattern persisted: parents still put off vaccination until their children reached school age. Nevertheless, another pattern had emerged: teenagers either got vaccinated or revaccinated, with the highest levels of vaccination in some northeastern cities finally reaching 96 percent among nineteen year olds. Education apparently achieved what compulsion could not—a heightened public awareness of the need to revaccinate. There were wide regional differences as well, with far greater proportions of the population avoiding vaccination in southern and western cities. See Collins and Councell, "Extent of Immunization," 14, Table 3, for immunization percentages by 1945.

35. Sixteen states allow exemptions for all three categories, forty-six states (also Washington, DC) allow medical and religious exemptions, and two states allow medical exemptions only. See the National Vaccine Information Center website, http://www.nvic.org/Vaccine-Laws/state-vaccine-requirements.aspx, accessed 1 May 2014. This is an advocacy group for skepticism about immunizations. See also the CDC website, http://www2a.cdc.gov/nip/schoolsurv/schImmRqmtReport.asp, accessed 5 May 2014, which also shows that every state allows for exemptions to its immunization requirements.

36. George J. Annas, "Puppy Love: Bioterrorism, Civil Rights, and Public Health," *Florida Law Review* 55 (2003): 1176.

Bibliography

Primary Sources

Archives

Legislative papers and unpassed legislation. Massachusetts State Archives.

Massachusetts State Board of Health. *Records of the State Board of Health of Massachusetts*. Massachusetts State Archives.

Swedish Evangelical Lutheran Augustana Church of Cambridge, Massachusetts, papers. Evangelical Lutheran Church in America (ELCA) Archives, Chicago, Illinois.

Faith Lutheran (formerly Swedish Evangelical Lutheran Augustana) Church of Cambridge, Massachusetts, records and papers. Lutheran Archives Center, Northeast Region Archives, Evangelical Lutheran Church of America, Germantown, Pennsylvania.

Aurin H. Hill Papers, 1887–1930 (MS 579). Special Collections and University Archives, University of Massachusetts Amherst Libraries.

Opposition to Vaccination Pamphlets file. Countway Library. Harvard University. Cambridge, Massachusetts.

Vaccination Pamphlet files. Ebling Library, University of Wisconsin–Madison.

Federal, State, and Municipal Documents

Bureau of the Census. *1880 United States Federal Census Record*.

———. *1900 United States Federal Census Records*.

———. *1910 United States Federal Census Records*.

———. *1920 United States Federal Census Records*.

Collins, Selwyn D., and Clara Councell. "Extent of Immunization and Case Histories for Diphtheria, Smallpox, Scarlet Fever, and Typhoid Fever in 200,000 Surveyed Families in 28 Large Cities." In *Illness and Medical Care among 2,500,000 Persons in 83 Cities, with Special Reference to Socio-Economic Factors*, 2–32. Washington, DC: Federal Security Agency, United States Public Health Service, 1945.

Commonwealth of Massachusetts. *Acts and Resolves Passed by the General Court of Massachusetts in the Year 1855*. Boston, 1855.

———. *Acts and Resolves Passed by the General Court of Massachusetts in the Year 1894*. Boston, 1894.

———. *Acts and Resolves Passed by the General Court of Massachusetts in the Year 1902*. Boston, 1902.

———. Joint Special Committee. *Senate . . . No. 155.* Report prepared by C. H. Stedman, chairman. Boston, 1855.

———. *Journal of the House of Representatives.* Boston, 1894–1903.

———. *Journal of the Senate.* Boston, 1894–1903.

———. *Manual for the Use of the General Court Containing the Rules of the Two Branches.* Boston, 1901, 1902, 1903.

———. *Documents Printed by Order of the Senate.* Boston, 1903.

Boston Board of Health. *Annual Reports.* Boston, 1873–1905.

Cambridge Board of Health. *Annual Reports.* Cambridge, 1901–5.

Massachusetts State Board of Health. *Annual Reports.* Boston, 1870–1905.

Massachusetts State Board of Prison Commissioners. *Annual Reports.* Boston, 1902–10.

New England Female Moral Reform Society. *Annual Reports.* Boston, 1893–1917.

Case Documents

Commonwealth v. Jacobson. 183 Mass. 242 (1903)

Ballard, Henry. "Additional Points and Considerations." In *Commonwealth v. Henning Jacobson,* vol. 183, *Massachusetts Reports: Papers and Briefs.*

Ballard, Henry, and J. W. Pickering. "Defendant's Exceptions." In *Commonwealth v. Henning Jacobson,* vol. 183, *Massachusetts Reports: Papers and Briefs.*

———. "Brief for Defendant." In *Commonwealth v. Henning Jacobson,* vol. 183, *Massachusetts Reports: Papers and Briefs.*

———. "Medical Authorities." In *Commonwealth v. Henning Jacobson,* vol. 183, *Massachusetts Reports: Papers and Briefs.*

Bancroft, Hugh. "Brief for the Commonwealth." In *Commonwealth v. Henning Jacobson,* vol. 183, *Massachusetts Reports: Papers and Briefs.*

Commonwealth v. Pear. 183 Mass. 242 (1903)

Ballard, Henry, and J. W. Pickering. "Defendant's Exceptions." In *Commonwealth v. Albert M. Pear,* vol. 183, *Massachusetts Reports: Papers and Briefs.*

———. "Brief for Defendant." In *Commonwealth v. Albert M. Pear,* vol. 183, *Massachusetts Reports: Papers and Briefs.*

———. "Medical Authorities." In *Commonwealth v. Albert M. Pear,* vol. 183, *Massachusetts Reports: Papers and Briefs.*

Bancroft, Hugh. "Brief for the Commonwealth." In *Commonwealth v. Albert M. Pear,* vol. 183, *Massachusetts Reports: Papers and Briefs.*

Commonwealth v. Mugford. 183 Mass. 249 (1903)

Davis, Frank M. "Defendant's Exceptions." In *Commonwealth v. John H. Mugford,* vol. 183, *Massachusetts Reports: Papers and Briefs.*

———. "Defendant's Brief." In *Commonwealth v. John H. Mugford,* vol. 183, *Massachusetts Reports: Papers and Briefs.*

Sughrue, M. J. "Brief for the Commonwealth." In *Commonwealth v. John H. Mugford,* vol. 183, *Massachusetts Reports: Papers and Briefs.*

Jacobson v. Massachusetts. 197 U.S. 11 (1905)

Lower court records. *Henning Jacobson, Plaintiff in Error, v. The Commonwealth of Massachusetts.* In *Supreme Court Records and Briefs, October Term, 1903.* Washington, DC: Judd & Detweiler, July 13, 1903.

Parker, Herbert, and Frederick H. Nash. "Brief for the Defendant in Error." *Henning Jacobson, Plaintiff in Error, v. The Commonwealth of Massachusetts.* In *Supreme Court Records and Briefs, October Term, 1904.* Washington, DC: Judd & Detweiler, 1904.

Williams, George Fred, and James A. Halloran. "Brief for the Plaintiff in Error." *Henning Jacobson, Plaintiff in Error, v. The Commonwealth of Massachusetts.* In *Supreme Court Records and Briefs, October Term, 1904.* Washington, DC: Judd & Detweiler, 1904.

Published Primary Sources

"A Further Object Lesson in Vaccination." *BMSJ* 146 (1902): 611.

Abbott, Samuel W., MD. "Vaccination and Its Results." *JMABH* 4 (1894): 20–23.

———. *The Past and Present Condition of Public Hygiene and State Medicine in the United States.* Boston: Wright & Potter, 1900.

———. "Legislation with Reference to Smallpox and Vaccination." *BMSJ* 147 (1902): 263–69.

Adams, George S. "Presidential Address." *The New England Medical Gazette* 10 (October 1902): 434–37.

Allen, Lyman, MD. "Two Cases of Tetanus following Vaccination." *BMSJ* 146 (1902): 544–45.

Amerige, C. W., MD. *Vaccination a Curse.* Springfield, MA, 1895.

Ames, Azel. "Letter to the Editor." *American Medicine* 4 (1902): 531–32.

"An Object Lesson in Anti-Vaccination." *JAMA* 38 (1902): 518–19.

"The Argument Relative to Vaccination." *BMSJ* 145 (1901): 632–35.

Babbit, George A. "Retirement of Dr. Samuel Holmes Durgin from the Boston Board of Health." *American Journal of Public Health* 2 (May 1912): 384–85.

Bacon, Edwin M. *Boston: A Guide Book to the City and Vicinity.* Boston: Ginn and Company, 1922. First published 1903.

Bacon, Francis, William A. Hammond, and David F. Lincoln. *Vaccination: A Report Read before the American Social Science Association, at New York, October 27, 1869.* New York: Nation Press, 1870.

Badcock, John. *A Detail of Experiments Confirming the Power of Cow Pox to Protect the Constitution from a Subsequent Attack of Small Pox* (Brighton, 1845). In Crookshank, *History and Pathology of Vaccination,* 515–27.

Baker, Henry B., MD. "Vaccination versus Compulsory Vaccination." *The American Lancet,* new series, 14 (1890): 281–85.

Ballard, Edward. *On Vaccination: Its Value and Alleged Dangers: A Prize Essay.* London: Longmans, Green, 1868.

Bannan, Theresa, MD. "The Vaccination Question." *New York Medical Journal* 76 (1902): 229–31.

Beckwith, D. H., MD. "Vaccination." Transcript of a paper given at the American Institute of Homeopathy, Indianopolis, IN, June 1882. Pittsburgh, PA: Stevenson & Foster, 1882.

Beebe, W. L., MD. "Smallpox—Old and New." *JAMA* 37 (1901): 299.

Bell, Clark. "Compulsory Vaccination: Should It Be Enforced By Law?" *JAMA* 28 (1897): 49–53.

Bergh, Henry. "The Lancet and the Law." *North American Review* 134 (February 1882): 161–69.

Boston Unversity. *Historical Register of Boston University*. Boston: University Offices, 1911.

Bracken, H. M., MD. "Pseudo, Modified, or True Smallpox—Which Is It?" *JAMA* 35 (1900): 608–10.

———. "Discussion of Papers of Drs. Doty and Iglesias." *Public Health Papers and Reports* 26 (1901): 244–53.

———. "Variola." *JAMA* 37 (1901): 307–10.

Brouardel, P., MD. "Vaccina." In Stedman, *Twentieth Century Practice*, 503–52.

Brummall, J. D., MD. "The Epidemic of So-Called Smallpox." *American Medicine* 3 (1902): 180.

Bryce, Peter H., MD. "Discussion of Papers of Dr. Bryce and Dr. Bernaldez." *Public Health Paper and Reports* 27 (1902): 339–43.

———. "Vaccinal Immunization from the Health Officer's Standpoint." *Public Health Papers and Reports* 27 (1902): 175–81.

Buist, John B. *Vaccinia and Variola: A Study of Their Life History*. London: J. & A. Churchill, 1887.

Bullard, John T., MD. "Smallpox: Its Diagnosis." *BMSJ* 147 (1902): 207–10.

"The Cambridge Smallpox Epidemic." *Medical News* 80 (1902): 1230–31.

"Caroline E. Hastings Report of Talitha Cumi Home." *Transactions of the American Institute of Homeopathy* 55 (1900): 141.

Carr, C. S., MD. "Smallpox Quarantine." *Medical Talk for the Home* 3 (1902): 393.

"The Case of Dr. Pfeiffer." *BMSJ* 146 (1902): 210–11.

"Cases of Tetanus following Vaccination." *American Medicine* 2 (1901): 801.

Chapin, Charles V. *Municipal Sanitation in the United States*. Providence, RI: Snow & Farnham, 1901.

———. "Justifiable Measures for the Prevention of the Spread of Infectious Diseases." In *Papers of Charles V. Chapin, M.D.*, edited by Clarence L. Scammon, 76–91. New York: Commonwealth Fund, 1934.

"The Choice of a Site for Vaccination." *JAMA* 35 (1900): 503.

Clymer, R. Swinburne, MD. "Smallpox and Vaccination." *The Medical Brief* 30 (1902): 1330–31.

———. *Vaccination Brought Home to You*. Terre Haute, IN: Press of G. H. Hebb, 1904.

———. *Nature's Healing Agents: the Medicines of Nature (or the Natura System)*. Quakertown, PA: Humanitarian Society, 1906.

———. *The Medicines of Nature: The Thomsonian System: A Course of Medical Treatment as Taught By Dr. Samuel Thomson*. Quakertown, PA: Humanitarian Society, 1926.

"Conference of State and Provincial Boards of Health of North America." *JAMA* 39 (1902): 1202–3.

"The Constitutionality of the Compulsory Asexualization of Criminals and Insane Persons." *Harvard Law Review* 26 (1912–13): 163–64.

Cooke, Willis S., MD. "Report of a Case of Tetanus following Vaccination." *New York Medical Journal* 77 (1903): 61–62.

Crandall, Floyd, MD. "A Century of Vaccination." *American Medicine* 2 (1901): 895–99.

Creighton, Charles. "Vaccination." In *The Encyclopedia Britannica*, 24:23–30. Edinburgh: Adam and Charles Buck, 1888.

———. "Vaccination: A Scientific Inquiry." *The Arena* 2 (September 1890): 422–40.

———. *A History of Epidemics in Britain.* 2 vols. Cambridge: Cambridge University Press, 1894.

———. *A History of Epidemics in Britain.* vol. 1. 2nd ed., with additional material by D. E. C. Eversley, E. Ashworth Underwood, and Linda Overall. London: Frank Cass & Co., 1965.

Crookshank, Edgar M. *The History and Pathology of Vaccination: A Critical Inquiry.* 2 vols. London: H. K. Lewis, 1889.

Cutler, William C., and J. F. Frisbie. *Variola and Vaccinia: History and Description.* Boston: New England Vaccine Company, 1897 [estimated].

Cutter, Ephraim. "Partial Report on the Production of Vaccine Virus in the United States." *Transactions of the American Medical Association* 23 (1872): 200–220.

Daland, Judson, MD. "The Technique, Value and Object of Vaccination." Report of a Paper Read before the North Branch of the Philadelphia County Medical Society, 20 December 1901. *JAMA* 38 (1902): 268.

Darling, Eugene, MD. "Vaccination: The Technique." *BMSJ* 147 (1902): 201–3.

Davis, William T. *Bench and Bar of the Commonwealth of Massachusetts.* New York: DeCapo Press, 1974. Reprint of 1895 edition.

De Bernaldez, Francisco, MD. "Human Vaccine as a Prophylactic of Smallpox: Its Advantages and Disadvantages." *Public Health Papers and Reports* 26 (1901): 87–91.

———. "Remarks Intended to Show the Innocuous Character of Humanized Vaccine as a Preventative of Smallpox." *Public Health Papers and Reports* 27 (1902): 182–83.

"The Diagnosis of Smallpox." *JAMA* 34 (1900): 368–69.

"The Diagnosis of Smallpox." *Medical News* 80 (1902): 943–45.

Dillingham, Frederick H., MD. "Some Observations in regard to Smallpox." *American Medicine* 4 (1902): 493–98.

Dock, George, MD. "The Works of Edward Jenner and Their Value in the Modern Study of Smallpox." *New York Medical Journal* 76, parts 1 and 2 (1902): 925–31, 978–84. Paper read before the Buffalo Academy of Medicine, 14 October 1902.

———. "Vaccine and Vaccination." *The Johns Hopkins University Bulletin* 15 (1904): 1–16.

———. "Compulsory Vaccination, Antivaccination, and Organized Vaccination." *The American Journal of the Medical Sciences* (February 1907): 218–33.

———. "Vaccination." In *Modern Medical Practice: Its Theory and Practice,* edited by Sir William Osler and Thomas McCrae, 822–48. Philadelphia: Lea & Febiger, 1913.

"Dr. Samuel H. Durgin." *American Journal of Public Health* 2 (May 1912): 357–58.

"Durgin, Samuel Holmes." *National Cyclopaedia of American Biography.* New York: James T. White & Co., 1906.

Durgin, S. H., MD. "Discussion of Papers of Drs. Doty and Iglesias." *Public Health Papers and Reports* 26 (1901): 244–53.

———. "Comments in Discussion of Papers of Dr. Bryce and Dr. Bernaldez." *Public Health Papers and Reports* 27 (1902): 339–43.

———. "Vaccination and Smallpox." *BMSJ* 146 (1902): 114–15.

Duxbury, Joseph E., MD. "Variola, or Smallpox." *BMSJ* 146 (1902): 165–67.

"The Early Recognition of Smallpox." *JAMA* 39 (1902): 83–84.

Edson, Cyrus, MD. "The Present and Future of Medical Science." *North American Review* 154 (1892): 117–19.

Edwardes, Edward J. *A Concise History of Small-Pox and Vaccination in Europe.* London: H. K. Lewis, 1902.

Elgin, W. F., MD. "Influence of Temperature on Vaccine Virus." *Public Health Papers and Reports* 26 (1901): 80–83.

———. "Comments in Discussion of Papers of Dr. Bryce and Dr. Bernaldez," *Public Health Papers and Reports* 27 (1902): 339–43.

———. "Some Facts That Physicians Should Know in Reference to Vaccine and Vaccination." Paper Read at the Semiannual Meeting of the Medical and Chirurgical Faculty at Annapolis, Maryland, 27–28 September 1906.

Fisher, William R., MD. "School Vaccinations." *American Medicine* 4 (1902): 508–9.

Fleisher, Steven M. "The Law of Basic Health Activities: Police Power and Constitutional Limitations." In *Legal Aspects of Health Policy: Issues and Trends*, edited by Ruth Roemer and George McKray, 3–32. Westport, CT: Greenwood Press, 1980.

Flexner, Abraham. *Medical Education in the United States and Canada.* New York: Arno Press, 1972. Reprint of 1910 edition.

Flower, Benjamin O. "How Cleveland Stamped Out Smallpox." *The Arena* 27 (1902): 426–29.

———. *Progressive Men, Women, and Movements of the Past Twenty-Five Years.* Boston: The New Arena, 1914.

Foster, Eugene, MD. "Report of the Committee on Compulsory Vaccination; also, a Supplementary Report on the Efficiency and Safety of Vaccination." *Public Health Papers and Reports* 9 (1883): 238–87.

Fourth Annual Announcement of the Woman's Hospital Medical College of Chicago, Illinois. Chicago: Fergus Printing Company, 1873.

Franklin, C. P., MD. "Vaccination Shield." *JAMA* (1901): 1691.

———. "Vaccination Shield." *American Medicine* 3 (1902): 57–58.

Freund, Ernst. *The Police Power: Public Policy and Constitutional Power.* Chicago: Callaghan & Company, 1904.

Friedrich, Martin, MD. "How We Rid Cleveland of Smallpox." *Cleveland Medical Journal* 1 (February 1902): 77–89.

Garciadiego, Salvador, MD. "The Only Certain Prophylaxis against Smallpox Is Human Vaccine Which, If Well Inoculated, Does Not Transmit Infectious Contagious nor Diathetic Disease." *Public Health Papers and Reports* 26 (1901): 84–86.

Giles, Alfred E. *The Iniquity of Compulsory Vaccination.* Boston: Colby & Rich, 1882.

"Glycerinated Virus versus Dried Vaccine Virus." *JAMA* 38 (1902): 1306.

Good, Charles, MD. "The Vexed Question of Vaccination." *American Medicine* 2 (1901): 777–80.

Greene, Joseph M. "In the Interests of Humanity, Should Vivisection Be Permitted, and If So, under What Restrictions and Limitations?" In *Vivisection: Five Hundred Dollar Prize Essays,* edited by George T. Angell, 7–25. July 1891.

———. "The Hearing on Vivisection." *The Animals' Defender* 5 (April 1900): 6–26.

———. "Beating Vaccination." *The Animals' Defender* 5 (October 1900): 4–5.

———. "Hearing on Vivisection." *The Animals' Defender* 6 (April 1901): 5–30.

———. "Lockjaw and Vaccination." *The Animals' Defender* 6 (August 1901): 15–16.

———. "Some Vaccination Triumphs." *The Animals' Defender* 6 (September 1901): 14.

———. "Vaccination Stopped." *The Animals' Defender* 6 (September 1901): 10.

———. "Facts about Vaccination." *The Animals' Defender* 6 (December 1901): 20–30.

———. "The Legitimate Result: Infant Slaughter in St. Louis." *The Animals' Defender* 6 (December 1901): 20–30.

———. "A Request." *The Animals' Defender* 6 (December 1901): 26.

———. "Some Fruits of Vaccination." *The Animals' Defender* 6 (December 1901): 31.

———. *Vaccination Is the Curse of Childhood.* Boston, 1901.

———. "The Vaccination Scourge." *The Animals' Defender* 7 (January 1902): 20–27.

———. "Notes on a Form of Animal and Human Vivisection Called Vaccination." *The Animals' Defender* 7 (February 1902): 11–17.

———. "Notes on Vaccination." *The Animals' Defender* 7 (February 1902): 11–17.

———. "Legal Blood-Poisoning in Massachusetts." *The Animals' Defender* 7 (March 1902): 17–36.

———. "Crime in Massachusetts." *The Animals' Defender* 7 (May 1902): 20–29.

———. "Law versus Order." *The Animals' Defender* 7 (August 1902): 16–22.

———. "A Great Medical Scandal." *The Animals' Defender* 7 (November 1902): 24–35.

———. "Mass. Anti-Compulsory Vaccination Society." *The Animals' Defender* 7 (November 1902): 26–27.

———. "A Medical Crime." *The Animals' Defender* 7 (December 1902): 21–35.

———. "Compulsory Vaccination." *The Animals' Defender* 8 (February 1903): 19.

———. "Vaccination." *The Animals' Defender* 8 (March 1903): 6.

———. "An Adverse Decision." *The Liberator* 3 (April 1903): 208.

———. "Eighty Victims." Parts 1–3. *The Liberator* 3 (April 1903): 211–13; (May 1903): 239–43; (June 1903): 271–72. *The Liberator* 4 (October 1903): 27–28.

———. "State House Hearing on Vaccination." *The Animals' Defender* 8 (April 1903): 23–25.

———. "State vs. Pear and Jacobson." *The Animals' Defender* 8 (April 1903): 27.

———. "Legislative Hearings on Vaccination." *The Animals' Defender* 8 (May 1903): 20–29.

———. "The Supreme Court Decision." *The Animals' Defender* 8 (June 1903): 19–24.

———. "Important Notice." *The Animals' Defender* 8 (June 1903): 26; (July 1903): 26; (November 1903): 31.

———. "Prosecution or Persecution?" *The Animals' Defender* 8 (December 1903): 5–6.

———. "The Test Case." *The Animals' Defender* 9 (January 1904): 13.

———. "A Progressive Body." *The Animals' Defender* 9 (April 1904): 11.

Greenleaf, Robert W. *An Historical Report of the Boston Dispensary for One Hundred and One Years, 1796–1897.* Brookline, MA: Riverdale Press, 1898.

Groff, George, MD. "Vaccine Production and Vaccination." *American Medicine* 2 (1901): 907–8.

Hamilton, Allan McLane, and Bache McE. Emmet, MDs. "Small-Pox and Other Contagious Diseases." In *A Treatise on Hygiene and Public Health,* edited by Albert H. Buck, 515–27. New York: William Wood & Company, 1879.

Hancock, John C., MD. "Some Aspects of the Present Smallpox Epidemic." *Medicine* 8 (1902): 807–18.

Happel, T. J., MD. "Pseudo (?) or Modified (?) Smallpox." *JAMA* 35 (1900): 600–607.

———. "A Further Study of Pseudo, or Modified Smallpox (?)." *JAMA* 37 (1901): 295–98.

Hardaway, William A. *Essentials of Vaccination.* Chicago: Jansen, McClurg, 1882.

Harlan, Justice John Marshall. "James Wilson and the Formation of the Constitution." *The American Law Review* (July–August, 1900): 481–504.

Hastings, Caroline Eliza. "Lecture II." In *Dress Reform: A Series of Lectures Delivered in Boston on Dress as It Affects the Health of Women,* edited by Abba Goold Woolson, 42–67. Boston: Roberts, 1874.

———. "The Indicated Remedy vs. the Knife." *Proceedings of the Massachusetts Homeopathic Medical Society* 14 (1900): 204–12.

"Hastings, Caroline." In *Daughters of America; or Women of the Century,* edited by Phebe A. Hanaford, 323. Augusta, ME: True & Co., 1882.

"Hastings, Caroline Eliza." In *The Biographical Cyclopedia of American Women,* edited by Mabel Ward Cameron, 240. New York: Halvord Publishing Company, 1924.

"Hastings, Caroline Eliza." In *Cleave's Biographical Cyclopedia of Homeopathic Physicians and Surgeons.* Philadelphia: Galaxy Publishing Company, 1873.

Hennessy, Michael E. *Twenty-Five Years of Massachusetts Politics.* Boston: Practical Politics, 1917.

Hibberd, James F., MD. "Propositions concerning Vaccination." *Public Health Papers and Reports* 8 (1882): 123–24.

Hodge, J. W., MD. *How Small-Pox Was Banished from Leicester.* Pamphlet reprinted from *Medical Century* (January 1911).

"How Anti-Vaccinists Are Made." *The Vaccination Inquirer* 24 (April 1902–March 1903): 249.

Hutchinson, Jonathan. *Illustrations of Clinical Surgery.* 2 vols. London: J. & A. Churchill, 1878–88.

Hyde, Alan. *Bodies of Law.* Princeton, NJ: Princeton University Press, 1997.

Hyde, James Nevins. "The Late Epidemic of Smallpox in the United States." *Popular Science Monthly* 59 (1901): 557–67.

Jacobson, Pastor H. *Historik Öfver Förberedelserna Och Organiseringen Af Svenska Ev. Luth. Augustana Församlingen I Cambridge, Massachusetts, Jemte Dess Tio-Åriga Verksamhet, Räknadt Från Den 21 Augusti 1892 Till Och Med Nyårsstämman 1902.* Boston: Svenska Tryckeriet, 1902.

"The Journal of Universal Antiism." *American Medicine* 3 (1902): 293.

Keath, J. W., MD. "The Proper Method of Vaccination." *JAMA* 38 (1902): 526.

Kelly, Michael, MD. "Smallpox: Its Medical Treatment." *BMSJ* 147 (1902): 236–41.

Keperling, Dr. I. L. "The Rights of the People." *Medical Talk for the Home* 7 (1906): 305–6.

King, Moses. *King's Handbook of Boston.* Boston: Moses King Corporation, 1889.

King, William Harvey. *History of Homeopathy and Its Institutions in America.* 4 vols. New York: Lewis Publishing, 1905.

Knowlton, Marcus Perrin. "Legislation and Judicial Decision: In Their Relations to Each Other and to the Law." *The Yale Law Journal* 11 (1901): 95–110.

Lawrence, William R. *A History of the Boston Dispensary.* Boston: John Wilson and Son, 1859.

Leavitt, Frederick, MD. "The Distinguishing Characteristics between Mild Discrete Smallpox and Chicken-Pox." *JAMA* 37 (1901): 305–7.

Liceaga, Eduardo, MD. "The Jenner Vaccine Well Preserved and Carefully Propagated Is a Permanent Preservative against Smallpox." *Public Health Papers and Reports* 26 (1901): 92–97.

"Life History of the Tetanus Bacillus." *American Medicine* 2 (1901): 840.

Little, Lora. "The Only Way: Educate." *The Liberator* 6 (1905): 158–59.

"Lockjaw in the Air." *Our Home Rights* 1 (December 1901): 1–4.

Marson, J. F., MD. "Smallpox." In Reynolds, *A System of Medicine,* 1:152.

Martin, Henry Austin, MD. "Anti-Vaccinism." *North American Review* 134 (1882): 368–78.

Martin, Stephen C., MD. "A Pregnant Cause of Failure in Vaccination." *BMSJ* 120 (1889): 398–99.

"Mayor Prince and the Board of Health." *BMSJ* 75–76 (1877): 659.

McAllister, Alex, MD. "The Cause of Sore Arms during the Recent Vaccinations" and "Cause of Tetanus following Vaccination." Papers read at the Medical Society of the State of New Jersey. Reported in *American Medicine* 4 (1902): 88, 89.

McCollom, John H., MD. "Deaths from Smallpox in Boston for Forty Years—1852–1871 and 1874–1893." *Journal of the Massachusetts Association of Boards of Health* 4 (April 1894): 6–7.

———. "Discussion of Smallpox in Massachusetts." *Journal of the Massachusetts Association of Boards of Health* 4 (April 1894): 2.

———. "Vaccinations: Accidents and Untoward Effects." *BMSJ* 147 (1902): 203–7.

McCormack, J. N., MD. "The Value of State Control and Vaccination in the Management of Smallpox." *JAMA* 38 (1902): 1434–35.

McFarland, Joseph, MD. "The Relationship of Tetanus to Vaccination." Paper given at the 2nd Annual Meeting of the American Association of Pathologists and Bacteriologists, 28 March 1902. *BMSJ* 146 (1902): 441–42.

———. "Tetanus and Vaccination—An Analytical Study of Ninety-Five Cases of This Rare Complication." *Medicine* 8 (June 1902): 441–56. Previously published as "Tetanus and Vaccination: An Analytical Study of Ninety-Five Cases of This Rare Complication," *Boston Journal of Medical Research* (May 1902).

McVail, John C. *Vaccination Vindicated: Being an Answer to the Leading Anti-Vaccinators.* London: Cassell & Company, 1887.

Medical Directory of Greater Boston. Boston: Boston Medical Publishing Co., 1906.

Mellish, Ernest J., MD. "Vaccination from the Standpoint of a Surgeon." *American Medicine* 3 (1902): 820–22.

Merrick, Sara Newcomb, MD. "Consumption, What Causes It and What Prevents It—Its Health Treatment at Home." *The Liberator* 4 (March 1904): 179.

———. "Review of the U.S. Supreme Court Decision in the Massachusetts Vaccination Case." *The Liberator* 7 (1905): 113–15.

———. "John and Simon Newcomb: The Story of a Father and Son." *McClure's Magazine* 35 (1910): 677–87.

Millard, C. Killick, MD. *The Vaccination Question in Light of Modern Experience.* London: H. K. Lewis, 1914.

Moore, John William, MD. "Smallpox." In Stedman, *Twentieth Century Practice,* 389–489.

"More Protest against Repeal of Law." *BG,* 3 February 1902, 4.

Morse, Frank, MD. "The Recent Smallpox Epidemic in Massachusetts." *Journal of the Massachusetts Association of Boards of Health* 13 (July 1903): 46–64.

Newcomb, Simon. *Reminiscences of an Astronomer.* Boston: Houghton, Mifflin, 1903.

New England Moral Reform Society. *Annual Report of the New England Moral Reform Society for 1917.* Boston: The Fort Hill Press, 1917.

Nichols, C. F., MD. *A Blunder in Poison.* Boston: Rockwell and Churchill Press, 1902.

———. *The Outrage Vaccination: The Arraignment of Vaccination By Eminent Men and By Medical Specialists.* Boston, 1908.

———. *Syphilis and Vaccination.* 4th ed. Boston, 1911.

"Nichols, Charles Fessenden." In *The Cyclopedia of American Biography,* 14:133–34. New York: James T. White & Co., 1917.

Osler, William, MD. *The Principles and Practices of Medicine.* New York: D. Appleton and Company, 1892.

Page, Charles E., MD. "Vaccination." *The Animals' Defender* 6 (July 1901): 14.

———. "Are Bacilli the Cause of Disease, or a Natural Aid to Its Cure?" Paper read before the American Social Science Association, Washington, DC, 8 May 1900. Reprinted in *The Liberator* 2 (1902): 67–69.

Peabody, Susan Wade. "Historical Study of Legislation regarding Public Health in the States of New York and Massachusetts." *Journal of Infectious Diseases,* Supplement No. 4 (February 1909): 1–158.

Pfeiffer, Immanuel, MD. "The Fruit of Vaccination." *Our Home Rights* 1 (1901): 9–10.

———. "Vaccination." *Our Home Rights* 1 (October 1901): 13–18.

———. "Justice! Justice! Justice!" *Our Home Rights* 2 (January 1902): 33.

———. "A Violent One of the Emma Goldman School." *Our Home Rights* 2 (January 1902): 32.

———. "Dr. Pfeiffer's Statement." *Our Home Rights* 2 (February–April 1902): 33–44.

———. "The Anti-Compulsory Vaccination Society of Massachusetts and the U.S. Supreme Court." *Our Home Rights* (June–July 1903): 10–11.

———. "Anti-Vaccination and the Supreme Court." *Our Home Rights* 3 (June–July 1903): 7–8.

"The Production of Vaccine Lymph." *BMSJ* 146 (1902): 22–25.

Rawlings, Issac D. *The Rise and Fall of Disease in Illinois.* 2 vols. Springfield, IL: State Department of Public Health, 1927.

"The Relative Immunizing Value of Human and Bovine Vaccine Virus." *BMSJ* 148 (1903): 24–25.

"Report of the Committee on the Value and Necessity of Vaccination and Revaccination for the Eradication of Smallpox." *Transactions of the American Medical Association* 16 (1866): 263–77.

"Report of the Committee on the Relative Immunizing Value of Human and Bovine Vaccine Virus." *BMSJ* 148 (1903): 40–42.

Reynolds, J. Russell, ed. *A System of Medicine*. vol. 1. Philadelphia: Henry C. Lea's Son & Co., 1880,

Rosenau, M. J., MD. "Dry Points versus Glycerinated Virus, from a Bacteriological Standpoint." *American Medicine* 3 (1902): 637–39.

———. *The Bacteriological Impurities of Vaccine Virus: An Experimental Study*. Hygenic Laboratory, Bulletin No. 12. Washington, DC: Government Printing Office, 1903.

Russell, F. H., MD. "A Case of Fatal Vaccination Infection Which Resembled Appendicitis." *JAMA* 38 (1902): 34–35.

"Sarah Newcomb Merrick." In *A Woman of the Century: Fourteen Hundred-Seventy Biographical Sketches Accompanied By Portraits of Leading American Women in All Walks of Life*, edited by Frances E. Willard and Mary A. Livermore, 500. New York: Charles Wells Moulton, 1893.

"Sara Newcomb Merrick, M.D." *The Liberator* 7 (August 1905): 112.

Schamberg, Jay F., MD. "The Diagnosis of Smallpox." *American Medicine* 2 (1901): 899–903.

———. "The Diagnosis of Smallpox." *JAMA* 38 (1902): 215–17.

Seaton, Edward Cator, MD. "Vaccination." In Reynolds, *A System of Medicine*, 1:158–82.

Sedgwick, William T. "Remarks on 'Opposition to Vaccination.'" *Journal of the Massachusetts Association of Boards of Health* 12 (April 1902): 5–19.

Shattuck, Lemuel. *Report of a General Plan for the Public and Personal Health, Devised, Prepared and Recommended by the Commissioners Appointed under a Resolve of the Legislature of Massachusetts, relating to a Sanitary Survey of the State*. 1850. Reprint, New York: Arno Press, 1972.

Shea, Thomas B., MD. "Smallpox and Vaccination." *Journal of the Association of Massachusetts Boards of Health* 12 (April 1902): 19–25.

Silver, William J. "How Utah Won Freedom." *The Liberator* 5 (1905): 121–22.

Simpson, C. Asbury. "Adverse Decision in Massachusetts." *The Liberator* 3 (1903): 265–69.

"The Smallpox Situation in Boston." *BMSJ* 145 (1901): 286–87.

"Smallpox and Vaccination—Mr. Shattuck's Memorial." *BMSJ* 54 (1856): 264–65.

Smith, Theobald, MD. "The Preparation of Animal Vaccine." *BMSJ* 147 (1902): 197–201.

Soiland, Albert, MD. "Notes on One Hundred and Fifty Cases of Smallpox in Private Practice." *JAMA* 37 (1901): 912–13.

Somerset, William L., MD. "The Course and Diagnosis of Variola—Based on Its Last Outbreak in New York City." *New York Medical Journal and Philadelphia Medical Journal* 78 (1903): 989–91.

Spalding, Heman, MD. "Differential Diagnosis between Chickenpox and Smallpox." *JAMA* 36 (1901): 497–500.

———. "Diagnosis of Mild and Irregular Smallpox as Found in the Present Outbreak in the United States." *JAMA* 37 (1901): 302–5.

———. "Some Facts about Vaccination." *JAMA* 39 (1902): 906–9.

Spencer, Herbert. *Facts and Comments.* New York: D. Appleton and Company, 1902.

Stedman, C. H. "Senate . . . No. 155." *Documents Printed By Order of the Senate of the Commonwealth of Massachusetts during the Session of the General Court, A.D. 1855.* Boston: Wright & Potter Printing Co., 1855.

Stedman, Thomas L., ed. *Twentieth-Century Practice: An International Encyclopedia of Modern Medical Science By Leading Authorities of Europe and America.* New York: William Wood and Company, 1898.

Suiter, A. Walter, MD. "Report of the Committee on the Cause and Prevention of Infectious Diseases." *Public Health Papers and Reports* 16 (1901): 69–79.

Tebb, William. "Anti-Vaccination in the United States and Canada." *The Vaccination Inquirer* 1 (April 1879–March 1880): 154–57.

"Tetanus after Vaccination." *JAMA* 38 (1902): 768–69.

"Tetanus and Vaccination." *BMSJ* 146 (1902): 639–40.

"Tetanus following Vaccination." American News and Notes. *American Medicine* 2 (1901): 889.

Thompson, Jerry D., ed. *From Desert to Bayou: The Civil War Journal and Sketches of Morgan Wolfe Merrick.* El Paso: Texas Western Press, 1991.

Toner, J. M., MD. "A Paper on the Propriety and Necessity of Compulsory Vaccination." *Transactions of the American Medical Association* 16 (1865): 307–30.

Towle, Harvey P., MD. "Vaccination Eruptions." *BMSJ* 147 (1902): 269–71.

"Tuberculosis Cows as Sources of Vaccine Lymph." *American Medicine* 3 (1902): 846–47.

"Two Bad Methods of Fighting the Antivaccination Craze." *American Medicine* 3 (1902): 294.

"Vaccination Opposed." *BET*, 4 February 1902, 3.

"Vaccination Upheld By Homeopathists." *BMSJ* 146 (1902): 181.

Wallace, Alfred Russel. *The Wonderful Century: Its Successes and Failures.* New York: Dodd, Mead, 1898.

Watson, Edward W., MD. "Some Experiences in Vaccination." *American Medicine* 2 (1901): 683.

Webster, Charles L., MD. "Some Proofs That Vaccination Prevents and Mitigates Smallpox." *Cleveland Journal of Medicine* 6 (1901): 131–41.

Wende, Ernest, MD. "The Smallpox Problem." *Medical News* 80 (1902): 1026–29.

White, Almira Larkin, ed. *White Family Quarterly: An Illustrated Genealogical Magazine.* 3 vols. Haverhill, MA: Almira Larkin White, 1903.

Wilgus, Sidney D., MD. "A Case of Generalized Vaccinia with Unusual Complications." *American Medicine* 3 (1902): 501–2.

Willson, Robert N., MD. "Tetanus Appearing in the Course of Vaccinia: Report of a Case." *American Medicine* 2 (1901): 903–7.

———. "An Analysis of Fifty-Two Cases of Tetanus following Vaccinia, with Reference to the Source of Infection: 1839–1902." Parts 1 and 2. *JAMA* 38 (1902): 1147–52, 1222–31.

Winslow, C.-E. A. "A Half-Century of the Massachusetts Public Health Association." *American Journal of Public Health and The Nation's Health* 30 (April 1940): 325–35.

Winterburn, George William, MD. *The Value of Vaccination: A Non-Partisan Review of Its History and Results.* Philadelphia: F. E. Boericke, Hahnemann, 1886.

Wolfe, Albert Benedict. *The Lodging House Problem in Boston.* Boston: Houghton, Mifflin, 1906.

Woodhouse, T. M., MD. "Medical Laws Not Constitutional." *Medical Talk for the Home* (January 1906): 304–5.

Woods, Robert, and Albert J. Kennedy. *The Zone of Emergence.* Abridged and edited by Sam Bass Warner, Jr. Cambridge, MA: Harvard University Press, 1962.

Wyeth, John Allen, MD. "The President's Address." *BMSJ* 146 (1902): 615–19.

Secondary Sources

Abraham, Henry J. "John Marshall Harlan: A Justice Neglected." *Virginia Law Review* 41 (November 1955): 871–91.

Albert, Michael R., Kristen G. Ostheimer, and Joel G. Breman. "The Last Smallpox Epidemic in Boston and the Vaccination Controversy, 1901–1903." *New England Journal of Medicine* 344 (2001): 375–79.

Allen, Arthur. *Vaccine: The Controversial Story of Medicine's Greatest Lifesaver.* New York: W. W. Norton, 2007.

Annas, George J. "Puppy Love: Bioterrorism, Civil Rights, and Public Health." *Florida Law Review* 55 (2003): 1171–90.

Augustana Lutheran Church. *After Fifty Years, 1892–1942.* Cambridge, MA: Augustana Lutheran Church, 1942.

Baldwin, Peter. *Contagion and the State in Europe, 1830–1930.* Cambridge: Cambridge University Press, 1999.

Baxby, Derrick. *Jenner's Smallpox Vaccine: The Riddle of Vaccinia Virus and Its Origins.* London: Heinemann Educational Books, 1981.

———. *Vaccination: Jenner's Legacy.* Berkeley, England: The Jenner Educational Trust, 1994.

Bell, Whitfield J., Jr. "Dr. James Smith and the Public Encouragement of Vaccination for Smallpox." *Annals of Medical History*, 3rd series, 2 (November 1940): 500–517.

———. *The College of Physicians of Philadelphia: A Bicentennial History.* Philadelphia, PA: Science History Publications, 1987.

Berman, Alex. "Neo-Thomsonianism in the United States." *Journal of the History of Medicine* 11 (1956): 133–55.

Berman, Joel, and D. A. Henderson. "Diagnosis and Management of Smallpox." *New England Journal of Medicine* 346 (2002): 1300–1308.

Beth, Loren P. *John Marshall Harlan: The Last Whig Justice.* Lexington: University Press of Kentucky, 1992.

Biskupic, Joan. *Congressional Quarterly's Guide to the United States Supreme Court.* 2nd ed. Washington DC: Congressional Quarterly, 1997.

Blake, John B. "The Inoculation Controversy in Boston, 1721–1722." In Leavitt and Numbers, *Sickness and Health in America*, 347–55. Originally published in the *New England Quarterly* 25 (1952): 489–506.

————. *Benjamin Waterhouse and the Introduction of Vaccination.* Philadelphia: University of Pennsylvania Press, 1957.

————. "Benjamin Waterhouse: Harvard's First Professor of Physic." *Journal of Medical Education* 33 (1958): 771–82.

————. *Public Health in the Town of Boston, 1630–1822.* Cambridge, MA: Harvard University Press, 1959.

Bliss, Michael. *Plague: A Story of Smallpox in Montreal.* Toronto: HarperCollins, 1991.

Bowers, John Z. "The Odyssey of Smallpox Vaccination." *Bulletin of the History of Medicine* 55 (1981): 17–33.

Boyd, Robert T. *The Coming of the Spirit of Pestilence: Introduced Infectious Diseases and Population Decline among the Northwest Indians, 1774–1874.* Seattle: University of Washington Press, 1999.

Brieger, Gert H. "Sanitary Reform in New York City: Stephen Smith and the Passage of the Metropolitan Health Bill." In Leavitt and Numbers, *Sickness and Heath in America*, 399–413. 3rd ed. Originally published in *Bulletin of the History of Medicine* 40 (1966): 407–29.

Burrage, Walter L. *A History of the Massachusetts Medical Society with Brief Biographies of the Founders and Chief Officers, 1781–1922.* Norwood, MA: The Plimpton Press, 1923.

Burrows, Paul. *Organized Medicine in the Progressive Era: The Move Toward Monopoly.* Baltimore, MD: The Johns Hopkins University Press, 1977.

Cassedy, James. *Charles V. Chapin and the Public Health Movement.* Cambridge, MA: Harvard University Press, 1962.

————. *Medicine in America: A Short History.* Baltimore, MD: The Johns Hopkins University Press, 1991.

Chase, Alan. *Magic Shots: A Human and Scientific Account of the Long and Continuing Struggle to Eradicate Infectious Disease.* New York: William Morrow and Company, 1982.

Colgrove, James. "Between Persuasion and Compulsion: Smallpox Control in Brooklyn and New York, 1894–1902." *Bulletin of the History of Medicine* 78 (2004): 349–78.

————. "'Science in a Democracy': The Contested Status of Vaccination in the Progressive Era and the 1920s." *Isis* 96 (2005): 167–91.

————. *State of Immunity: The Politics of Vaccination in Twentieth-Century America.* Berkeley: University of California Press, 2006; New York: Milbank Memorial Fund, 2006.

Cordasco, Francesco. *Homeopathy in the United States: A Bibliography of Homeopathic Medical Imprints, 1825–1925.* London: Junius-Vaughan Press, 1991.

Crosby, Alfred W. *The Columbian Exchange: Biological and Cultural Consequences of 1492.* Westport, CT: Greenwood, 1972.

Currier, Isabel. "A Worcester College That Grew Up in Waltham." *Worcester Sunday Telegram*, 10 December 1933.

Curry, Lynne, ed. *The Human Body on Trial: A Sourcebook with Cases, Laws, and Documents.* Indianapolis, IN: Hackett, 2002.

Davidovitch, Nadav. "Negotiating Dissent: Homeopathy and Anti-Vaccinationism at the Turn of the Twentieth Century." In *The Politics of Healing: Histories of Alternative Medicine in Twentieth-Century North America*, edited by Robert D. Johnston, 11–28. London: Routledge, 2004.

Deutsch, Sarah. *Women and the City: Gender, Space, and Power in Boston, 1870–1940*. Oxford: Oxford University Press, 2000.

Dixon, C. W., MD. *Smallpox*. London: J. & A. Churchill, 1962.

Dubber, Marcus. *The Police Power: Patriarchy and the Foundations of American Government*. New York: Columbia University Press, 2005.

Dubos, René, and Jean Dubos. *The White Plague: Tuberculosis, Man, and Society*. New Brunswick, NJ: Rutgers University Press, 1996 [1952].

Duffy, John. *A History of Public Health in New York City, 1625–1866*. New York: Russell Sage Foundation, 1968.

———. *A History of Public Health in New York City, 1866–1966*. New York: Russell Sage Foundation, 1974.

———. "School Vaccination: The Precursor to School Inspection." *Journal of the History of Medicine and Allied Sciences* 3 (July 1978): 344–55.

———. *The Sanitarians: A History of American Public Health*. Urbana: University of Illinois Press, 1990.

Durbach, Nadja. "'They Might as Well Brand Us': Working-Class Resistance to Compulsory Vaccination in Victorian England." *Social History of Medicine* 13 (2000): 45–62.

———. "Class, Gender, and the Conscientious Objector to Vaccination, 1898–1907." *Journal of British Studies* 41 (January 2002): 58–83.

———. *Bodily Matters: The Anti-Vaccination Movement in England, 1853–1907*. Durham, NC: Duke University Press, 2005.

Feldberg, Georgina D. *Disease and Class: Tuberculosis and the Shaping of Modern North American Society*. New Brunswick, NJ: Rutgers University Press, 1995.

Fenn, Elizabeth. *Pox Americana: The Great Smallpox Epidemic of 1775–82*. New York: Hill and Wang, 2001.

Fleisher, Steven M. "The Law of Basic Health Activities: Police Power and Constitutional Limitations." In *Legal Aspects of Health Policy: Issues and Trends*, edited by Ruth Roemer and George McKray, 3–32. Westport, CT: Greenwood Press, 1980.

Fowler, William. *Smallpox Vaccination Laws, Regulations, and Court Decisions*. Washington, DC: Treasury Department, United States Public Health Service, 1927.

Fraser, Stuart M. F. "Leicester and Smallpox: The Leicester Method." *Medical History* 24 (1980): 315–32.

Friedman, Leon, and Fred L. Israel, eds. *The Justices of the United States Supreme Court, 1789–1969: Their Lives and Major Opinions*. vols. 2 and 3. New York: Chelsea House Publishers, 1969.

Galishoff, Stuart. "Public Health in Newark, 1832–1918." PhD diss., New York University, 1969.

———. *Safeguarding the Public Health, Newark, 1895–1918*. Westport, CT: Greenwood Press, 1975.

———. *Newark: The Nation's Unhealthiest City, 1832–1895*. New Brunswick, NJ: Rutgers University Press, 1988.

Gevitz, Norman. "Osteopathic Medicine: From Deviance to Difference." In Gevitz, *Other Healers*, 124–56.

———, ed. *Other Healers: Unorthodox Medicine in America*. Baltimore, MD: The Johns Hopkins University Press, 1988.

Gostin, Lawrence O. *Public Health Law: Power, Duty, Restraint.* New York: The Milbank Memorial Fund, 2000.

Häggland, S. G. "Jacobson, Henning." *My Church: An Illustrated Manual* 17 (1931): 160–61.

Haller, John S., Jr. *Medical Protestants: The Eclectics in American Medicine, 1825–1939.* Carbondale: Southern Illinois University Press, 1994.

Hobson, Barbara Meil. *Uneasy Virtue: The Politics of Prostitution and the American Reform Tradition.* Chicago: University of Chicago Press, 1987.

Hopkins, Donald R. *The Greatest Killer: Smallpox.* Chicago: The University of Chicago Press, 2002. Originally published as *Princes and Peasants: Smallpox in History.* Chicago: The University of Chicago Press, 1983.

Howard, William Travis, Jr., MD. *Public Health Administration and the Natural History of Disease in Baltimore, Maryland, 1797–1920.* Washington, DC: The Carnegie Institution, 1924.

Hyde, Alan. *Bodies of Law.* Princeton, NJ: Princeton University Press, 1997.

"Jacobson, Henning." *Korsbaneret: Kristlig Kalendar för Året 1932.* Rock Island, IL: Augustana Book Concern, 1932.

Johnston, Robert D. *The Radical Middle Class: Populist Democracy and the Question of Capitalism in Progressive Era Portland, Oregon.* Princeton, NJ: Princeton University Press, 2003.

———. "Introduction." In *The Politics of Healing: Histories of Alternative Medicine in Twentieth-Century North America,* edited by Robert D. Johnston, 1–8. London: Routledge, 2004.

Jordan, Phillip D. *The People's Health: A History of Public Health in Minnesota to 1948.* St. Paul: Minnesota Historical Society, 1953.

Kaufman, Martin. "The American Anti-Vaccinationists and Their Arguments." *Bulletin of the History of Medicine* 41 (1967): 463–78.

———. "Homeopathy in America: The Rise and Fall and Persistence of a Medical Heresy." In Gevitz, *Other Healers,* 99–123.

Kirschmann, Anne Taylor. *A Vital Force: Women in American Homeopathy.* New Brunswick, NJ: Rutgers University Press, 2004.

Latham, Frank B. *The Great Dissenter: John Marshall Harlan, 1833–1911.* New York: Cowles Book Company, 1970.

Leavell, Byrd S., MD. "Thomas Jefferson and Smallpox Vaccination." *Transactions of the American Clinical and Climatological Association* 88 (1977): 119–27.

Leavitt, Judith Walzer. *The Healthiest City: Milwaukee and the Politics of Health Reform.* Princeton, NJ: Princeton University Press, 1982; Madison: University of Wisconsin Press, 1996.

———. "'Be Safe. Be Sure.': New York City's Experience with Epidemic Smallpox." In *Hives of Sickness: Public Health and Epidemics in New York City,* edited by David Rosner, 95–114. New Brunswick, NJ: Rutgers University Press, 1995.

———. *Typhoid Mary: Captive to the Public's Health.* Boston: Beacon Press, 1996.

Leavitt, Judith Walzer, and Ronald L. Numbers, eds. *Sickness and Health in America: Readings in the History of Medicine and Public Health.* 2nd ed., revised. Madison: University of Wisconsin Press, 1985.

Liebenau, Jonathan. *Medical Science and Medical Industry: The Formation of the American Pharmaceutical Industry.* Baltimore, MD: The Johns Hopkins University Press, 1987.

Lombardo, Paul A. "Medicine, Eugenics, and the Supreme Court: From Coercive Sterilization to Reproductive Freedom." *Journal of Contemporary Health Law and Policy Issues* 13 (1996–97): 1–25.

MacLeod, R. M. "Law, Medicine and Public Opinion: The Resistance to Compulsory Health Legislation, 1870–1907." Parts 1 and 2. *Public Law: The Constitutional and Administrative Law of the Commonwealth* (Spring 1967): 107–28, and (Summer 1967): 189–211.

Markel, Howard. *Quarantine!: East European Jewish Immigrants and the New York City Epidemics of 1892.* Baltimore, MD: The Johns Hopkins University Press, 1997.

McFarland, Gerald W. *Mugwumps, Morals and Politics, 1884–1920.* Amherst: University of Massachusetts Press, 1975.

Miller, Genevieve. *The Adoption of Inoculation for Smallpox in England and France.* Philadelphia: University of Pennsylvania Press, 1957.

Mortimer, Philip. "Robert Cory and the Vaccine Syphilis Controversy: A Forgotten Hero?" *Lancet* 367 (2006): 1112–15.

Mott, Rodney L. *Due Process of Law: A Historical and Analytical Treatise of the Principles and Methods Followed By the Courts in the Application of the Concept of the "Law of the Land."* Indianapolis, IN: The Bobbs-Merrill Company, 1926.

Moyer, Albert E. *The Scientist's Voice in American Culture: Simon Newcomb and the Rhetoric of Scientific Method.* Berkeley: University of California Press, 1992.

Novak, William J. "Intellectual Origins of the State Police Power: The Common Law Vision of a Well-Regulated Society." *Legal History Program Working Papers.* Series 3. Madison: University of Wisconsin–Madison Law School, 1989.

———. *The People's Welfare: Law and Regulation in Nineteenth-Century America.* Chapel Hill: University of North Carolina Press, 1996.

Numbers, Ronald L. "The Making of an Eclectic Physician: Joseph M. McElhinney and the Eclectic Medical Institute of Cincinnati." *Bulletin of the History of Medicine* 47 (1973): 155–66.

———. "The Fall and Rise of the American Medical Profession." In Leavitt and Numbers, *Sickness and Health in America,* 185–96.

Parmet, Wendy. "From Slaughter-House to Lochner: The Rise and Fall of the Constitutionalization of Public Health." *American Journal of Legal History* 40 (1996): 476–505.

———. *Populations, Public Health, and the Law.* Washington, DC: Georgetown University Press, 2009.

Paul, Arnold M. "David J. Brewer." In Friedman and Israel, *Justices of the United States Supreme Court, 1789–1969,* 2:1515–34.

Pernick, Martin. *The Black Stork: Eugenics and the Death of "Defective" Babies in American Medicine and Motion Pictures since 1915.* New York: Oxford University Press, 1996.

Porter, Dorothy, and Roy Porter. "The Politics of Prevention: Anti-Vaccinationism and Public Health in Nineteenth-Century England." *Medical History* 32 (1988): 231–52.

Przybyszewski, Linda. *The Republic according to John Marshall Harlan.* Chapel Hill: The University of North Carolina Press, 1999.

Roettinger, Ruth Locke. *The Supreme Court and State Police Power: A Study in Federalism.* Washington, DC: Public Affairs Press, 1957.

Rosenburg, Charles E. "Social Class and Medical Care in 19th-Century America: The Rise and Fall of the Dispensary." In Leavitt and Numbers, *Sickness and Health in America*, 273–86. First published in the *Journal of the History of Medicine and Allied Sciences* 29 (1974): 32–54.

——. *The Care of Strangers: The Rise of America's Hospital System*. New York: Basic Books, 1987.

Rosenkrantz, Barbara. *Public Health and the State: Changing Views in Massachusetts, 1842–1936*. Cambridge, MA: Harvard University Press, 1972.

——. "The Search for Professional Order in Nineteenth-Century American Medicine." In Leavitt and Numbers, *Sickness and Health in America*, 219–32.

Rothenberg, Mikel A, MD, and Charles F. Chapman. *Dictionary of Medical Terms for the Nonmedical Person*. 3rd ed. Hauppauge, NY: Barron's Educational Series, 1994.

Ross, Steven J. "Single-Tax Movement." In *Oxford Companion to American History*, edited by Paul Boyer, 709. Oxford: Oxford University Press, 2000.

Rothstein, William G. *American Physicians in the Nineteenth Century: From Sects to Science*. Baltimore, MD: The Johns Hopkins University Press, 1972.

——. "The Botanical Movements and Orthodox Medicine." In Gevitz, *Other Healers*, 29–51.

Scanlon, Dorothy Therese. "The Public Health Movement in Boston, 1870–1910." PhD diss., Boston University, 1956.

Schwartz, Bernard. *A History of the Supreme Court*. New York: Oxford University Press, 1993.

Skolink, Richard. "Rufus Peckham." In Friedman and Israel, *Justices of the United States Supreme Court, 1789–1969*, 3:1685–1703.

Smillie, Wilson G. *Public Health: Its Promise for the Future; A Chronicle of the Development of Public Health in the United States, 1607–1914*. New York: The Macmillan Company, 1955.

Spector, Benjamin. "The Growth of Medicine and the Letter of the Law." *Bulletin of the History of Medicine* 26 (November–December 1952): 499–521.

Starr, Paul. *The Social Transformation of American Medicine: The Rise of a Sovereign Profession and the Making of a Vast Industry*. New York: Basic Books, 1982.

Stevens, Rosemary. *In Sickness and in Wealth: American Hospitals in the Twentieth Century*. New York: Basic Books, 1989.

Thernstrom, Stephan. *The Other Bostonians: Poverty and Progress in the American Metropolis, 1880–1970*. Cambridge, MA: Harvard University Press, 1973.

Tobey, James. "Vaccination and the Courts." *JAMA* 83 (1924): 462–64.

——. *Public Health* Law. 2nd ed. New York: The Commonwealth Fund, 1939. First published as Public *Health Law: A Manual for Sanitarians*. Baltimore, MD: The William & Wilkins Company, 1926.

Tomes, Nancy. *The Gospel of Germs: Men, Women, and the Microbe in American Life*. Cambridge, MA: Harvard University Press, 1998.

Tucker, David M. *Mugwumps: Public Moralists of the Gilded Age*. Columbia: University of Missouri Press, 1998.

Underwood, E. Ashworth. "Charles Creighton, the Man and His Work." In Creighton, *A History of Epidemics in Britain* (1965), 1:43–135.

Verbrugge, Martha H. *Able-Bodied Womanhood: Personal Health and Social Change in Nineteenth-Century Boston*. New York: Oxford University Press, 1988.

Vogel, Morris. *The Invention of the Modern Hospital: Boston, 1870–1930*. Chicago: University of Chicago Press, 1980.

Waite, Frederick C. "American Sectarian Medical Colleges before the Civil War." *Bulletin of the History of Medicine* 19 (1946): 148–66.

Walsh, Mary Roth. *"Doctors Wanted: No Women Need Apply": Sexual Barriers in the Medical Profession, 1835–1975*. New Haven, CT: Yale University Press, 1977.

Warner, Sam Bass, Jr. *Streetcar Suburbs: The Process of Growth in Boston (1870–1900)*. 2nd ed. Cambridge, MA: Harvard University Press, 1978. Originally published in 1962.

Warren, Charles. "The Progressiveness of the United States Supreme Court." *Columbia Law Review* 13 (1913): 294–313.

Westin, Alan. "John Marshall Harlan and the Constitutional Rights of Negroes: The Transformation of a Southerner." *The Yale Law Journal* 66 (April 1957): 637–710.

Whipple, George Chandler. *State Sanitation: A Review of the Work of the Massachusetts State Board of Health*. 2 vols. Cambridge, MA: Harvard University Press, 1917.

White, G. Edward. "John Marshall Harlan I: The Precursor." *The American Journal of Legal History* 19 (1975): 1–21.

Wiebe, Robert. *The Search for Order, 1877–1920*. New York: Hill and Wang, 1967.

Willrich, Michael. *Pox: An American History*. New York: Penguin Press, 2011.

Wing, Kenneth R. *The Law and the Public's Health*. 4th ed. Ann Arbor, MI: Health Administration Press, 1995.

Winslow, Ola. *A Destroying Angel: The Conquest of Smallpox in Colonial Boston*. Boston: Houghton Mifflin, 1974.

Wolff, Eberhard. "Sectarian Identity and the Aim of Integration." *British Homeopathic Journal* 85 (April 1996): 95–114.

———. "Sectarian Identity and the Aim of Integration: Attitudes of American Homeopaths toward Smallpox Vaccination in the Late Nineteenth Century." In *Culture, Knowledge and Healing: Historical Perspectives of Homeopathic Medicine in Europe and North America*, ed. Robert Jütte, Guenter B. Risse, and John Woodward, 217–50. Sheffield, England: European Association for the History of Medicine and Health Publications, 1998.

Yarborough, Tinsley E. *Judicial Enigma: The First Justice Harlan*. New York: Oxford University Press, 1995.

Index

1855 Massachusetts vaccination law, 20–21, 104, 147–48
1894 Massachusetts vaccination law, 105, 147, 262n9, 262n10
1902 vaccination bill: analysis of votes, 160–62; first vote, 160, 286n78; second vote, 160, 286n81
1902 vaccination hearings, 147–57, 283n26, 285n57, 285n58
2003 Bush smallpox vaccination program, 219–20

Abbott, Samuel W., 16, 17, 32–33, 45, 49; on local health boards' delays in ordering vaccination, 164; on Massachusetts vaccination law, 147–48
Adams, Horatio, 32
Adams, Samuel Hopkins, and *The Great American Fraud*, 130–31
Alexander, H. M., 34–35, 46; contamination, 94, 248n197; and dispute with H. K. Mulford Company over tetanus, 97, 248n197; and tetanus contamination of its vaccine, 260n91; and Wyeth Laboratories, 46
Allen, Lyman, comments on tetanus following vaccination, 92
Allgeyer v. Louisiana (1897), and Justice Rufus Peckham opinion, 206
American Medical Liberty League, 5
American Medical Association: and antivaccination, 112–15; campaign to reform and reorganize medical profession, 130–31; cultural authority, 233n38; membership in 1901, 132
Amerige, Charles Wardell, 105–6, 262–63n12

Angell, George Thorndike, 106
Animals' Defender, The, 6, 106; circulation, 265n43; relationship with *Our Home Rights*, 110
antivaccination: and disease theories, 114; and homeopathy, 115; and *Jacobson v. Massachusetts*, 216–18; in late nineteenth-century Massachusetts, 104–12; in the medical and popular press, 114–15; opposition to medical monopoly, 113–14; physicians, 267n72
antivaccinationists, 9, 102–3; 1902 campaign to amend the Massachusetts vaccination law, 148, 151–52; critique of medical monopoly, 113; in the medical and popular press, 114–15; and public health authorities in 1902, 103–4
Anti-vaccination League of America, 4, 217
Anti-vaccination League of New York, 4
Anti-vaccination Society of America, 4, 274n146
antivivisection: and antivaccinationists, 95, 106, 111, 115, 120, 173; support, 265n44
Arena, The, 89

Back Bay, and compulsory vaccination sweeps, 179
Bactil Chemical Company, 95
Badcock, John, 32, 33
Baker, Ezra H., 111
Ballard, Henry, 189, 299–300n57; arguments in Jacobson and Pear appeal, 189–90; and special section apended to Jacobson appeal, 191

Bancroft, Hugh, 185; arguments for the state in Jacobson and Pear appeals, 191–92; biographical details, 191, 298n24

Bannon, Theresa, 81, 84

Bassett, William, 111, 157

Beacon Hill, and vaccination sweeps, 179

Beckwith, D. H., 46

Bedford: and quarantine of Immanuel Pfeiffer, 67–68, 138–40; reaction to Pfeiffer's illness and quarantine, 141

Bell, James Batchelder, 111, 265n45

Bigelow, Henry J., 106

Biggs, Herman, and compulsory vaccination, 218

Biologics Control Act (1902), 10, 55, 94, 214–15, 260n95

Blake, John, 19

Blue, Frank D., 4; and Rosicrucian Order, 274n146

Blue v. Beach (1900), 4; and Frank D. Blue, 274n146

Blunder in Poison, A, 7, 122–23

Boardman, Mrs. S. I., 136

Boston: 1901–2 smallpox epidemic, 63–74, 286n84; socioeconomic description of, 62; smallpox mortality rates, 252n63; student population, 256n7; vaccination order in 1901, 74, 165; vaccination rates, 18–26; vaccination sweeps in 1902, 171–73

Boston Board of Health: origin, 60; and quarantine policy, 63; vaccination campaign in 1901–2, 73–74; vaccination order in 1901, 74, 165

Boston Elevated Railroad Company vaccinations, 86–87, 88, 97–98, 167; and Benjamin F. Thurston vaccination, 87; honoring unfitness certificates, 110

Boston Police Department vaccination policy, 83

Boston University School of Medicine, 118–19

Boylston, Zabdiel, 12

bovine lymph, 27, 32; commercialization, 43–46; introduction, 43; problems with, 46–58; and the Union army, 43

Brewer, Justice David J.: biographical details and previous opinions, 206; dissent without comment in Jacobson v. Massachusetts, 205

Brookline, smallpox and vaccination in 1901, 164

Brouardel, Paul, 30, 35, 41, 236n41

Bryce, Peter, 52

Buck v. Bell (1927), 219

Buist, John, 35

Cabot's Supho-Napthol, 83

Cambridge: 1901–2 smallpox epidemic, 75–78, 179–86; 1902 vaccination order, 77, 165; compulsory vaccination enforcement, 179–86; as hotbed of antivaccination, 181; population in 1902, 256n121; socioeconomic description of, 62; vaccination stations, 255n112

Canning, Henry, 55

Caswell, Annie, tetanus death, 94

Cate, Charles E., 176–78, 291n91, 291n93

Cates, Dr., testimony at 1902 vaccination hearings, 159

Ceely, Robert, 32

Chapin, Charles V., 36, 44, 53, 147; and compulsory vaccination, 218

Clement, Edward, 106

Cleveland 1901 smallpox epidemic, in A Blunder in Poison, 123

Clymer, Rueben Swinburne: and Annie Shore vaccination complications, 86; biographical information, 123–25, 273n138, 274n146; comments on Camden, New Jersey, tetanus cases, 92; hired by Immanuel Pfeiffer, 136; and Immanuel Pfeiffer, 123

Codman & Shurtleff, 45, 46

coerced and forced vaccinations, 166–70; in Philadelphia, 289n41

Coffey, James C., 68, 69

Coleman, William H., 181
Commonwealth v. Albert M. Pear, 189–95
Commonwealth v. Henning Jacobson,
  189–95
compulsory vaccination: and Herman
  Biggs, 218; in Boston, 170–79; in
  Cambridge, 179–86; and Charles V.
  Chapin, 218; in East Boston, 171–72;
  exemption laws in US as of 2014,
  307n35; and focus on lodging houses
  in Boston, 171; lack of enforcement
  in wealthy Boston districts, 179; laws
  in the US in 1927, 306n32–33; laws in
  Massachusetts after *Jacobson*, 217–18;
  laws in other states around 1900,
  232n26, 232n27, 232n28, 232n29,
  301n84; in Massachusetts, 20–22,
  104, 105, 254n96; and the medical
  profession, 17–18; and the "new
  public health," 9; in Roxbury, 171;
  violations in 1902, 287n2
Cone, Frank W., 183
Connecticut Anti-compulsory
  Vaccination Society, 5
Cooke, Willis S., comments on tetanus
  following vaccination, 92–93
Coomb's Germicide Tablets, 101
Cope, Sir Monkton, 47
Cory, Robert, 42
cowpox, 31, 32, 242n38
Coxe, John Redman, 14–15
Creighton, Charles, 3, 229n3
Crookshank, Edgar, 32
Cutler, William C. and Frisbie, J. F., and
  New England Vaccine Company, 46
Cutter, Ephraim, 32, 34

Darling, Eugene, 38–39, 40, 41;
  testimony at the 1902 vaccination
  hearings, 155
Davis, Frank M., 176
Day, Sen. Cornelius R., abstention on
  1902 vaccination bill vote, 161
Diaz, Abby Morton, 106
Dillingham, Frederick, 70, 79
dispensaries, 64–65
Dixon, Cyril, 38

Dock, George, 37, 38, 39, 40, 41, 54,
  243n77; and proper vaccination
  technique, 243n84; reaction to
  Jacobson decision, 211–12
Draper, Francis, 66; testimony at 1902
  vaccination hearing, 157
Dreyfus, Carl, 83
Dudley, Charles, vaccination of Annie
  Caswell, 94
Durgin, Mary Bradford Davis, 60–61
Durgin, Samuel Holmes, 7, 38; and
  1901 vaccination order, 74, 95–96,
  163; and 1902 vaccination bill,
  146, 150, 156–60, 285n57, 285n58;
  attitude toward antivaccinationists,
  163, 278n41; biographical
  information, 59–61, 249n4,
  250n9; and campaign for state-
  run vaccine facility, 56–58, 95,
  248n201, 249n207–9; and Charles
  E. Cate case, 177; comments on
  antivaccinationists, 104, 127;
  comments on use of 1894 law to
  evade vaccination, 107; comments
  on lax vaccination among Boston
  schoolchildren, 81; comments on
  Immanuel Pfeiffer's issuance of
  unfitness certificates, 110, 158;
  comments on proper vaccination,
  82; comments on fear of tetanus
  following vaccination, 97; conflict
  with Dr. Immanuel Pfeiffer, 132–
  33; conflict with Dr. Caroline E.
  Hastings, 154, 158, 283n43, 283n44;
  criticism of dispensaries, 64–65;
  and criticism of his management
  of the epidemic, 152–53, 253n77;
  and Pfeiffer's visit to the isolation
  hospital, 133–35; and policy for
  dealing with smallpox outbreak, 63;
  on propriety of allowing Pfeiffer to
  visit the isolation hospital, 135–36;
  on public fear of isolation hospitals,
  72–73; and refusal to quarantine
  in Boston, 69; and transmission of
  smallpox via clothing, 66, 251n37;
  and virus squads, 169–70

East Boston: description, 172;
vaccination sweep, 172–73
Elgin, W. F., 38, 47–48
Eliot, Charles W.: comments on
tetanus and antivaccinationists,
95; comments on wealthy families'
avoidance of vaccination, 98,
179; comments on homeopathic
physicians and antivaccination, 107;
letter supporting vaccination, 157;
and vaccination at Harvard, 179
Emmons, Judge William H. H., 173;
decisions on vaccination refusals, 175
erysipelas, 31
Evans, John M., 175
Evans, Kate, 175

Fenger, Christian, 84
Fisher, William R., 79
Fitz, Reginald H., 66, 252n40
Flower, Benjamin Orange: on
antivaccination and criticism of
medical monopoly power, 113; article
on Martin Friedrich and Cleveland
vaccination, 89; on George Fred
Williams, 199
Flynn, Councilman George A., 73,
98–99, 169
forced vaccinations, 163
Foster, Rep. John F., 111; 1902
vaccination bill, 151, 282n22;
commenting on Immanuel Pfeiffer's
illness, 144; testimony at 1902
vaccination hearings, 159
Fourteenth Amendment, 187–88; and
police power, 188–89
Frederick Stearns and Company, 34
Frederickson, A. P., 65
Friedrich, Martin: comments on
vaccination complications in
Cleveland, 88–89; decision to
suspend vaccination in Cleveland,
90, 258n60; in Charles Fessenden
Nichols, *A Blunder in Poison*, 123
Fuller Court, 205

G. G. Disinfectant, 101

Gahan, P. F., 66
Galvin, George W., offer of free
vaccinations, 95
Garrison, Francis J., testimony at 1902
vaccination hearings, 159
Garrison, William Lloyd, 105
generalized vaccinia, 28
germ theory, 8
Giles, Alfred Ellingwood, 104–5,
262n6
Giles, S. R. H., 231n22
Gilpatric, Rep. Fred C., 1902 vaccination
bill, 151
glycerin, 246n162
glycerinated lymph, 27, 246n162;
addition to bovine lymph, 47; lack
of state control in its production, 49;
problems with, 48–52
Good, Charles, 70
Goodwin, George H., 111
Gostin, Lawrence, on *Jacobson* decision,
212
Gould, Ephraim, 183
Gould, George M.: comments on
tetanus and vaccination, 91–92; on
Our Home Rights, 130
Gould, Maggie, 183
Grainger, William H., 158
Greene, Edward M., 158
Greene, Joseph M., 7; as author of
Vaccination is the Curse of Childhood,
263n20; comments on Dr. Towle's
report on vaccination complications,
85; criticism of virus squads, 170; as
founder of the New England Anti-
vivisection Society, 106, 257n40; as
a leading antivaccination organizer,
106–7, 111, 257n40; reaction to
Jacobson decision, 195; reporting
on vaccination hearings, 283n26;
reporting on vaccination tragedies,
87; reports on tetanus following
vaccination, 94–95; and Annie Shore
vaccination complications, 85, 86;
on unfitness certificates, 110; on
vaccination sweeps, 174
Gunn, Robert A., 4

H. K. Mulford Company, 34, 50–51, 248n197; and tetanus contamination of its vaccine, 94, 260n91

Hale, George Carlton, testimony at 1902 vaccination hearings, 159, 286n73

Harlan, Justice John Marshall: biographical details and previous opinions, 207–8; opinion in *Jacobson v. Massachusetts*, 208–11; research for his ruling in *Jacobson v. Massachusetts*, 304n132, 304n134, 304n135; ruling in *Jacobson v. Massachusetts*, 205

Harris, Charles, 181

Hart, Thomas M., 83

Hartshorne, Henry, 36

Harvell, Sen. Elisha T., and 1902 vaccination bill, 162

Hastings, Caroline Eliza, 7, 111: biographical information, 116–17, 268n76, 268n80, 268n82, 268n84; and *Boston Courier* editorial, 155–56; conflict with Samuel Durgin, 117, 154, 284n43, 284n44; position on vaccination, 154–55; questioning Samuel Durgin's testimony about unfitness certificates, 158; testimony at the 1902 vaccination hearing, 153–54

Hatch, Fred W., testimony on vaccination, 86

Henderson, Mrs. Jessica L. C., 161, 287n85; and MACVS, 161

Higgins, Benjamin, tetanus death lawsuit, 90

Higgins, Charles M., 4, 217–18

Hill, Aurin F., 106, 112, 265n50

Hill, Hibbert W., 147

Hollis, Stanley, vaccination complications, 87

homeopathic antivaccination physicians, 115–16

homepaths' attitudes about vaccination, 3, 246n155, 267n69, 267n70

homeopathy: and official stance on vaccination, 115; and women physicians, 116

Howard Health Company, 83, 84

humanized lymph, 27, 52–53, 247–48n186; and syphilis transmission, 42–43

Hutchinson, Jonathan, 42

Hyde Park, and vaccination in 1901, 165

Iniquity of Compulsory Vaccination, The, 104–5, 262n6

isolation hospitals, 71–73

Issacs, Mary, 178–79

J. A. Dreyfus & Sons, 83

Jacobson, Henning, 1, 112; appeal of guilty verdict, 185–86; biographical information, 182, 184, 212–14, 294n157, 294n159, 295n160, 295n162; criminal complaint against, 182; initial appearance in court, 183; jury trial and arguments, 185; and preferential treatment by health authorities, 168; receiving financial aid for legal fees from the MACVS, 184

Jacobson v. Massachusetts (1905), 1–2; arguments, 196–205; and continued opposition to vaccination, 216–18; decision, 205; effect on other states' passage of compulsory vaccination laws, 219; effect on vaccination efforts, 212; and eugenics laws, 219; Harlan's opinion, 208–11; reaction to decision, 211–12

Jefferson, Thomas, 14

Jenner, Edward, 13; as an icon of scientific medicine, 114; and original strain of vaccine lymph, 31

Johnston, Robert D., 112

Joint Committee on Public Health: and Caroline Hastings, 117; and hearings on bills to change compulsory vaccination laws, 146–47; members, 283n33

Jorgenson, Christina, tetanus death following vaccination, 94

Journal of the Massachusetts Association of Boards of Health, 250n14

Judge, James D., 153, 284n37

Justices of the Supreme Court of the United States in 1904–5, 303n105

Keating, Marjorie, 110
Kirschmann, Anne Taylor, 116
Knight, Samuel, 32
Knowlton, Chief Justice Marcus Perrin: biographical details, 192; decision in Jacobson and Pear appeals, 192–94; on unconstitutionality of forcible vaccination, 194
Koch, Robert, and tuberculin, 266n59

Ladies Physiological Institute, 133n38, 278n38
Lafollette, Gov. Robert, veto of compulsory vaccination law, 200
Langtry, Lily, 82
Lawrence, Mortimer W., 179
Leavitt, Annie, 85–86; in *Vaccination Brought Home to You*, 124
Leicester method, 272n129
Liberator, The, 217
Lifebuoy Soap, 100, 101
Little, Lora C. W., 5, 217; and *Jacobson v. Massachusetts*, 216; and Joseph Greene, 87; and Sara Newcomb Merrick, 120
Lochner v. New York (1905), and Justice Harlan dissent, 207
Logan, D. W., 110
Lohan, Thomas B.: letter about vaccination at the Parker House Hotel, 86; use of unfitness certificate, 110
Loud, Hulda B., 162, 283n34
Loyster, James, 217

MACVS (Massachusetts Anti-Compulsory Vaccination Society), 102, 111–12
Malden, and quarantine, 67
Marson, J. F., 13, 28, 241n13
Martin, Francis C., 45–46
Martin, Henry Austin, 30, 32, 45–46
Martin, John C., 32

Massachusetts Anti-Compulsory Vaccination Society, 5, 102, 111–12; at the 1902 vaccination hearings, 150; decision to hire Henry Ballard for the Jacobson and Pear appeals, 189; formation of Cambridge branch, 182; mission statement, 112; origin, 111; payment of court costs and fines for Jacobson and Pear, 212; support for Henning Jacobson and Albert Pear appeals, 186, 295n173, 299n53
Massachusetts, legislative procedure, 151
Massachusetts Association of Boards of Health, 7, 61, 147, 233n34; 1902 annual meeting, 147, 281n1
Massachusetts Homeopathic Medical Society, resolution supporting vaccination, 98
Massachusetts State Board of Health, 16; circular recommending general vaccination in 1899 and 1901, 164
Mather, Cotton, 12
McCollom, John H., 13, 31, 40, 42–43, 80, 284n52; debate with Immanuel Pfeiffer, 132–33; testimony at the 1902 vaccination hearing, 156
McCormick, Joseph N., 39, 45, 53
McFarland, Joseph: analysis of tetanus contamination of vaccines, 93–94; used in argument for Jacobson and Pear appeals, 190
McGee, Anita Newcomb, 118
McGinley, Maria, tetanus death lawsuit, 90
McKay, Duncan, 175
McKenna family, 64
McNamee, Mayor John H. H., 67; criticism of E. Edwin Spencer's vaccination policy, 180–81
Mead, Master, testimony at 1902 vaccination hearings, 158
Medford, smallpox and vaccination in 1901, 164
medical registration laws, 276n11
Medical Rights League of Massachusetts, 129

Mellish, Ernst, 39, 41
Merrick, Morgan Wolfe, 118, 269n94, 269n98
Merrick, Sara Newcomb, 7, 111; biographical information, 117–20, 269n94, 269n98; reaction to *Jacobson* decision, 211, 216
Miller, A. E., 56
Miller, Charles Ransom, friendship with George Fred Williams, 197
Milwaukee 1894 smallpox riots, 3
Montagu, Lady Mary Wortley, 12
Moore, John William, 41, 234n2
Morse, Frank, 16; and Immanuel Pfeiffer, 139
Mott, Frederick, 174
Mugford, Bessie, 172, 290n73
Mugford, Eva, 172, 176, 196
Mugford, John: appeal, sentence, and fine, 196; biographical information, 172, 290n73; prosecution for vaccination refusal, 172–75; trial and appeal, 176, 295n173
Mugler v. Kansas (1887), and Harlan opinion, 207–8
Munn v. Illinois (1877), 188
Murphy, Father J. J., neglect to vaccinate, 98

NEAVS (New England Anti-compulsory Vaccination Society), 105
Negri, Pietro, 43
New England Anti-compulsory Vaccination Society, 5
New England Anti-vivisection Society: and Joseph Greene, 106, 257n40; origins, 106
New England Female Reform Society, 117
New England Vaccine Company, 27, 38, 40, 41, 44, 46, 47
new public health, 8; and compulsory vaccination, 9; definition, 60
Newcomb, Simon, 118, 120
Newton: and quarantine, 68; and vaccination in 1901, 165

Nichols, Charles Fessenden, 7; biographical information, 121–22, 271n114, 271n115, 272n122; comments on Immanuel Pfeiffer, 144
Nichols, Rep. Walter F., 283n31; comments on Immanuel Pfeiffer, 144; dissent on Durgin's vaccination bill, 159; position on vaccination at 1902 vaccination hearings, 152
North Adams, and vaccination in 1901, 165
Novak, William J., 54, 187
Noyes, D. K., 110–11
Nugent, Bridget, 85

Osler, William, 30, 43
Our Home Rights, 6, 110, 130; and *The Animal's Defender*, 264n29

Packard, Horace, 115; testimony at 1902 vaccination hearing, 157
Page, Charles, E.: commenting on Immanuel Pfeiffer's smallpox attack, 141; biographical information, 120–21, 270n109; letter on Charles E. Cate, 178; letter on Martin Friedrich and Cleveland vaccinations, 89; testimony at the 1902 vaccination hearings, 153
Palmer, L. M., 65
Park, Davis, and Company, 34
Parker, Herbert, arguments in *Jacobson v. Massachusetts*, 203–5
Parker House Hotel, and vaccination of its employees, 86
Pasteur, Louis, as orginator of the term "vaccination," 266n61
Peabody, Philip G., 106
Peabody, William Rodman, 76, 181
Pear, Albert M.: biographical details, 182; initial court appearance, 183; jury trial and appeal, 184–85; and the MACVS, 185; and special treatment from the Cambridge Board of Health, 182–83

Peckham, Justice Rufus: biographical details and previous opinions, 206–7; dissent without comment in *Jacobson v. Massachusetts*, 205

Pennsylvania State Board of Health, resolution on tetanus following vaccination, 92

pesthouse, aversion to, 71–73

Pfeiffer, Alice, 137, 140

Pfeiffer, Hannah, 137

Pfeiffer, Immanuel, 6–7; 1902 vaccination bill, 151, 283n25; and the AMA, 131–32; biographical information, 128–30, 275n5, 275n7, 275n8; comments on Annie Shore and Annie Leavitt vaccination complications, 85; comments on the 1894 vaccination exemption law, 110; conflict with United States Postal Service, 131, 277n27; depiction as an example of the folly of antivaccination, 142–43; disappearance, 135–36; on fasting, 129; hiring Reuben Swinburne Clymer, 136; and Howard Health Company, 131; and MACVS, 112; opposition to medical registration laws, 129, 276n11; political and social ideals, 127–28; and rationale for evading the Boston Health department, 139; recounting cases of vaccination injury, 86–87; reaction to *Jacobson* decision, 195; reaction to quarantine by Bedford, 140; as smallpox victim, 137; as "special champion" of antivaccination, 127; suggestion of George Fred Williams for Jacobson appeal, 196; testimony at the 1902 vaccination hearing, 135, 153; unfitness certificates, 110, 131, 158; visit to the isolation hospital, 133–35

Pfeiffer, Immanuel, Jr., 140; conversation with Thomas B. Shea, 141

physician registration laws, 129

Pickering, James W., 151: argument in Jacobson and Pear appeal, 189–90; as attorney for Henning Jacobson and Albert Pear at jury trials and appeals, 183–86; defense of Frank Cone, 183

Piehn, L. H., 4; and Rosicrucian Order, 274n146

Pilsbury, Edwin L., 150

Pitcairn, John, 4, 217–18

Plessy v. Ferguson (1896), and Justice Harlan's dissent, 207

Plummer, Julia Morton, 117, 268n81, 268n82

police power, 5, 187; and the Fourteenth Amendment, 188–89

Poole, Mary, 174

Poole, Frederick B., 174

Porter, Sen. J. Frank: amendment to restore original vaccination law, 160; as chair of Joint Committee on Public Health, 160

Powell v. Pennsylvania (1888), and Justice Harlan's opinion, 208

quarantine, rules of, 63

Quincy, and vaccination in 1901, 165

Radam's Microbe Killer, 99, 101

Reeve, Ada, 82

Republican Party, domination of Massachusetts legislature, 160

retrovaccination, 32

revaccination, 30–31

Rich, Zoeth, vaccination complications, 87

Righter, Harvey M., 85

Rivalta incident, 42

Roche, Richard, 169

Rosenau, M. J., 48–49; report on tetanus contamination, 94

"Rose's vaccinator," 37

Roxbury Homeopathic Dispensary, 119–20

Rush, Benjamin, 15

Sacco, Luigi, 32

Salem, and quarantine, 67

Sanders, William B., 104, 107, 262n9, 264n25; testimony at the 1902 vaccination hearing, 153

school vaccination rates, 158
Seaton, Edward Cator, 28, 37–38, 42, 240n4
Seaver, Edwin P., 65
Sedgwick, William T., 127, 147; on antivaccinationists at Massachusetts Association of Boards of Health meeting, 148–50; testimony at the 1902 vaccination hearing, 156
Shattuck, Lemuel, 20, 21, 238n64
Shea, Thomas B., 63, 67; on antivaccinationists, 103–4; commenting on Pfeiffer's smallpox attack, 137, 140; conversation with Immanuel Pfeiffer, Jr., 141; examination of Pfeiffer, 139; talk at January 1902 Massachusetts Association of Boards of Health meeting, 147–48; testimony at the 1902 vaccination hearing, 156
Sheldon, Judge Henry N., 176
Shore, Annie, 85–86; in *Vaccination Brought Home to You*, 124
Simpson, Charles Asbury, 112, 265n51; comments on *Jacobson* decision, 194–95
Simpson, William F., 111
single tax, 128n4, 275n4
Small, Joshua T., 111, 112
Small, Rep. Issac M., 281n18; and 1901 abolition bill, 162
smallpox: cases in Massachusetts in 1901, 286n84; description of signs and symptoms, 11–12; diagnosis in 1902, 70–71; epidemics before and after inoculation, 235n14; immunity from second attack, 234n7, 234n8; inoculation, 12–13; mortality rates, 233n1, 252n63; and physicians' precautions against spreading it, 66; and quarantine in 1902, 67–68; role in American history, 12–13; and transmission via clothing or by a vaccinated person, 66–67; and vaccination in Massachusetts in 1901, 164–65; variola major, 11; variola minor, 11; varioloid, 11; virus, 235n18

Smith, James, 14
Smith, Theobald, 50, 56, 147
Somerville, smallpox and vaccination in 1901, 164
South Boston: description, 173; vaccination sweep, 173–74
Southbridge, and vaccination in 1901, 165
Spalding, Heman, 39
Spencer, E. Edwin, 7; biographical information, 75–76, 255n99, 255n100, 255n107; decision to prosecute vaccination refusals, 182; policy on vaccination, 77, 163, 179–80; policy on vaccination refusals, 180; and quarantine in Cambridge, 67, 77; vaccination order, 77; and vaccination rate in Cambridge, 81
Spencer, Herbert, 3
Starr, Paul, 113
Stedman, Charles H., 14; 1855 vaccination report, 20–21
Stevens, Edmond H., 56
substantive due process, 10, 188–89
Sullivan, Joseph, and vaccination complications, 87
Sullivan, Sen. Charles S., abstention on 1902 vaccination bill vote, 161
Swartz, Gardner T., 68

Talitha Cumi Home, 117, 268n84
Taylor, Major, 82
Temple, William F., 158
tetanus, 90, 259n77; and diphtheria antitoxin deaths in St. Louis, Missouri, 90–91, 259n73; and vaccination deaths in Camden, New Jersey, 260n91
Thirteenth Amendment, 187
Thurston, Benjamin F., vaccination complications, 87
Tierney, Sarah, 175
Toner, Joseph M., 16, 36, 37, 38, 43, 234n8
Towle, Harvey P., 85
tuberculin, 266n59

unfitness certificates, 110, 131, 158
United States Public Health and Marine
    Hospital Service, Rosenau report on
    tetanus contamination, 94

"Vaccinated, The," 82–83
vaccination: arm-to-arm, 35; aversion
    for, 81–89, 97–101; Boston campaign
    in 1901–2, 73–74; Boston Police
    Department policy, 83; in Cleveland,
    87–88; commercialization of, 43–46,
    245n136, 245n138; complications,
    28–31, 241n26; and cowpox,
    32; description, 27; and French
    Canadians, 22, 239n82; of homeless
    men in Boston, 168–69; and Edward
    Jenner, 13; laws in Massachusetts
    before *Jacobson*, 254n96; laws in
    Massachusetts after *Jacobson*, 217–18;
    lawsuits, 90, 167, 179; lichen, 28;
    and local health departments'
    avoidance of compulsion, 164; on
    leg vs. arm, 40–41; in Massachusetts,
    18–26; origin of the word, 266n61;
    physicians' trust in, 66; prices, 22;
    primary vs. secondary, 16–17; rates
    in Boston, 21–26; requirements
    for Massachusetts businesses, 166;
    and revaccination, 24–25; and
    Rivalta incident, 42; shields, 38–39,
    244n92, 244n100; and smallpox in
    Massachusetts in 1901, 164–65; spread
    of, 14–16; sweeps in Boston, 163, 171–
    73; and syphilis, 8, 42–46, 245n129;
    techniques, 37–41; and tetanus, 8,
    90–97, 259n77; versus traditional
    public health measures, 68–69, 155–
    56; and transition to bovine lymph,
    42–46; in the Union army, 43
Vaccination a Curse, 105–6
Vaccination Brought Home to You, 124–25
Vaccination Is the Curse of Childhood,
    107, 108–9; and Joseph Greene's
    authorship, 263n20
vaccination laws: in Massachusetts, 102,
    147; Utah, 5–6; in various states,
    232n26, 232n27, 232n28, 232n29

vaccinia: and cowpox, 242n38;
    definition of, 13; generalized, 27;
    virus, 242n36
vaccine manufacture: differences among
    producers, 50; and state control, 49,
    52–58
"Vaccine Point, A" 83
vaccine roseola, 28
vaccine virus: and argument for
    return to humanized lymph,
    53–54; Beaugency strain, 33–34, 45;
    methods of lymph extraction and
    preservation, 35–37; nineteenth-
    century sources of, 31–35; transition
    to bovine lymph, 42–46
Van Bibber, C., 32
variola: major, 11; minor, 11, 70
variolation, 14
Vaughan, Samuel, vaccination
    complications, 87
vote on 1902 vaccination bill, 160

Waite, Chief Justice Morrison R.,
    188
Wakefield, and quarantine, 67
Walcott, Henry P., 49, 50, 55;
    complaining of general neglect of
    vaccination, 164; and state control of
    vaccine production, 248n201
Wallace, Alfred Russel, 3, 149n8, 281n8
Waltham Watch Company, and
    vaccinations, 87
Waterhouse, Benjamin, 14
Watson, Rep. James A., 64–65
Weeks, C. T., and Annie Caswell death,
    94
Wesselhoeft, Conrad, 115, 267n73;
    comments on fine for refusing
    vaccination, 163
West Roxbury, and vaccination sweeps,
    179
Wheeler, Dr. Morris P., 286n74;
    testimony at 1902 vaccination
    hearings, 159
Wilder, Alexander, 4
Williams, Sen. Chester B.: amendment
    to Durgin's vaccination bill, 159–60;

dissatisfaction with Samuel Durgin's management of the smallpox epidemic, 152–53; dissent on Durgin's vaccination bill, 159; interrogation of Samuel Durgin, 156; position on vaccination at the 1902 hearings, 152; reason for proposing amendment to allow adult exemption, 162; representing Wayland, 161, 287n85

Williams, G., and vaccination complications, 87–88

Williams, George Fred, 112; as advocate for progressive reform, 199, 299n55, 299n56; arguments in *Jacobson v. Massachusetts*, 200–203; biographical details, 196–200, 299n54, 300n59, 301n77, 301n80; and friendship with Charles Ransom Miller, 197, 300n69;

support for William Jennings Bryan, 199, 301n73

Williams, Ralph B., 111

Willson, Robert: article on fifty tetanus cases, 92; comments on tetanus following vaccination, 91

Winslow, C.-E. A., 147

Winterburn, George, 15, 16, 28, 32, 34, 37, 38, 41, 42, 44–45

women physicians, 7, 267n74; and homeopathy, 116

Wonderful Century, The, 149n8, 281n8

Woolson, Abba Gould, 116

Worcester, and vaccination in 1901, 165

Wyeth, John Allen, 130

Yee Kee, John, 168

Young, Master, testimony at 1902 vaccination hearings, 158

Lightning Source UK Ltd.
Milton Keynes UK
UKHW021904200622
404706UK00004B/498